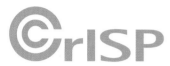

FOURTH EDITION

# Care of the Critically Ill Surgical Patient®

## Student Handbook

Edited by
**John Jameson and Danny Bryden**

First published in Great Britain in 1999 by the Royal College of Surgeons of England
Second edition 2003
Third edition 2010
This fourth edition published in 2017 by
The Royal College of Surgeons of England
35-43 Lincoln's Inn Fields, London, WC2A 3PE

www.rcseng.ac.uk

British Library Cataloguing in Publication Data

A catalogue record for this book is available from the British Library

Library of Congress Cataloging-in-Publication Data

A catalogue record for this book is available from the Library of Congress

ISBN 978-1-904096-32-0

Typeset by Prepress Projects Ltd

# Contents

# 4th edition contributors

## Editors

| | | |
|---|---|---|
| Dr Daniele Bryden | MB ChB, FRCA, FFICM, LLB(Hons), MML | Consultant in Intensive Care Medicine and Anaesthesia, Sheffield Teaching Hospitals, Sheffield, England |
| Mr John S Jameson | MA(Cantab), MB BS, FRCS, MD | Consultant Colorectal Surgeon, University Hospitals of Leicester NHS Trust, Leicester General Hospital, Leicester, England |

## Steering group members

| | | |
|---|---|---|
| Dr Philip Buckley | MBChB, FRCA | Consultant Anaesthetist, Hull & East Yorkshire Hospitals NHS Trust, Kingston upon Hull, England |
| Dr Joseph F Cosgrove | MB BS, FRCA, FFICM | Consultant in Anaesthesia and Intensive Care Medicine, Freeman Hospital, Newcastle upon Tyne, England |
| Dr Sarah Gillis | FRCA | Consultant Anaesthetist with an interest in ICM, Whittington Hospital, London, England |
| Mr Brian Johnson | MD, FRCS | Consultant Vascular Surgeon, Hull Royal Infirmary, Kingston upon Hull, England |
| Mr Andy Kordowicz | MA, MB, BChir, MEd, MRCS | Specialist Registrar in Vascular Surgery, Hull Royal Infirmary, Kingston upon Hull, England |
| Mr Ben Lindsey | FRCS | Consultant Vascular and Renal Transplant Surgeon, The Royal Free London NHS Foundation Trust, London, England |
| Dr Jon Walton | MBChB, MRCP, FRCA DipICM | Consultant in Critical Care Medicine and Anaesthesia, Freeman Hospital, Newcastle upon Tyne, England |

# Contributors

| | | |
|---|---|---|
| Dr Shyam Balasubramanian | MB BS, MD, MSc, FRCA FFPMRCA | Consultant in Pain Medicine and Anaesthesia, UHCW NHS Trust, Coventry, England |
| Mr Marius Berman | MD, FRCS (CTh) | Consultant Cardiothoracic and Transplant Surgeon, Papworth Hospital, Cambridge, England |
| Dr Mike Fried | BSc(Hons), MB BS, MRCGP, FRCA, FFARCSI | Consultant in Anaesthesia and Critical Care Medicine, St John's Hospital, Livingston, Scotland |
| Dr Simon Gabe | MD, MSc, MBBS, BSc(Hons), FRCP | Consultant Gastroenterologist & Honorary Senior Lecturer and Co-Chair of the Lennard-Jones Intestinal Failure Unit, St Mark's Hospital, Harrow, England |
| Dr Debbie Kerr | MB ChB, FRCA, MCEM | Advanced Trainee in Intensive Care Medicine, Sheffield Teaching Hospitals NHS Foundation Trust, Sheffield, England |
| Dr Karen Kerr | MBChB, FRCA | Consultant Anaesthetist, Sheffield Teaching Hospital NHS Foundation Trust, Sheffield, England |
| Dr Mathew V Patteril | MD, DA, FRCA, DipClinEdu(RCS) | Consultant Cardiothoracic Anaesthetist, Department of Anaesthesia, Critical Care and Pain Management, University Hospitals of Coventry and Warwickshire, Coventry, England |
| Dr Thanthullu Vasu | MB BS, MD, DNB, FRCA, FFPMRCA, Dip Pain Mgt | Consultant and Head of Pain Service, University Hospitals of Leicester NHS Trust, Leicester, England |
| Dr Arunan Yogasundaram | MB ChB(Hons), FRCA | Post CCT Fellow in Intensive Care Medicine, The Alfred Hospital, Melbourne, Australia |

# Contributors to previous editions

## Contributors to the 3rd edition

Mr Ian Loftus FRCS

Mr Iain Anderson FRCS

Dr Daniele Bryden FRCA

Mr Francis Calder FRCSEd

Dr Joe Cosgrove FRCA

Dr Sarah Gillis FRCA

Dr Jonathan Goodall FRCA

Mr John Jameson FRCS

Mr Brian Johnson FRCS

Mr Keith Jones FRCS

Dr Philip Newman FRCA

Dr Declan O'Brian FRCA

Professor Rob Sayers FRCS

Mr Mark Taylor FRCS

## Contributors to the 2nd edition

Mr G L Carlson

Dr M Hunter

Dr B Riley

Professor B J Rowlands

Dr G B Smith

Professor M M Thompson

## Contributors to the 1st edition

Dr T N Appleyard

Professor K Fearon

Mr D R Griffin

Professor D J Leaper

Dr G Ramsay

Mr R C G Russel

Professor J M Ryan

Dr A I K Short

Dr S W Turner

Dr R G Wheatley

# Acknowledgements

Peter Loader MSc

Senior Project Manager

Royal College of Surgeons of England

# Dedication

Leon Grant and the late Mrs Grant

# Foreword to 4th Edition

In my foreword to the first edition, written in 1999, I referred to the tragedy that took place on 15th April 1989 at Hillsborough Football Ground when 96 spectators, who were mainly young people, were crushed to death.

Twenty-seven years later, a coroner's inquest has concluded that the victims were unlawfully killed, primarily as a result of compression asphyxia. Although, in the main, it was observed that most of the deaths were unavoidable, there was a suggestion that, given better and more prompt treatment, fewer might have died.

In November 1994, the Trustees of the Hillsborough Disaster Charitable Trust issued the following statement: 'We have agreed to support the development by the Royal College of Surgeons of England of a training programme for doctors and other medical staff directed at improving medical care in the immediate aftermath of injury and trauma'.

The College readily accepted this generous offer and its Education Department, under the leadership of Iain Anderson, produced a course called Care of the Critically Ill Surgical Patient (CCrISP). CCrISP rapidly became popular among surgical trainees, both in the United Kingdom and overseas, and the continuing demand for places has shown that it continues to fill a gap in surgical training programmes.

This 4th edition by Daniele Bryden and John Jameson has radically restructured the scope and presentation of the course, while retaining the underlying educational approach.

It is the hope of the College and all involved with this 4th edition that the CCrISP course will, by continuing to bring high-quality surgical care to patients today, remain a valuable memorial to those who died at Hillsborough in 1998.

Professor Sir Miles Irving
DSc(Hon), MD, ChM, FRCS, FMedSci
Emeritus Professor of Surgery Manchester University

# Preface

Medical training today is very different from the training that present-day consultants received when they were surgical junior doctors (as they were called then) working for a small number of consultants and often on call with the same team at nights and weekends. Trainees now report times when they feel disengaged from their trainers and their patients, as a result of shiftworking patterns that have an adverse effect on continuity. Moreover, because of a lack of clinical exposure, surgical trainees can feel unprepared to deal with emergencies and the routine day-to-day planning of care for the unwell ward patient. These changes have occurred against a background of increasing expectations of patients and their relatives and ever greater scrutiny of the healthcare system. As a result, it is more difficult than in the past to develop a sense of belonging to a team and an ability to recognise a job done well and learn where improvements can be made.

The Care of the Critically Ill Surgical Patient (CCrISP) course is a valuable adjunct to traditional ward-based experiential training and provides young surgeons with the structure and confidence they require to safely and effectively care for their patients on the wards. The 4th edition of this course was developed during the 20th anniversary year of the Hillsborough football stadium tragedy. Money from the Hillsborough Disaster Charitable Trust contributed to the development of the original CCrISP course, and this edition remains true to those original aims of encouraging surgeons to take responsibility for critically ill surgical patients, to 'predict and prevent' problems that patients might encounter while in hospital, to function well within the surgical team and to communicate effectively with colleagues from other disciplines.

The majority of UK surgical trainees take the CCrISP course, which is available in over 40 centres and has become a requirement for higher specialist training in several surgical specialties. It is also compulsory in Australasia and is taught in Italy, Malaysia and Singapore. More recently, the START (Systematic Training in Acute Illness Recognition and Treatment) Surgery course has successfully adopted some of the CCrISP principles for training foundation year doctors and provides a useful introduction to CCrISP principles. A CCrISP instructor's course also runs at the Royal

College of Surgeons of England to prepare senior surgeons, all of whom have taken the CCrISP course during their training, for providing the course nationwide. Similar arrangements exist in Australasia. The new edition of the course, the 4th edition, continues to reinforce the clinical application of the theoretical basis provided in this manual. The manual has been updated to reflect developments in the understanding of some subjects and how the organisation of the delivery of healthcare has changed. The principles remain the same however – to encourage the development of practical skills, improve patient management and develop the interpersonal skills required to work effectively and confidently within the multidisciplinary team. The need to master these skills early in training has never been more pressing, given the changes to working patterns and demands on trainee surgeons' time and morale.

The CCrISP algorithm for simultaneous assessment and resuscitation has become the benchmark for the management of surgical patients and is used by even the most senior and experienced surgeons on a daily basis. The emphasis is on supporting the patient's abnormal physiology while a credible reason for the patient's deterioration is found and a definitive management plan is formulated and enacted.

As with previous editions, this review is based on the opinions of a multidisciplinary steering group that has worked tirelessly to ensure that it represents the needs of current surgical trainees. Acknowledgement and our thanks must also be given to faculty who have helped in developing the pilot courses, proofread materials and contributed to book chapters.

It is important that you use this manual to adequately prepare yourself for the face-to-face element of the course. You will have access to a number of senior doctors experienced in the management of surgical patients. Ensure that you make the most of this valuable opportunity.

We hope, therefore, that you will find the CCrISP manual and subsequent course instructive and beneficial in the care you provide to your patients, but most of all we hope it helps you to appreciate what a vital role you play in good surgical outcomes. You really can and do make a difference.

Danny Bryden and John Jameson

# Course objectives

- Develop the theoretical basis and practical skills necessary to manage the critically ill surgical patient.

- Be able to assess critically ill patients accurately and appreciate the value of using a system of assessment.

- Understand the subtlety and variety of presentation of critical illness and the methods available for improving detection.

- Appreciate that complications tend to occur in a cascade and realise that prevention of complications is fundamental to a successful outcome.

- Be aware of multidisciplinary teamworking and understand how members of the team interact to support the patient who is at the centre of the process.

- Be aware of the importance of the lead role the surgeon needs to assume in coordinating this care and making decisions as necessary.

- Understand the importance of a plan of action in order to achieve clinical progress, accurate diagnosis and early definitive treatment.

- Be able to ensure that the plan of action is carried out accurately and in a timely manner and that it is communicated to all the relevant people, including the patient and relatives.

- Ensure that the assessment, decision-making process and communication are accurately and adequately documented in the patient's case notes.

- Understand the requirements of the patient and his or her relatives during critical illness and be able to inform, involve and support the patient and relatives appropriately.

An aide-memoire for success is to:

- ACCEPT responsibility for patient management.

- ADOPT a systematic approach to patient assessment.

- APPRECIATE that complications tend to cascade rapidly.

- ANTICIPATE and prevent complications with simple, timely actions.

- APPLY effective communication skills to facilitate patient care.

- ASK for appropriate assistance in a timely manner.

## About the Royal College of Surgeons

The Royal College of Surgeons (RCS) is a professional membership organisation and registered charity, with over 25,000 members in the UK and internationally. We provide support for our members across all career stages, specialties and locations, enabling them to drive the profession forward and achieve our vision of advancing surgical care. Membership benefits include:

- Resources to help you stay up to date in this fast-moving profession, including invaluable career-development events, access to e-journals, publications and regular e-newsletters.

- Standards and guidance, research fellowships and leadership opportunities to support your development, in addition to a 10% discount on selected courses.

- Careers advice, support and access to new opportunities including bursaries, a regional network with key contacts, and confidential support service.

Find out more at www.rcseng.ac.uk/join.

# Abbreviations

| | |
|---|---|
| ABG | arterial blood gas |
| ACE | angiotensin-converting enzyme |
| ACS | acute coronary syndrome |
| ACTH | adrenocorticotrophic hormone |
| ADH | antidiuretic hormone |
| A&E | accident and emergency department |
| AF | atrial fibrillation |
| AKIN | Acute Kidney Injury Network |
| AP | anteroposterior |
| APTT | activated partial thromboplastin time |
| ARDS | acute respiratory distress syndrome |
| ASA | American Society of Anaesthesiology |
| ASB | assisted spontaneous breathing |
| ATN | acute tubular necrosis |
| *ATLS®* | *Advanced Trauma Life Support®* |
| AV | atrioventricular |
| BAL | bronchoalveolar lavage |
| BBB | bundle branch block |
| bd | twice daily |
| BE | base excess |
| BIPAP | bilevel positive airway pressure |

| | |
|---|---|
| BMI | body mass index |
| BMR | basal metabolic rate |
| CCrISP | Care of the Critically Ill Surgical Patient |
| CI | cardiac index |
| CKD | chronic kidney disease |
| CNS | central nervous system |
| COAD | chronic obstructive airways disease |
| COX-2 | cyclo-oxygenase 2 |
| COPD | chronic obstructive pulmonary disease |
| CPAP | continuous positive airway pressure |
| CPET | cardiopulmonary exercise testing |
| CPR | cardiopulmonary resuscitation |
| CRBSI | catheter-related bloodstream infection |
| CRP | C-reactive protein |
| CSM | carotid sinus massage |
| CT | computed tomography |
| CTPA | CT pulmonary angiography |
| CURB | Confusion, Urea, Respiratory rate, Blood pressure |
| CVC | central venous catheter |
| CVP | central venous pressure |
| CVS | cardiovascular system |
| CVVH | continuous veno-venous haemofiltration |
| CXR | chest X-ray |
| DKA | diabetic ketoacidosis |

| | |
|---|---|
| 2,3-DPG | 2,3-diphosphoglycerate |
| DVT | deep vein thrombosis |
| EBD | external biliary drainage |
| ECF | extracellular fluid |
| ECG | electrocardiography |
| EE | energy expenditure |
| EEG | electroencephalography |
| EGDT | early goal-directed therapy |
| ENT | ear, nose and throat |
| ERAS | enhanced recovery after surgery |
| ERCP | endoscopic retrograde cholangiopancreatography |
| FBC | full blood count |
| $FEV_1$ | forced expiratory volume in 1 second |
| FRC | functional residual capacity |
| FTc | corrected flow time |
| GCS | Glasgow Coma Scale |
| GFR | glomerular filtration rate |
| GH | growth hormone |
| GI | gastrointestinal |
| $[H^+]$ | Hydrogen ion concentration |
| HDU | high-dependency unit |
| HR | heart rate |
| 5-HT | 5-hydroxytryptamine (serotonin) |
| IAH | intra-abdominal hypertension |

| | |
|---|---|
| IAP | intra-abdominal pressure |
| ICU | intensive care unit |
| ICP | intracranial pressure |
| IgE | immunoglobulin E |
| IL | interleukin |
| IVU | intravenous urography |
| JVP | jugular venous pressure |
| LFT | liver function test |
| LiDCO™ | lithium dilution cardiac output |
| LMWH | low-molecular-weight heparin |
| LVF | left ventricular failure |
| MAC | mid-arm circumference |
| MAMC | mid-arm muscle circumference |
| MAP | mean arterial pressure |
| MEWS | Modified Early Warning Score |
| MI | myocardial infarction |
| MRSA | methicillin-resistant *Staphylococcus aureus* |
| MUST | Malnutrition Universal Screening Tool |
| NCEPOD | National Confidential Enquiry into Patient Outcome and Death |
| NELA | National Emergency Laparotomy Audit |
| NEWS | National Early Warning Score |
| NGT | nasogastric tube |
| NICE | National Institute for Health and Care Excellence |
| NIDDM | non-insulin-dependent diabetes mellitus |

| | |
|---|---|
| NIV | non-invasive ventilation |
| NOAC | novel oral anticoagulants |
| NOTSS | non-technical skills for surgeons |
| NPSA | National Patient Safety Agency |
| NRS | numerical rating scale |
| NSAID | non-steroidal anti-inflammatory drug |
| OSA | obstructive sleep apnoea |
| PA | posteroanterior |
| PCA | patient-controlled analgesia |
| PCIRV | pressure-controlled inverse ratio ventilation |
| PCV | pressure-controlled ventilation |
| PE | pulmonary embolism |
| PEEP | positive end-expiratory pressure |
| PEG | percutaneous endoscopic gastrostomy |
| PICC | peripherally inserted central catheter |
| PiCCO | pulse contour cardiac output with indicator dilution |
| PPN | peripheral parenteral nutrition |
| PSV | pressure support ventilation |
| PTC | percutaneous trans-hepatic cholangiography |
| PTSD | post-traumatic stress disorder |
| qSOFA | quick Sequential Organ Failure Assessment |
| qds | four times a day |
| RIG | radiologically inserted gastrostomy |
| RR | respiratory rate |

| | |
|---|---|
| RRT | renal replacement therapy |
| rTPA | recombinant tissue plasminogen activator |
| SA | sinoatrial |
| SIMV | synchronised intermittent mandatory ventilation |
| SIRS | systemic inflammatory response syndrome |
| SOFA | Sequential Organ Failure Assessment |
| SSC | Surviving Sepsis Campaign |
| STEMI | ST elevation myocardial infarction |
| SVC | superior vena cava |
| SVR | systemic vascular resistance |
| SVT | supraventricular tachycardia |
| tds | three times a day |
| TNF | tumour necrosis factor |
| TOD | trans-oesophageal Doppler |
| TSF | triceps skinfold thickness |
| U&Es | urea and electrolytes |
| VAS | visual analogue score |
| VEs | ventricular ectopics |
| VF | ventricular fibrillation |
| VRIII | variable-rate intravenous insulin infusion |
| VRS | verbal rating scale |
| VT | ventricular tachycardia |
| WCC | white cell count |
| WPW | Wolff–Parkinson–White syndrome |

# Normal laboratory values

| Measurement | Normal range |
|---|---|
| Sodium (Na$^+$) | 135–145 mmol/L |
| Potassium (K$^+$) | 3.5–5.0 mmol/L |
| Chlorine (Cl$^-$) | 95–108 mmol/L |
| Urea | 3.1–7.9 mmol/L |
| Creatinine | 75–155 μmol/L |
| Total protein | 58–78 g/L |
| Albumin | 34–50 g/L |
| Calcium (Ca$^{2+}$) | 2.12–2.60 mmol/L |
| Phosphate (PO$_4$$^{3-}$) | 0.80–1.44 mmol/L |
| Bilirubin | 0–19 μmol/L |
| Alkaline phosphatase (ALP) | 35–120 units/L |
| Alanine aminotransferase (ALT) | 0–45 units/L |
| Creatine kinase | |
|     Male | 38–174 units/L |
|     Female | 96–140 units/L |
| Haemoglobin (Hb) | 130–180 g/L |
| Platelets | 150–450 × 10$^9$/L |
| White cell count (WCC) | 4.0–11.0 × 10$^9$/L |
| Prothrombin time (PT) | 11.0–13.0 seconds |
| Activated partial thromboplastin time (APTT) | 24–39 seconds |
| Fibrinogen | 1.5–4.0 g/L |
| pH | 7.35–7.45 |
| $PaCO_2$ | 4.5–6.0 kPa (34–42 mmHg) |
| $PaO_2$ | 11.0–14.0 kPa (83–105 mmHg) |
| HCO$_3$$^-$ | 24–28 mmol/L |

| Measurement | Normal range |
|---|---|
| Base excess | –2 to +2 mmol/L |
| Lactate | 0.4–1.7 mmol/L |
| Glucose | <11.1 mmol/L random |
| C-reactive protein (CRP) | 0–5 mg/L |
| Amylase | 28–100 units/L |

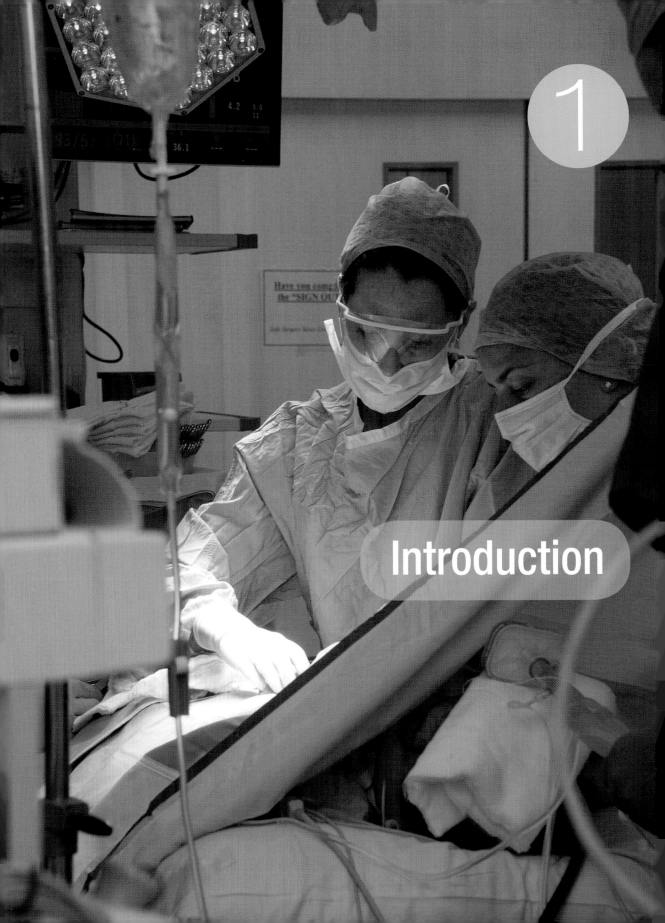

1

Introduction

## Why have CCrISP?

To the non-medical population, surgeons are doctors who perform operations of varying complexity under general or regional anaesthesia. Much of the initial motivation for people like you who enter surgical specialties focuses on an interest in anatomy and pride in the technical skill of operating and how surgery can qualitatively and quantitatively improve people's lives. In isolation these motivations form only part of the role of a surgeon working within the multidisciplinary environment of perioperative medical care. Regardless of whether an operation is a technical success, the majority of complaints made by patients and their families relate to either poor communication or real or perceived inadequacies in ward-based care rather than the nature of the surgery and technical skill of the operator. In other words, as a surgeon, you are only as good as the team around you (Box 1.1). Therefore, it is imperative that surgeons and those looking after surgical patients are aware of the interactions between these factors and have the skills to deal with them.

Increasingly, surgical patients are likely to have prolonged inpatient stays, as they are elderly, have undergone major surgery or are emergency admissions. Out-of-hours duty arrangements may mean that the initial medical responder is not immediately from the base specialty and may be a doctor, nurse or allied health professional from

### Box 1.1 Risk and stress factors in surgical care

- Ageing population
- Concomitant chronic disease processes (often severe and associated with several years of functional decline)
- Expectations: patients', relatives', staff's, society's
- Increasing complexity and specialisation of surgery
- Greater number of postoperative interventions and therapies
- Higher standards of monitoring
- Shortage of permanent and experienced nurses
- Altered patterns of doctors' duty hours

a medical response or hospital at-night team. As a trainee surgeon, you must be aware of this and your ability to respond and plan patient care in order to minimise the rate and severity of complications is vital.

Many of these patients can deteriorate rapidly when their chronic disease processes combine with a perioperative complication to cause a massive imbalance in oxygen demand, oxygen delivery and oxygen utilisation. The subsequent development of multiorgan dysfunction is likely to precipitate critical care referral and admission, with in-hospital mortality rates in excess of 50%. Furthermore, an absolute failure to recognise and manage an acute deterioration in the perioperative period can result in cardiorespiratory arrest, the nature of which is frequently asystole or PEA (pulseless electrical activity), which carries a mortality rate of > 85%. Even if the patient survives to hospital discharge, there are likely to be significant rehabilitation consequences, which can in turn be catastrophic for patients and their families. This phenomenon is often described as failure to rescue (FTR) and is recognised throughout multiple healthcare systems. Early recognition is vital for effective care. In most cases it can save lives and reduce perioperative complication rates and hospital length of stay, and in a minority of circumstances may save a dying patient from futile, torturous treatments (Figure 1.1)

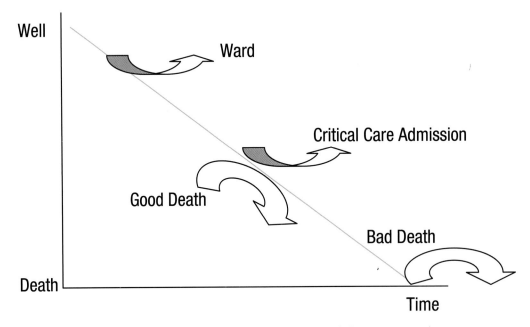

Figure 1.1 Physiological derangement (timely intervention vs. failure to rescue). CCrISP®, RCS Eng.

At ward level, efforts to reduce FTR have included marrying standard nursing observations to illness severity or so-called early warning scores, eg in the NHS the National Early Warning Score (NEWS) has been introduced to enable rapid measurement and scoring of baseline, bedside clinical measurements. The measurements (respiratory rate, heart rate, blood pressure, oxygen saturation, temperature, consciousness level, urine output and the presence of supplementary oxygen) reflect oxygen delivery and oxygen utilisation, and are easily reproducible and documented in a numeric and colour-coded score designed to illicit a so-called graded track and trigger response according to severity (Figure 1.2).

Increasingly, the response to the deteriorating patient is being used as a quality indicator for healthcare. However, although observation charts encompassing early warning scores have become best practice, the systems are designed as safety nets in the first stages of preventing FTR – they are not substitutes for good medical and nursing care. Therefore, the challenge for surgeons like you is to use them in processes that deal with patients who may become critically ill, thereby developing your practice and interpretation skills to allow early identification and correction of complications. This comes not only through direct application of care but also through education, training and leadership of others in the principles of dealing with the acutely ill (Box 1.2). The strategies outlined are complementary, applied in differing proportions to different patient groups and in modern surgical practice they are arguably more important than heroic last-ditch efforts to rescue the patient in extremis.

Box 1.2  Complementary approaches to critical care

- Prediction: identifying an at-risk population
- Prevention
- Prompt identification and early adequate treatment

## Aims of training in surgical critical care

The beginnings of critical illness are detectable and treatable long before a patient arrives in the critical care unit, with the majority of abnormal clinical signs being measureable at the bedside. In the UK the three most common abnormalities in the

# Care of the Critically Ill Surgical Patient®

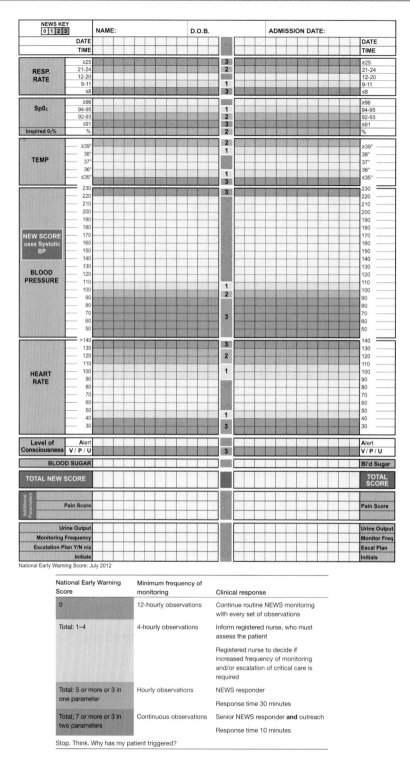

Figure 1.2 National Early Warning Score (NEWS).
Newcastle upon Tyne Hospitals NHS Foundation Trust, November 2014

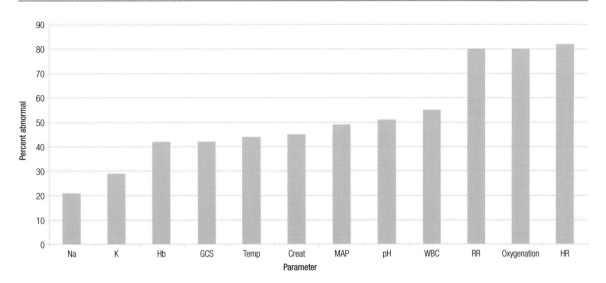

Figure 1.3 Abnormal parameters in the 24 hours before intensive care admission.
*Quarterly Journal of Medicine* 2001; 94: 507–510
*British Journal of Anaesthesia* 2004; 92: 882–884

24 hours before emergency admission to intensive care are abnormalities in heart rate, oxygen saturation and respiratory rate (Figure 1.3), all easily measureable and recognisable. The objective of CCrISP, therefore, is to equip you to predict and prevent deterioration, and to treat deteriorating patients in a timely and effective manner so that they have the best chance of a good recovery if complications occur. The course offers you an opportunity to practise and develop your management skills for ward and critical care practice.

When you come to the course, the faculty will help you combine your clinical skills and professional behaviours to identify at-risk patients and take the necessary steps to prevent complications (Box 1.3).

Many adverse episodes can be terminated by the immediate provision of simple support (eg oxygen or intravenous fluids) and by the early attainment of a diagnosis enabling early definitive treatment (eg antibiotics, provision of usual cardiac medications or drainage of an abscess). The course will ensure that the basics are done properly every time, because they are important.

## Box 1.3 Objectives of the CCrISP course

### Clinical skills

- Identify at-risk patients
- Manage critically ill surgical patients:
  - marry theory to practice
  - clinical assessment
- Prevent the 'complications cascade' and minimise 'failure to rescue'
- Learn to play your part in surgical critical care, understanding your role and the roles of others in the multidisciplinary team

### Professional behaviours

- Lead the ward team in surgical critical care
- Organise and communicate:
  - colleagues: own specialty/other specialties
  - patients and relatives
- Assume increasing responsibility
- Be aware of limitations:
  - others' and yours
  - treatments.

- Avoidable problems occur either because simple measures are not taken or because their effectiveness and adequacy is not checked, eg failure to ensure effective support for a postoperative woman with retained sputum on a quick Saturday morning ward round by following through that the patient has actually had physiotherapy and is improving at the end of your shift may result in that patient having established pneumonia by the time you return on Monday morning. Patient survival will be threatened and her length of stay certainly prolonged. Implementing simple interventions such as humidified oxygen and physiotherapy can be life saving, if not very glamorous, and requires the same skills and professional behaviours necessary for instituting more complex treatments at consultant level. They include clinical examination, judicious investigation, formulating and communicating a plan of action, reviewing it and, if necessary, invoking greater degrees of timely support. Workload and the ability to prioritise can also have a bearing on patient outcome and you should learn to recognise when you may need assistance, so that patient care is not compromised (see case scenario 1.1, below).

## Case scenario 1.1

A 68-year-old man (with mild chronic obstructive airways disease smoking 20 cigarettes per day) underwent a robotically assisted laparoscopic cystectomy and ileal conduit formation for transitional cell carcinoma of the bladder on a Thursday. By Friday he was mobilising but becoming breathless. No formal request for physiotherapy had been made and the on-call team was informed that he was 'progressing'. At 10pm on Friday evening he complained of abdominal pain and was noted to have a NEWS of 7 (respiratory rate (RR) 33/min, HR 103 bpm, urine output < 30 ml/h).

The foundation year 2 (FY2) doctor covering urology was informed and told the nursing staff to 'check the PCA', saying that she would review the patient when she had a chance but was currently being trained (in emergency theatre) to insert a ureteric stent. The nursing staff informed the FY2 that 'the PCA had been taken down and the patient was drinking and taking oral analgesia'. The FY2 asked the nursing team to contact the pain team, unaware that the pain team (out-of-hours) is represented by the anaesthetic specialty trainee currently anaesthetising the patient with ureteric obstruction, who afterwards had to join his consultant in the A&E resuscitation room. The FY2 said that she would 'review the patient when she got a chance'. The FY2 did not communicate any specifics to the anaesthetic specialty trainee throughout the case. The anaesthetic specialty trainee made no further enquiries.

The ureteric stent insertion was difficult, taking a further 90 minutes. The urology specialty trainee went home and the FY2 completed reviewing an 18-year-old male with testicular pain. During this time the 68-year-old man developed pyrexia (39.1°C) and hypotension; his pain and tachypnoea worsened. He was reviewed at 3am on Saturday and after oxygen, intravenous fluids and antibiotics he underwent computerised tomography (CT) and was found to have a rectal perforation. He had an emergency laparotomy and Hartmann's procedure and spent 10 days in intensive care and a further 2 weeks in hospital.

## Learning points

- New breathlessness on initial mobilisation should be queried and investigated.
- New or worsening abdominal pain 24–48 hours after major surgery requires early review and possible investigation, particularly where pain control was previously good.
- When problems arise out of hours and resources are more stretched, extra care must be taken to ensure details are communicated appropriately.
- Improved communications could have led to an earlier assessment and, although subsequent emergency surgery and intensive care admission may have been unavoidable, the severe consequences of rectal perforation and intra-abdominal sepsis could have been minimised and length of stay reduced.

## Practice points

- Prompt, simple actions save lives and prevent complications.
- Reassess your treatment plan. Has your intervention been effective?
- Further prompt and simple actions (or more advanced ones) may be necessary.

## Patients to be considered at risk

Patients and practices associated with increased risk are summarised in Box 1.4 and the patients affected fall into three broad categories:

- the elective preoperative patient;
- the emergency admission;
- the postoperative ward patient.

## Box 1.4  At-risk patients

### At-risk patients

- Emergencies
- Elderly patients
- Patients with coexisting disease
- Non-progressing patients
- Severity of acute illness (including shock) or magnitude of surgery (including re-bleeding and the need for massive transfusion)
- Failure/delay in diagnosis and treatment

### Practices that increase risk

- Incomplete or infrequent assessment
- Failure to act on abnormal findings
- Failure to check on outcomes of interventions
- Failure of continuity of care (poor communication)
- Failure of nursing support: insufficient numbers, wrong ward, etc.

### The elective preoperative patient

The presence of coexisting disease (and treatments of such disease) can play a significant role in the development of postoperative complications and optimisation is necessary (see case scenario 1.2, below). Careful specialist preoperative assessment should occur (see Chapter 16). This may include active testing of functional status, eg cardiopulmonary exercise testing (CPET), postoperative planning and (especially) in high-risk patients a discussion of risk via a shared decision-making process.

## Case scenario 1.2

A male patient presents on the day of surgery for elective repair of an inguinal hernia. He describes himself as being fit and well but ECG shows left bundle branch block. He smokes 20 cigarettes a day, admits to drinking in excess of 20 units of alcohol per week and has occasional nocturia.

Does this man need a plan for his surgical care?

If anaesthesia and surgery proceed without further investigation and planning, a predictable chain of minor events could occur that have the potential to prove fatal. For example, a simple hernia repair can lead to urinary retention; a subsequent urinary tract infection could contribute to an acute confusional state (exacerbated by alcohol withdrawal). The patient fails to cough adequately, leading to atelectasis and pneumonia, and subsequent hypoxaemia compounds coronary artery perfusion.

### Learning points

- It is crucial to predict and prevent problems.
- Consider the pros and cons of surgery on a case-by-case basis. Elective patients need to have plans for their perioperative care.
- Review comorbidities and their potential impact in the perioperative period.
- Optimise appropriately if surgery is essential.

### *The emergency admission*

Emergency admissions present with a variety of underlying diseases and comorbidities that may be unrecognised (eg occult ischaemic heart disease) or recognised but with significant surgical implications (eg anticoagulant therapies). Many of these patients may also be inherently unstable and at risk of further complications. Prompt and effective resuscitation can reduce this, but the consequences of general anaesthesia in the shocked patient must also be considered, ie the risks of vasodilation and reduced contractility. Simultaneous resuscitation and surgery may be necessary. Furthermore, emergency surgery frequently takes place out of hours, taxing organisational and communication skills and professional behaviours rather than clinical skills.

### The ward patient

On business ward rounds, many apparently stable patients will need to be reviewed quickly: this is potentially one of the most effective ways of practising good critical care by conducting systematic and thorough reviews using the CCrISP approach. A standardised approach like this can identify many problems, allowing them to be corrected before significant upset occurs.

When ward patients develop complications, the major pitfall is usually a failure to take further prompt action when initial interventions have proved insufficient to rescue the patient. Therefore, clear plans that are communicated and followed up are very important.

More difficult ward patients to deal with are those 'who fail to progress'. In such circumstances there is a high probability of an underlying problem eluding detection, especially if you are unfamiliar with the usual postoperative time course for the surgical procedure. These types of patients are often elderly and failure to progress can be easy to miss either because changes in their clinical and laboratory indices are subtle and/or because they have associated delirium. Thorough assessment with subsequent investigation and follow-up can prevent major problems occurring, so your level of clinical suspicion must be high unless you use a system like CCrISP to ensure that you do not cut corners and miss things.

## Why the CCrISP method of approach works

As you progress in seniority throughout your career, your role changes as your responsibilities develop. The requirement to make decisions that have a direct bearing on patient management and outcome increases. Using the skills and approaches developed on the CCrISP course assists you in this process and encourages reflection that further aids the development of decision-making. All clinicians find the management of emergencies stressful and will have experienced occasions when the stress has been compounded by limited information, disorganisation and a lack of appreciation of the severity of the situation. CCrISP provides templates for trainee surgeons to deal with these dilemmas by rapidly assessing the situation and the patient, responding to the immediate problem and initiating treatment. The CCrISP algorithm (Figure 1.4) and simple immediate thoughts can help set your assessment off on the right foot (Box 1.5).

## What the CCrISP course is not

The main ethos of the course is the prevention of further deterioration through accurate and prompt ASSESSMENT and TREATMENT, minimising the need for, or impact of, critical care admission. CCrISP takes a practical, management-orientated approach to surgical critical care. The manual is not designed as a comprehensive textbook for intensive care and will not teach candidates on the CCrISP course to become specialists in intensive care medicine. There is overlap between surgical care and the principles applied day to day by the intensive care team, and surgeons should therefore be aware of the nature and principles of intensive care, the support it provides, when such support should be sought and what the limitations of that support may be. They should also be aware of the support and advice that intensive

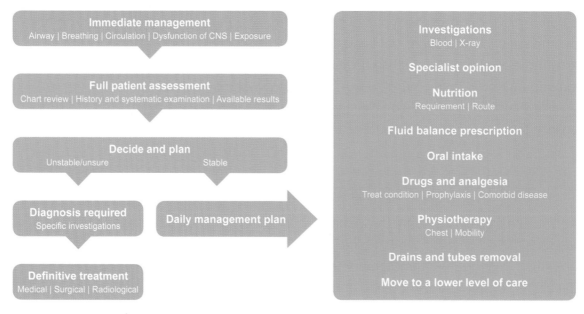

Figure 1.4 The CCrISP algorithm.
CCrISP®, RCS Eng.

Box 1.5 Thinking on the run

- Think early: when the phone call comes
  - Instructions to the caller
  - What do I know about?
  - What will I do when I arrive?

- Think basics: when I arrive
  - Check and secure ABCs
  - What system has failed?
  - What observations are available?
  - What observations can I make quickly?

- Think simply
  - How quickly must I act?
  - Do I have a diagnosis?
    - How will I get the diagnosis safely
    - What help do I need?

Box 1.6 Basic summary of levels of patient care

- Level 3: invasive organ support (nurse–patient ratio of 1:1)
- Level 2: no invasive respiratory support required (nurse–patient ratio of 1:2)
- Level 1: ward levels of care
- Level 0: self-caring patients

care requires from them and the impact of intensive care on patients that survive. Use the course as an opportunity to explore this interface and your role as a surgeon in patient care on an HDU or ICU.

Increasing surgical input

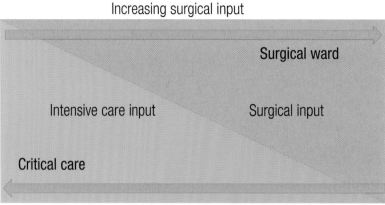

Surgical ward

Intensive care input                    Surgical input

Critical care

Increasing intensive care input

Figure 1.5  Interplay between intensive care and surgical care.
CCrISP®, RCS Eng.

Following discharge from intensive care, a further range of skills are necessary to ensure that the patient does not fall into the trap of early deterioration and re-admission. Much of this relates to the assessment principles of CCrISP, it may also include difficult discussions about the possible futility of further intensive care treatments and the appropriateness of advanced organ support in a deteriorating patient. These topics will be dealt with on the course and will contribute towards making you a better practitioner, marrying clinical skills to professional behaviours.

## Summary

- Preventing deterioration is more effective than attempting salvage at a later stage.

- Surgical critical care includes prediction and prevention of problems as well as investigation and intervention in the acutely unwell.

- There is a continuum in surgical critical care extending from the surgical ward (prediction, prevention) to critical care and back again.

- Simple logical thought and actions utilising systematic guidance will often be effective.

## Further reading

American College of Surgeons. *Surgical Traits*. https://www.facs.org/education/resources/residency-search/traits (accessed November 2015).

Bismark MM, Spittal MJ, Gurrin LC et al. Identification of doctors at risk of recurrent complaints: a national study of healthcare complaints in Australia. *BMJ Qual Saf* 2013; 22: 532–540.

Department of Health. *A Review of the NHS Hospitals Complaints System: Putting Patients Back in the Picture*. Department of Health, London; 2013.

Department of Health. *Comprehensive Critical Care: a Review of Adult Critical Care Services*. Department of Health, London; 2000.

Goldhill DR, McNarry AF, Mandersloot G, McGinley A. A physiologically-based early warning score for ward patients: the association between score and outcome. *Anaesthesia* 2005; 60: 547–553.

Goldhill DR, McNarry AF. Physiological abnormalities in early warning scores are related to mortality in adult inpatients. *Br J Anaesth* 2004; 92: 882–884.

Health and Social Care Information Centre. *NHS Outcomes Framework Indicators*. http://www.hscic.gov.uk/nhsof (accessed November 2015).

Intensive Care Society and Department of Health. *Levels of Critical Care for Adult Patients*. Intensive Care Society and Department of Health, London; 2009.

Nolan JP, Soar J, Smith GB et al. Incidence and outcome of in-hospital cardiac arrest in the United Kingdom National Cardiac Arrest Audit. *Resuscitation* 2014; 85: 987–992.

Ou L, Chen J, Hassan A, Hollis SJ et al. Trends and variations in the rates of hospital complications, failure-to-rescue and 30-day mortality in surgical patients in New South Wales, Australia, 2002–2009. *PLoS One* 2014; 9: e96164.

Royal Australian College of Surgeons. Interviews with surgeons. http://www.surgeons. org/becoming-a-surgeon/surgery-as-a-career/videos/ (accessed November 2015).

Royal College of Anaesthetists. *Perioperative Medicine. The Pathway to Better Surgical Care*. Royal College of Anaesthetists, London; 2014.

Royal College of Physicians. *National Early Warning Score (NEWS)*. Royal College of Physicians, London; 2012.

Stringer W, Casaburi R, Older P. Cardiopulmonary exercise testing: does it improve perioperative care and outcome? *Curr Opin Anaesthesiol* 2012; 25: 178–184.

Subbe CP, Kruger M, Rutherford P, Gemmel L. Validation of a modified Early Warning Score in medical admissions. *Q J Med* 2001; 94: 521–526.

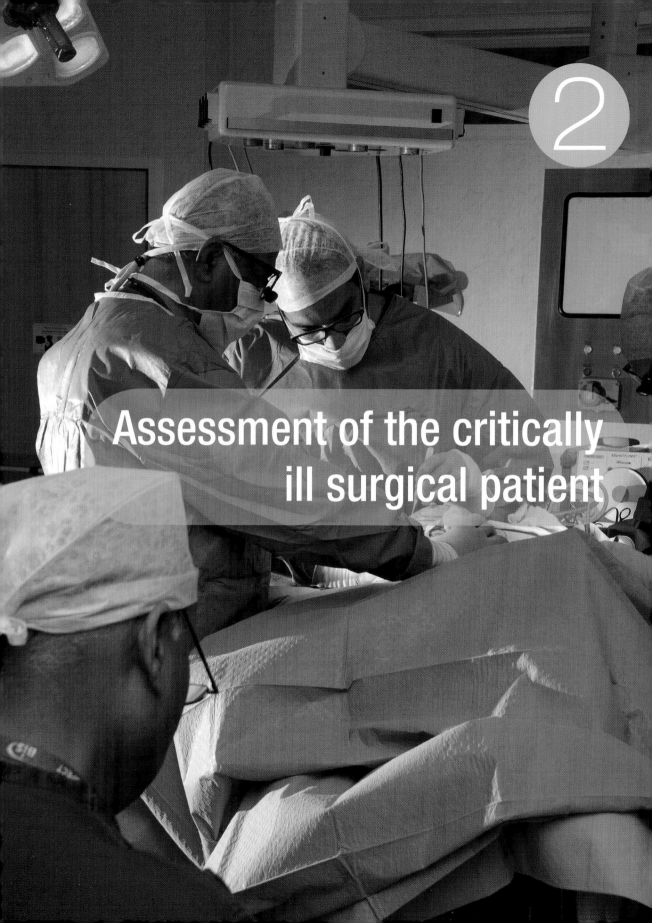

2

Assessment of the critically
ill surgical patient

## Learning outcomes

This chapter will help you to:

- recognise the critically ill patient who must undergo simultaneous examination and resuscitation when first seen;

- assess and manage critically ill patients systematically;

- recognise that examination and resuscitation must be performed in a systematic manner;

- understand why abnormal physiology needs to be treated irrespective of the cause;

- recognise the importance of finding an underlying explanation for deterioration in a patient's condition;

- formulate management plans for patients irrespective of physiological stability.

## Introduction

All patients in hospital should have a management plan. This plan will differ depending on the underlying problem and degree of physiological instability of the patient.

The CCrISP three-stage assessment process will help you to define the acuity of your patients, what the underlying problems are, what interventions are needed and how frequently the patients should be reviewed. Most UK hospitals now use 'track and trigger' systems, such as the National Early Warning Score (NEWS), to aid the recognition of the deteriorating patient. The role of the CCrISP course and three-stage assessment process is to allow you to assess these patients properly when called to see them and to plan their subsequent care.

Most often, surgical patients who end up requiring critical care will either have been admitted acutely unwell or will have suffered an acute deterioration on the ward following admission or elective or emergency surgery. These patients require simultaneous resuscitation and diagnosis, followed by definitive treatment, and CCrISP helps you to do this in an organised manner.

Other patients will be relatively more stable but remain at risk of deterioration, either on the ward or in an HDU setting. These patients need to be re-evaluated, and their management plan updated, at least twice daily. The aim is to ensure that the patient is getting better. It is better to prevent morbidity by detecting problems as early as possible; failure to progress is an important sign that an incipient problem is present. If you fail to diagnose and treat that problem until it has resulted in a major deterioration in the patient's condition, then the patient's chance of survival is dramatically reduced. Case reviews of patients who have apparently undergone an acute deterioration often reveal evidence of subtle signs of impending problems that were not dealt with promptly and correctly. This is our challenge as surgeons: to minimise the risk of adverse events and to give each patient the best chance of experiencing a good outcome.

The CCrISP system of assessment is shown in Figure 2.1. It is the system that many experienced doctors use. The same system is used for all patients to help determine whether they are stable or unstable. In this context, it needs to be recognised that stability is a relative term and often a patient will be stable but ill and needs to be treated with great attention to detail, something which the three-stage assessment process will guide.

The CCrISP ethos therefore is to apply the three-stage assessment process to all patients both during scheduled ward rounds and in the event of deterioration.

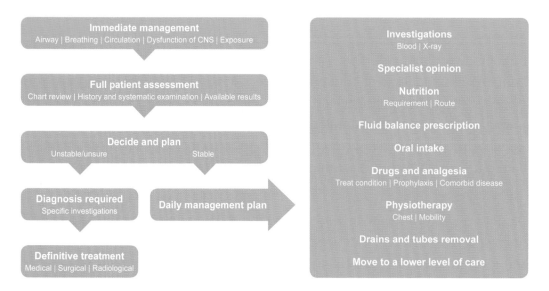

Figure 2.1 The CCrISP system of assessment.

## Immediate assessment and treatment of the acutely ill patient

When assessing a patient, your goal is to determine whether the patient is acutely unwell and, if so, what is making the patient ill and, having identified any life-threatening problem, to treat it immediately. Life-threatening illnesses kill in a predictable and reproducible pattern. When viewed in isolation, a disease process that produces an obstructed airway will kill more quickly than a problem in the lungs, which, in turn, kills more quickly than isolated haemorrhage. Many critically ill surgical patients have abnormalities of more than one system and it is important therefore that you are not distracted by obvious, and potentially minor, factors but assess and treat patients systematically.

## Immediate management

A      Airway assessment and treatment.

B      Breathing assessment and treatment.

C      Circulation assessment and treatment.

D      Dysfunction of the CNS and treatment.

E      Exposure of the patient sufficient for full assessment and treatment.

This process prioritises the order in which assessment and treatment is carried out; although represented as a sequence, such information can often be obtained virtually simultaneously. For example, the patient's response to the question 'How are you?' can be very revealing. A patient who is able to reply in a coherent manner has, at least at that moment, sufficient airway control to allow an adequate intake of breath, adequate respiratory function to produce oxygen transfer, adequate circulatory function to perfuse the brain and adequate CNS function to formulate a reply. While this is encouraging, it does not relieve you of the need to perform a detailed assessment of each of the ABCDE components of the immediate assessment; detailed examination picks up the subtle abnormalities that are not always obvious unless specifically sought out.

**Practice point**

Do not be falsely reassured by patients who look well from the end of the bed.

## A: Airway

Recognition that airway obstruction is present is based on a simple 'Look, Listen and Feel' clinical assessment, with immediate treatment if there is airway compromise.

- LOOK for the presence of central cyanosis, an obstructed 'see-saw' pattern of respiration or abdominal breathing, the use of accessory muscles of respiration, tracheal tug, alteration of level of consciousness and any obvious obstruction by foreign body or vomitus.

- LISTEN for abnormal sounds such as grunting, snoring, gurgling, hoarseness or stridor.

- FEEL for air flow on inspiration and expiration.

- TREAT. If objective signs of airway obstruction are present, the immediate goals are to obtain and secure the airway to provide for adequate oxygenation and prevent hypoxic brain damage. Administer high-flow oxygen (12–15 L/min, preferably humidified, via a reservoir bag).

Often, only simple methods are required to obtain an airway, such as chin lift or jaw thrust to open the airway, suction to remove secretions and the insertion of either an oral Guedel airway (if tolerated) or a soft nasopharyngeal airway (if the gag reflex is present). Problems with the airway are covered in Chapter 3. If you cannot maintain the airway by the simple measures outlined as above, you need to call for help.

Remember that patients can be maintained with an airway, plus bag and mask ventilation as required while waiting for the anaesthetist – this is often a better option for the non-expert, particularly in a hospital, where skilled help is usually rapidly available.

Patients who are not fully conscious may be unable to protect their airway with the result that it is patent only intermittently. These patients may tolerate and benefit from airway manoeuvres while the cause of their reduced consciousness level is addressed.

Although unusual in the non-trauma situation, if there is a risk of coexisting pathology of the cervical spine, all airway manoeuvres should be performed while maintaining manual in-line immobilisation of the cervical spine.

### Practice point

Get help from an anaesthetist early to secure a compromised airway.

## B: Breathing

Objective evidence of respiratory distress or inadequate ventilation can also be determined using the clinical 'Look, Listen and Feel' technique, followed by immediate treatment of life-threatening conditions:

- LOOK for central cyanosis, use of accessory muscles of respiration, respiratory rate, equality and depth of respiration, sweating, raised jugular venous pressure (JVP), patency of any chest drains and the presence of any paradoxical abdominal movement. Note the inspired oxygen concentration ($FiO_2$) and saturation. Pulse oximetry should be in use but remember that pulse oximetry does not detect hypercarbia.

- LISTEN for noisy breathing, clearance of secretions by coughing, the ability of the patient to talk in complete sentences (evidence of confusion or decreased level of consciousness may indicate hypoxia or hypercarbia, respectively) or change in percussion note and auscultate for abnormal breath sounds, heart sounds and rhythm.

- FEEL for equality of chest movement, the position of the trachea, the presence of surgical emphysema or crepitus, paradoxical respiration and tactile vocal fremitus if indicated. Percuss the chest superiorly and laterally. Abdominal distension may limit diaphragmatic movement and should be looked for as part of respiratory assessment.

- TREAT. The precise resuscitative treatment will be determined by the cause of the respiratory embarrassment and will be discussed later in the chapter on respiratory failure (Chapter 4). During the immediate assessment, you should specifically look for signs of the immediately life-threatening conditions: tension pneumothorax, massive haemothorax, open pneumothorax, flail chest and cardiac tamponade should be identified and treated without delay. Consider the diagnoses of bronchial obstruction, bronchoconstriction, pulmonary embolism (PE), cardiac failure (see C: Circulation) and unconsciousness (see D: Dysfunction of the nervous system). Simple manoeuvres such as sitting the patient up can help. However, if the patient is tiring to the point of incipient respiratory arrest, assisting ventilation by bag/mask is obligatory, in conjunction with whatever airway manoeuvres have been necessary, until help arrives.

## C: Circulation

Hypovolaemia should always be considered to be the primary cause of circulatory dysfunction in the surgical patient until proven otherwise. Haemorrhage (overt or covert) must be rapidly excluded. Furthermore, unless there are obvious signs of cardiogenic shock (particularly raised JVP), you should regard any patient who is cool and tachycardic to have hypovolaemic shock, so establish and secure adequate venous access with at least one large (16G) cannula, send off blood for cross-matching and other routine tests, and initiate appropriate fluid replacement.

Start with a rapid fluid challenge of 10 ml/kg warmed crystalloid in the normotensive patient or 20 ml/kg if the patient is hypotensive. You should be more tentative in patients with known cardiac dysfunction, starting with an initial bolus of 5 ml/kg. Closer monitoring may be needed in these patients.

Having identified and treated airway and breathing abnormalities that can compromise the circulation, life-threatening circulatory dysfunction is recognised by looking for:

- reduced peripheral perfusion (prolonged capillary refill time, pallor, coolness, collapsed or underfilled veins – remember that blood pressure can be normal in the shocked patient);

- obvious external haemorrhage from either wounds or drains;

- evidence of concealed haemorrhage: (i) thoracic or abdominal, even when an empty drain is present; (ii) into the gut or from pelvic or femoral fractures.

Initially, you should assess perfusion and the simplest way of doing this is to measure capillary refill time. Institute management with a fluid bolus based on your findings. Check the blood pressure at an early point; it can often be preserved in a patient with significant circulatory problems. Marked hypotension can be a late sign in a young, fit person and needs rapid correction.

Feel for pulses, both peripheral and central, assessing for rate, quality, regularity and equality. Treatment and monitoring are covered in detail in Chapters 6 and 7 and should be directed towards haemorrhage control and restoration of tissue perfusion.

No amount of fluid replacement will be of use in the face of on-going severe haemorrhage. Immediate surgery to control haemorrhage may be required at this stage as the only effective form of resuscitation. More frequently, urgent but non-immediate surgery will be needed to stop lesser degrees of continued haemorrhage.

Shocked patients fall into three categories and fluid challenges can be both diagnostic and therapeutic, helping you to determine into which category the patient falls:

- In obviously exsanguinating patients, immediate definitive treatment (usually surgery) is required to save the patient's life.

- Unstable patients need rapid resuscitation and repeated reassessment over a short period while the cause is identified and treatment planned. Such patients may appear to respond transiently to aggressive fluid resuscitation. Urgent definitive treatment is essential.

- Patients with a relatively minor problem will respond rapidly and adequately to a fluid challenge and remain stable on reassessment.

Reassessment (which should be performed after each intervention) determines whether or not a patient is responding to treatment. If there is no response (or only a transient or inadequate response), different treatment is needed immediately. Patients requiring large and on-going volumes of fluid are not stable, even if reasonable vital signs are maintained.

Occasionally is it necessary to give uncross-matched blood as type-specific blood is relatively safe and can be obtained within 20 minutes. Blood is presently the best resuscitation fluid for the bleeding patient who has cardiovascular instability and who requires, as a guide, more than 1500–2000 ml of resuscitation fluid.

Avoid 'blindly' continuing to transfuse the patient who, in reality, needs surgery. Bleeding patients who need immediate surgery are encountered on the ward as well as in the emergency room – patients with postoperative bleeding or recurrent bleeding from a peptic ulcer who are pale and shocked are typical examples. Once you have determined that a patient is not responding to resuscitation, you should call for senior help, cross-match 6 units of blood and alert theatre, the anaesthetist and the porters. Shocked or hypotensive patients who are not bleeding are also seen regularly – do not continue to 'blindly' fill up a patient with litres of fluid without a clear diagnosis, a clear plan or senior review. The message is to use the assessment process, come to a sensible conclusion, carry out an intervention, review the patient and seek help if the patient is not responding as expected.

Most surgeons have failed to respond adequately to continuing haemorrhage at some point during their career – so reassess and reconsider and do not leave a patient with inadequate perfusion without further adequate treatment.

## Practice points

- Most unwell surgical patients benefit from administration of oxygen and fluids while further assessment is undertaken.

- Reassess as resuscitation proceeds – it often takes more than one assessment to decide on all aspects of the problem.

## D: Dysfunction of the CNS

In the initial assessment, a rapid determination of neurological status is performed by examining the pupils and by using the AVPU system:

- A – Alert.

- V – responds to Verbal stimulus.

- P – responds only to Pain.

- U – Unresponsive to any stimulus. Remember that in surgical patients alteration of consciousness level can be due to causes other than a primary brain injury. Hypoxia and cerebral underperfusion due to shock should have already been detected.

Recent administration of sedatives, analgesics or anaesthetic drugs may be responsible. Hypoglycaemia is a common (and sometimes overlooked) cause that you should look for and treat. If you have thought of all these and the patient is still not fully conscious, reassess and review the ABCs: you might have missed something.

### E: Exposure

In order to make accurate diagnoses and allow access to the patient for therapeutic manoeuvres, it is essential that the patient is adequately exposed. However, be aware that the patient may become cold and preserve the patient's dignity at all times.

## End of immediate management

By the end of the phase of immediate assessment and management, the patient will hopefully be showing signs of improvement and progressing out of immediate danger; if not, you need help. You may have called for help and the patient may have been to theatre or moved to intensive care before this point is reached.

By this stage, the patient should be receiving oxygen and IV fluids. If not done already, establish monitoring by attaching a pulse oximeter, check the blood pressure and confirm that oxygen saturation ($SaO_2$) is above 94% and determine the frequency of on-going observations. Arrange pressing investigations that you know have not been done recently and that are targeted and integral to the immediate assessment (perhaps arterial blood gases (ABGs), chest X-ray or ECG), insert a urinary catheter (if appropriate) and, if necessary, alert senior colleagues (if you have not already done so). Before you start the next phase, quickly reassess the ABCs.

### Practice point

If, at any time during the immediate assessment, the patient's condition deteriorates, you must reassess the ABCs.

Having started resuscitative manoeuvres, it will often take a few minutes for their effects to become apparent. Vital signs may not yet be normal but, provided the patient's condition is not deteriorating, you should use the time to continue with the next stage of assessment in order to determine the underlying cause of deterioration. However, if the patient is deteriorating, then quickly reassess, get help and arrange for further immediate treatment as appropriate.

## Assessment of the 'stable' surgical patient

In many surgical patients, particularly during ward rounds, the vital signs will be normal. Often this can be determined simply by looking at the patient, by asking how they are, asking the nurse how the patient is doing, and reviewing the observation charts and recent results. If any abnormality is spotted, a detailed immediate assessment should be performed, which with practice can be done very quickly. Using the system in this way can avoid simple errors, particularly when you are tired or stressed.

## Full patient assessment

Now that the immediate management phase has been completed, the aim is to gather all available information from a variety of sources, which will lead to a diagnosis of current or potential problems and, hence, to a plan of action. The full assessment incorporates a review of the charts and available results plus a full history and examination.

### Chart reviews

Inspection of the observation and fluid charts, preferably at the end of the bed, together with discussion with nursing and other junior medical staff, may bring to light any recent or outstanding problems. It also allows a more focused clinical assessment to be carried out. Charts, particularly those in HDU or ICU, may appear to carry an overwhelming amount of information, but this too can be handled by breaking the chart into sections and systematically noting both absolute values and trends (Box 2.1), together with the degree of intervention needed to maintain physiological stability.

It is not possible to give a comprehensive account of management for every potential scenario, but you should consider both general and specific aspects of care. For example, general care includes cardiorespiratory function and fluid balance;

## Box 2.1 Logical approach to charts

### Respiratory

Respiratory rate

Inspired oxygen concentration ($FiO_2$)

Oxygen saturation ($SaO_2$)

### Circulation

Heart rate and rhythm

Blood pressure

Urinary output

Fluid balance

Intravenous lines

Cardiac output measurements

### Surgical

Special requirements of this operation

Temperature

Drainages (nature and volume)

alternatively, following liver surgery, one might look specifically for production or drainage of bile, liver function tests, albumin, glucose and clotting factor levels.

Check the drug chart to see what new drugs have been given, and which of the patient's usual drugs might have been forgotten: either may be influencing the current clinical findings. Also consider whether drugs given prophylactically and any prescribed antibiotics are still needed.

## *History and systematic examination*

The history of the patient's present illness and subsequent treatment is just as important in critical illness as in the rest of clinical practice. However, the impact of comorbid conditions is almost as great and these are overlooked or underestimated at considerable peril. The patient, the case note and nursing and junior medical staff are the main sources of these types of information and the appropriate source will vary from case to case, depending on your prior knowledge of the patient. On occasion, family and other professional staff can also supply useful information.

The patient is then examined fully, paying particular attention to vital systems, the systems or regions involved by surgery or underlying disease and to potential problems already highlighted. This should follow the standard format, beginning with the hands, and include neck, chest, abdomen and limbs. Wounds or stomas may also require examination. The importance of clinical examination is often underestimated by inexperienced staff, particularly when it comes to diagnosing incipient problems in silent areas; for example, early signs of atelectasis are much more likely to be detected clinically than radiologically (case scenario 2.1).

Case scenario 2.1

You are on the orthopaedic ward at 3am with a trauma case when you are asked to see a 48-year-old male patient who is tachycardic (HR 110), 12 hours after he underwent fixation of shaft of femur following a motorcycle accident. The main ward lights are not on, the patient is distressed and in pain and the foundation year doctor has just started a 500 ml bolus fluid challenge and prescribed more analgesia. The patient's blood pressure is 105/75 mmHg. His capillary refill time before the fluid challenge was 3 seconds and you are not unduly concerned. You have a cup of coffee and then review the patient again. You realise that, despite 500 ml of saline, his perfusion is worse, he is oliguric and he has a tender, slightly distended abdomen. It is now clear to you that the patient may well have continuing bleeding from an occult abdominal injury and that more intensive resuscitation and consideration of urgent operation or imaging is required.

*Review of available results*

Available investigation results should now be reviewed (Box 2.2). With emergencies, a great deal of useful data may be available from reviewing any previous routine blood results, microbiology samples or imaging requests, so do not overlook this important source of information.

## Box 2.2  Review available results

- Biochemistry profile
  - ABGs
  - Glucose level

- Haematology
  - Blood count
  - Clotting
  - Cross-matched blood available

- Microbiology
- Radiology
  - Review reports or examine films

- ECG
- Other tests, eg echocardiography
- Return to charts and review any necessary points

Ensuring that all results are reviewed on routine ward rounds is also very important, and not doing so is a classic source of error. Most hospitals now have electronic systems. It is also important to check what has been requested so that you can chase results and avoid repeating tests unnecessarily.

## Decide and plan – stable or unstable?

Once you have assessed the patient and the available information, you need to make a decision – is the patient stable or unstable? Patients about whom you are unsure should be managed as if they were unstable. Also, you should be very cautious about being too quick to assign patients who were previously unstable but who have responded to treatment to the stable group. Instability is a relative term, but training yourself to make this decision is important as it will focus your mind on one of two very different subsequent approaches.

### *Stable patients – daily plan*

Stable patients have normal signs and are progressing as expected. No major interventions will be required to maintain normal physiological parameters and they will not have experienced any recent untoward events. This will apply to most patients seen on the daily ward round and so the immediate management phase of the three-stage assessment process can be completed quickly. Once the charts and results have been reviewed to confirm that there are no significant abnormalities, the patient can be considered to be stable. It is then your duty to formulate a management plan. On the ward this will be daily (Box 2.3); however, in the HDU, 12-hourly or more frequent assessment and planning will be needed.

In particular:

1  Ensure that necessary therapeutic drugs, including analgesia, are prescribed (modify these as the patient recovers).

2  Check that appropriate prophylaxis, particularly against venous thromboembolism, is prescribed.

3  Check that any antibiotic prescriptions are still required and the drug prescribed is appropriate to the sensitivities of the organism in question.

4  Verify that routine medications are being given (if necessary by an alternative route).

5  Consider what implications comorbid conditions or treatment might have for present management or prognosis.

Speak to patients, to encourage and reassure them, to ensure that they know what is happening, when they can expect to go home and what they need to achieve to be able to be discharged. Sum up your plan with clear instructions for your nursing colleagues and junior staff and make (or supervise) an entry in the notes so that this is clear to someone reading the notes who has no knowledge of the patient.

## Practice point

Plan and sum up, communicate and document.

## Box 2.3  Daily plan

- Investigations
    - Blood tests and imaging, specialist opinions
- Removal of drains/tubes
- Oral intake
- Fluid balance and prescription
- Nutrition
    - Requirement
    - Route
    - Is it being given?
- Physiotherapy
    - Chest and mobility
- Drugs and analgesia
    - Therapeutic (eg antibiotics, analgesia)
    - Preventative (eg subcutaneous heparin)
    - Routine (eg cardiac)
- Consider level of care

*Unstable patients*

If progress is not satisfactory, further investigation or definitive treatment will be needed. If a cause is already evident from your evaluation, treatment can be planned directly. Inform your senior and consider whether a higher level of care is needed.

## Specific targeted investigations

These are carried out as necessary to find out why the patient is unstable and to let you or others do something about it subsequently.

These range from the simple to the very complex. Usually, simple blood tests will have already been sent off during the immediate management phase but now is the time to check. Likewise, chest radiographs, ECGs and cultures may have already been done or may be needed now.

The safest way to accomplish more complex and specific investigations will differ between patients depending on the test required, the degree of urgency and how sick the patient is. Remember that the radiology department is an unsafe place for sick patients unless they have adequate support from medical and nursing staff.

The ideal test may have to be forgone in some circumstances, or it may be better to transfer the patient to critical care for full support before a planned transfer to the radiology department. Specialist opinions (eg cardiology, anaesthesia, intensive care) may be required. If you reach an impasse (either a diagnostic or organisational), involve your senior colleagues. If you are unsure at this stage how to make things happen, ask for help. However, do not give up on a necessary investigation or treatment just because it is difficult to arrange or beyond your expertise, or the timing is not convenient (case scenario 2.2).

Be careful to maintain momentum; on busy wards, multiple small delays at each stage can add up to a lengthy delay in treating the underlying cause, which can result in your previous resuscitation being in vain. Making things happen is an important skill.

Investigations may take time, during which you must ask yourself repeatedly:

- Is the present level of physiological support optimal?

- Are we reaching a diagnosis and a definite plan of action?

- Are we doing so quickly enough?

If not, a change of plan is needed.

## Case scenario 2.2

An elderly patient with known mild heart failure underwent endoscopy and diathermy of a bleeding duodenal ulcer at 8pm. He became steadily oliguric from 11pm and received two cautious fluid challenges from the junior ward doctor. You are asked to see him at 3.35am and note that he is not well perfused and mildly dyspnoeic. You give a further 350 ml of saline over 15 minutes without any change in his condition. You are unsure what fluids are required and feel that more invasive monitoring and assessment may be needed. You are aware that the patient needs to be reviewed by the critical care team, but they are already busy and you do not explain the full extent of your concerns. You elect to continue with maintenance fluids until the 8am ward round and do not arrange any further review. By then, the patient is anuric and has evidence of acute kidney injury.

## Learning points

- Unstable patients require diagnosis and definitive treatment without undue delay.
- Involve senior staff if you think patients do not appear to be receiving the care you feel they require.

When you have attended a patient, you must record the event in the case notes (Box 2.4). This serves several functions: writing your assessment helps clarify your thoughts, your note tells other staff what happened and lets them gauge the response, you can define clear criteria for further interventions and the note can be of medicolegal importance.

It should be clear from the note who saw the patient and when, why they were seeing them (routine review or called to see), what information was gathered, how that information was interpreted, what the decision was, what the plan was, who was to carry it out and when the patient is to be reviewed. Depending on the situation, it may also be prudent to record what was said to the patient and any concerns they have.

## Box 2.4 Writing your notes

- Name in capitals, date and time, contact details
- Assessment and findings
- Brief summary of past and present events
  - Present clinical features
  - Interventions performed
  - Response to any treatment already given
- Summary of current abnormalities
- Differential diagnosis if relevant
- Plan
  - Further investigations
  - Other specialist opinions
  - Treatment
- Communications to relatives, staff, seniors, etc.
- Review
  - By you
  - By others
- Parameters for change

## Definitive treatment

The underlying aim of critical care practice is to begin definitive treatment of life-threatening pathology or complications as quickly as possible. Steps taken in the immediate management phase keep the patient alive: however, unless you treat the underlying problem adequately, the patient will deteriorate again and may die. Once the need for intervention is clear to all, the situation may be irretrievable, so speed is of the essence.

Treatment may be medical, surgical or radiological or all three, so coordination is important. When the patient has a surgical problem, you will need to play a leading role in coordinating efforts. Consider where non-operative treatment should best be carried out, by whom, and what support will be necessary. If the patient is transferred, especially to an area unfamiliar with surgical patients (eg the coronary care unit), detailed instructions will need to be written in the case notes and frequent review will be necessary to ensure that other surgical aspects of care continue to be delivered even though the staff members are unfamiliar with them.

## Reassessment

Finally, once any treatment has been instituted, whether simple fluid therapy or a complex surgical operation, you must reassess the patient to ensure that he or she has responded to the treatment. The necessary time frame for doing this will depend on the urgency of the case.

If the patient has not responded adequately, then you need to look all the harder for a different cause to treat. Reassessment is the final step – and, if necessary, the first step in repeating the whole process.

## Summary

The CCrISP system encourages you to assess all your patients in a similar way to determine whether they are stable or unstable and to guide appropriate interventions. It is the system that many senior surgeons and intensivists use instinctively. With practice, the use of a system will allow you to assess patients without overlooking simple and potentially disastrous abnormalities and it will serve as a framework whereby you can apply your theoretical knowledge to clinical problems.

The CCrISP course encourages you to:

- use a structured system to assess patients and reduce serious omissions;

- identify those in need of immediate life-saving resuscitation – assess and treat them simultaneously;

- reach a diagnosis that accounts for clinical deterioration;

- formulate and institute a plan of definitive treatment;

- plan investigations to be selective and carried out in a safe environment;

- utilise repeated clinical assessment as the cornerstone of good practice – it identifies things missed first time around and tells you whether the patient is getting better in response to your interventions;

- inform and involve your senior colleagues as appropriate;

- consider the level of care necessary at each stage of the process;

- communicate and document clearly.

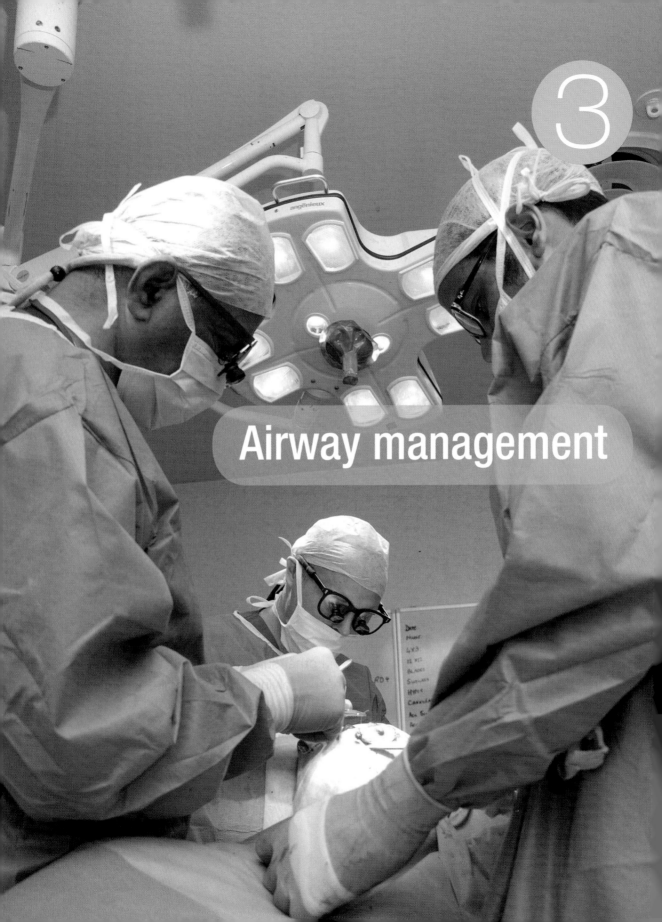

3

Airway management

## Learning outcomes

This chapter will help you to:

- describe the principles behind airway management;

- outline the indications for tracheostomy in critically ill patients;

- outline the key elements of tracheostomy care;

- model how to deal with common tracheostomy emergencies.

The most common reason for admission to a critical care unit is the provision of airway management and ventilatory care to critically ill patients.

The early recognition and treatment of an airway or ventilatory problem will often prevent further patient deterioration and is the basis of effective resuscitation. Many patients on surgical wards exhibit signs of respiratory compromise and their effective management in the ward environment is an important part of surgical critical care.

As outlined in Chapter 2, you should exclude an airway problem when assessing every patient. Often the patient will respond to you verbally but, if not, suspect airway compromise.

Alteration in the level of consciousness for any reason can result in loss of airway control. The decreased protective gag and laryngeal reflexes that accompany significant reductions in consciousness level also increase the risk of aspiration of gastric contents into the lungs.

Whilst significant airway problems are not particularly common on a general surgical ward, they are more commonly encountered in other surgical specialties and are generally quite intimidating for surgical trainees. Applying basic principles is vital.

It is important to remember that the 'ABCDE' approach of the CCrISP algorithm also applies in cases of apparent airway problems. The signs of an obstructed airway are noisy breathing including inspiratory stridor. Remember that complete obstruction will be silent. Other signs include seesaw breathing and indrawing of the suprasternal, supraclaviclar and intercostal spaces on attempted inspiration.

The signs of breathing difficulties include:

- dyspnoea, tachypnoea or apnoea

- inability to speak in complete sentences

- wheezing

- use of accessory muscles of respiration

- central cyanosis

- sweating and tachycardia

- showing a decreased level of consciousness or becoming agitated and difficult to control.

There are two golden rules to airway management:

- Always give oxygen in the highest concentration possible.

- Use simple methods of airway management first.

## Techniques of airway control

If the patient is breathing spontaneously, administer the highest flow rate of oxygen possible using a mask with a reservoir bag (Figure 3.1). This increases the available inspired oxygen concentration during inspiration by filling the reservoir with oxygen during expiration.

During resuscitation, you should not worry about the possibility of depressing ventilation by giving high concentrations of oxygen. Although some patients may have a hypoxic drive to control respiratory rate in the face of chronic hypercapnia, hypoxia kills people quicker than loss of respiratory drive and the condition is relatively rare in surgical patients. Apply a pulse oximeter to allow you to assess that oxygen administration is improving the patient's oxygen saturation level. Once the patient has stabilised, the oxygen concentration can be decreased to maintain adequate saturations (>94% unless there is clear evidence of a hypoxic drive, in which case the British Thoracic Society recommends a target saturation range of 88–92%).

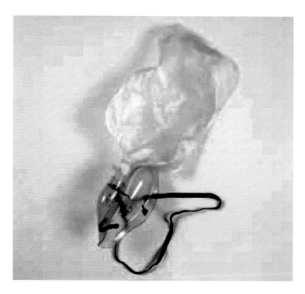

Figure 3.1  Facemask with reservoir bag.

Remember that pulse oximetry does not give an indication of hypercapnia or the effectiveness of ventilatory effort. Be very wary of any signs that the patient may be tiring.

## Escalating airway support

In increasing measure, airway support can be achieved by using:

- chin lift/jaw thrust

- suction

- airway adjuncts such oropharyngeal (Guedel) or nasopharyngeal airways

- a laryngeal mask or endotracheal tube

- a surgical airway.

Basic manoeuvres without airway adjuncts are often sufficient to improve gas exchange through a compromised airway. If not, an oral Guedel airway should be inserted (Figure 3.2). If the patient tolerates a Guedel airway, you need someone with advanced airway skills to attend the patient immediately.

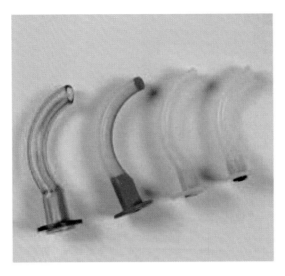

Figure 3.2 Oropharyngeal (Guedel) airways.

Neither technique should be attempted by the inexperienced or untrained practitioner.

The Guedel airway is sized from the tragus of the ear to the angle of the mouth and in adults is inserted upside down and rotated into place over the tongue.

Ensure that suction is present. If the patient has a gag reflex, it may be easier to insert a nasopharyngeal airway, but this carries a risk of epistaxis. Never force insertion of an oropharyngeal or nasopharyngeal airway.

In situations of airway compromise, call for help early. Seek anaesthetic/critical care help at any point if you are unable to cope or think you may reach the limits of your competence.

If the patient is apnoeic or has very shallow respiration, then ventilation using a bag/valve/mask system is necessary (Figure 3.3). This will usually maintain sufficient oxygenation until an anaesthetist arrives. Take every opportunity you can to practise your basic airway skills. One way is to ask the anaesthetist if you can practise manual ventilation under supervision in the anaesthetic room prior to elective surgery.

Patients who are semiconscious and unable to tolerate an oral airway will not tolerate endotracheal intubation or laryngeal mask insertion without additional sedation and so you must seek additional help to secure the airway.

With appropriate training, attempting to insert a laryngeal mask airway can often be simpler, quicker and easier than attempting intubation.

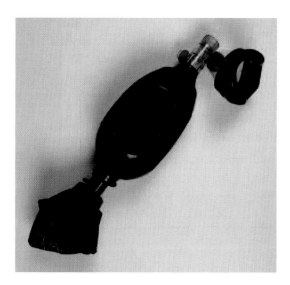

Figure 3.3 Bag/valve/mask.

If you try to intubate the patient and fail, or if you are unable to ventilate the patient manually or with a laryngeal mask airway, then you are committed to performing a surgical airway by surgical cricothyroidotomy in order to ensure life-saving oxygenation and ventilation. Emergency front of neck access is beyond the scope of the CCrISP course but should be practised in simulation.

## Tracheostomy

A tracheostomy is a hole in the trachea through which a person can breathe or be ventilated and can be required for various reasons (Box 3.1). There are two distinct types of tracheostomy.

1   Upper airway absent. Tracheostomy after laryngectomy: this is an end stoma formed when a patient has had a laryngeal resection. There is no upper airway connection to the lungs.

2   Upper airway present:

    a   Surgical tracheostomy: this is performed under direct vision and involves making a surgical cut in the trachea.
    b   Percutaneous dilational tracheostomy: this is performed using a Seldinger technique to dilate a needled hole in the trachea.

It is important to identify which type of tracheostomy a patient has as it affects the management of tracheostomy difficulties.

Practice point

The most important difference is between a laryngectomy stoma, in which case there is no remaining upper airway, and those forms of tracheostomy that allow management of the upper airway if problems arise.

Box 3.1 Reasons for a tracheostomy

- Upper airway obstruction
- Post laryngectomy/upper airway surgery
- Musculoskeletal disorders affecting ventilation (eg muscular dystrophy, spinal cord injury, motor neurone disease, post-traumatic brain injury)
- To assist weaning from ventilation on critical care
    - Reduced airway resistance
    - Improved airway toilet
    - Allows reduction in sedation as better tolerated than an oral tube
- Incompetent swallow/impaired upper airway reflexes

Tracheostomy is often performed on long-stay ICU patients, and in some hospitals patients with tracheostomies are managed on non-ENT wards following discharge from critical care. It is therefore important for surgeons to have knowledge of, and be able to deal with, common complications of tracheostomies.

Tracheostomy tubes come in a variety of types and sizes, and in the practical sessions of the CCrISP course you will have the opportunity to examine a number of them. The type of tube inserted, and its size, should be documented in the patient's notes. To facilitate this, specific documentation is being developed (eg the Trachi-pass), and an example of this will be shown on the course. Many hospitals are now developing local guidelines for managing patients with a tracheostomy tube, and a

National Tracheostomy Safety Project initiative is also on-going (www.tracheostomy. org.uk).

Other features of tracheostomy tubes are listed in Box 3.2 and different types are shown in Figure 3.4.

## Box 3.2 Types of tracheostomy tubes

Tracheostomy tubes are available in a number of sizes and types. The choice of tracheostomy tube depends on the needs of the patient and the clinical situation.

Inner tubes are usually recommended, to facilitate cleaning, unless the tube will be required for only a very short time.

- Cuffed: used if an airway seal is required (eg for intermittent ventilation in critical care)
- Uncuffed: primarily used in patients requiring a tracheostomy long term as they are less likely to cause trauma, which is usually due to cuff pressure
- Unfenestrated: usually used in association with a cuffed tracheostomy tube when intermittent ventilation is required, eg in surgical patients
- Fenestrated: allow upper airway flow for phonation, designed for medium- to long-term use

Information on tube size should be located on the flange. There is no uniformity of tracheostomy tube size with regard to length and dimensions so this needs to be checked for each type of tube. Most females will accommodate an internal diameter tube of 7–8 mm and males usually 8–9 mm. Selecting a tube of the appropriate size is important to maximise the internal tube dimensions and reduce the work of breathing through the tube. However, an oversized tube can cause pressure necrosis and damage the tracheal mucosa. If the tracheostomy tube is too small, the cuff will need to be overinflated to prevent accidental displacement of the tube or leakage during positive-pressure ventilation. Cuffed tracheostomy tubes available in critical care have an aspiration port above the cuff that is used to keep this area clear of secretions, thus reducing the risk of ventilator-acquired pneumonia.

Management of tracheostomies on the ward is usually straightforward, provided simple principles are followed.

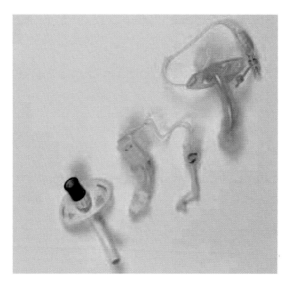

Figure 3.4 Types of tracheostomy tube.

## General management

- Humidification and regular suction are essential: blockage of the tracheostomy tube is often due to failure to carry out basic toileting of the airway.

- Tubes should not be changed within 3 days of a surgical procedure, and ideally not within 7–10 days of a percutaneous procedure, to ensure that the tract has formed properly.

- On the wards, single lumen tubes are generally undesirable because of the risk of blockage. These should be replaced with a tracheostomy tube with a removable inner tube to facilitate cleaning as soon as it is safe to do so. Use the CCrISP algorithm to determine whether the tracheostomy tube is still required.

## Practice point

Tracheostomy tubes should be changed only by staff who have the necessary skills. If you have not had training you should not plan to undertake the procedure unsupervised.

## Problems with tracheostomies

The commonest problems with tracheostomies are:

- displacement

- obstruction

- haemorrhage.

These can easily be remembered with the mnemonic: DOH!

## Critical incidents

- Apply the CCrISP algorithm when asked to deal with a tracheostomy problem.

- Determine when the procedure was performed and what type of tracheostomy tube the patient received. Specifically, check if the patient has an existing upper airway.

- The National Tracheostomy Safety Project (www.tracheostomy.org.uk) publishes algorithms to deal with tracheostomy critical incidents.

- The management of tracheostomy problems is logical once a general understanding has been achieved. Think clearly and do not panic.

## Desaturation with a tracheostomy with an existing airway: follow the CCrISP algorithm

This is generally due to displacement or obstruction.

- Call for help.

- Recognise that the patient has a patent upper airway.

- Recognise that the patient is breathing but that this is suboptimal.

- Administer 100% oxygen via facemask and tracheostomy tube.

- Assess tracheostomy patency assessing for improving ventilation after each step:

  - remove inner cannula
  - apply suction
  - deflate cuff

- remove tracheostomy tube
- manage upper airway with bag and mask ventilation plus airway adjuncts (remembering to temporarily cover the tracheostomy hole with a dressing)
- attempt bag and mask ventilation at tracheostomy stoma site (this can be difficult)
- perform upper airway intubation (this should only be done by a clinician skilled in the technique).

## Haemorrhage from a tracheostomy tube: follow the CCrISP algorithm

- Bleeding from a tracheostomy is generally due to erosion into blood vessels at or under the tracheostomy site. It can be life-threatening, particularly if there is significant haemorrhage into the airway. Most tracheostomy bleeds are minor and can be managed conservatively.

- Erosion into the innominate artery or vein at the superior end of the sternum, whilst rare, can be catastrophic and will need specialist assistance if the patient is to survive.

- Call for help: anaesthetic and surgical airway specialists may be needed.

- Follow the CCrISP algorithm; apply 100% oxygen to tracheostomy and face. Gain large-bore IV access.

- Inspect the stoma site without dislodging the tracheostomy and apply manual pressure to any obvious bleeding sites.

- Infiltration of dilute adrenaline (1:80,000 to 1:200,000 with or without local anaesthetic) can be attempted if there is diffuse bleeding. Application of adrenaline-soaked swabs may also be effective.

  - If the bleeding is significant, gentle pressure to the sternal notch and hyperinflation of the tracheostomy cuff may alleviate the situation temporarily until specialist help arrives.
  - Do not deflate the cuff or remove the tube.
  - A blood sample should be taken for full blood count (FBC), ABG analysis and cross-matching, but this should not be prioritised over securing the airway.

## Removal of a tracheostomy tube

Daily assessment of the continuing need for a temporary tracheostomy should always form part of a patient's management plan. Removal of a tracheostomy tube is usually called decannulation. This should be done only by someone with the relevant skills and should involve assessment of:

- neurological status

- ventilation and oxygenation needs

- quality of upper airway (including cord function and assessment of upper airway oedema)

    - ability to cough and clear secretions
    - confirmation that the original indication for tracheostomy has been successfully treated
    - confirmation that the patient is generally stable

Most dilational percutaneous tracheostomies require only an occlusive stoma site dressing after removal. Surgical tracheostomies may require formal operative closure.

After decannulation, a period of close monitoring and observation is necessary. Failure to successfully decannulate may present as rapid airway failure and it is therefore vital that specialist airway equipment and expertise are available.

Many patients require formal speech and language therapy and swallowing assessments prior to commencing oral diet.

## Summary

- Airway management should always follow two simple rules:

    - Always administer the highest oxygen concentration possible.
    - Use the simplest methods of airway control first.

- Seek specialist airway help early.

- Tracheostomy complications are usually due to **d**isplacement, **o**bstruction or **h**aemorrhage (DOH).

## Further reading

National Tracheostomy Safety Project (www.tracheostomy.org.uk).

Resuscitation Council UK. Advanced life support (ALS) guidelines and guidance 2015 (www.resus.org.uk/resuscitation-guidelines/).

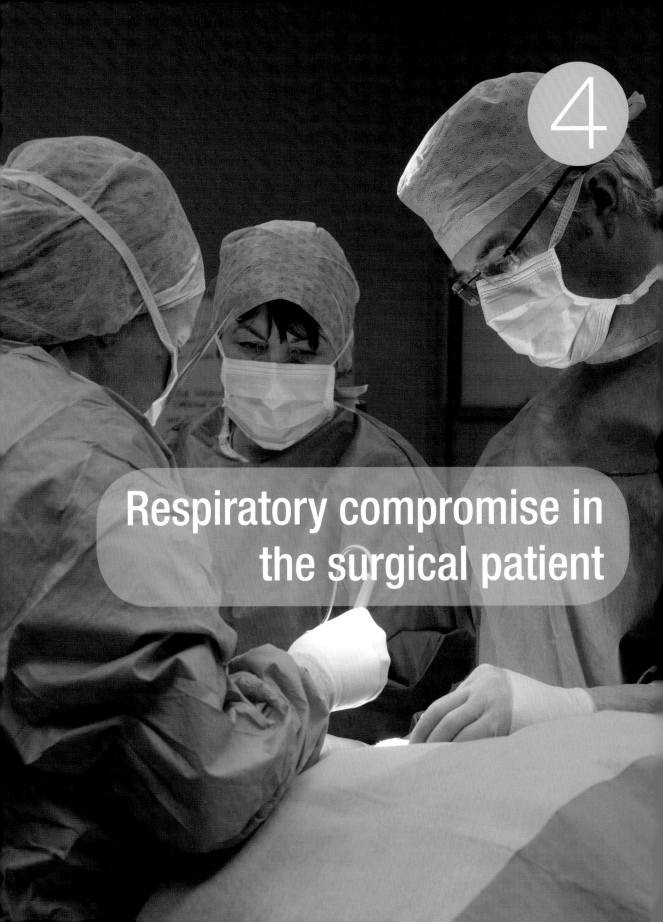

4

# Respiratory compromise in the surgical patient

## Learning outcomes

This chapter will help you to:

- understand the importance of respiratory failure and its prevention for good surgical outcomes;

- recognise the patient with respiratory failure and provide a management approach to respiratory failure;

- be familiar with common methods of providing respiratory support;

- understand the basic concepts of mechanical ventilation.

## Introduction

Respiratory failure occurs when there is inadequate pulmonary gas exchange such that blood oxygen and carbon dioxide cannot be maintained at normal levels. A $PaO_2$ of 8 kPa is the point on the oxygen dissociation curve when rapid desaturation occurs if there is any further fall in $PaO_2$ (Figure 4.1).

Respiratory failure is the commonest cause of a decreased level of consciousness in general surgical patients and is classified in accordance with the $CO_2$ level:

- Type 1 failure. Failure of oxygen uptake leads to hypoxia ($PaO_2$ of less than 8 kPa: normal range 10.6–13.3 kPa) but normal or reduced $PaCO_2$ (normal range 4.7–6.0 kPa).

- Type 2 failure. Failure of oxygen uptake and of carbon dioxide removal leads to hypoxia and hypercarbia ($PaCO_2$ of greater than 6.7 kPa).

Type 2 failure may be acute or may have a chronic element. This is determined by looking at the bicarbonate level and also from the patient's history. Bicarbonate levels are high in patients with a chronic degree of type 2 respiratory failure, eg those with chronic obstructive pulmonary disease (COPD).

Respiratory failure is more likely where surgery is prolonged and painful. Inadequate analgesia is an important contributor to respiratory failure; however, opiates also increase that risk.

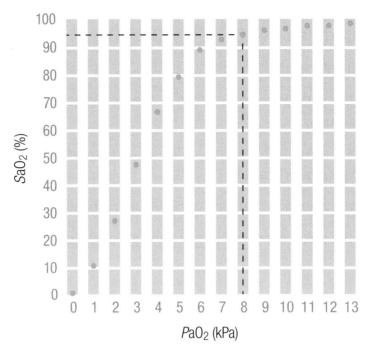

Figure 4.1 The oxygen–haemoglobin dissociation curve. Below a $PaO_2$ of 8 kPa the slope drops away steeply. Keep the saturation >94% to ensure that the $PaO_2$ is above 8 kPa.

There are a number of common causes of respiratory failure in the surgical patient, which can be classified into three broad groups:

1   Acute fall in functional residual capacity (FRC) without pulmonary vascular dysfunction:

- failure of chest mechanics after trauma or other processes that render the lungs stiff and non-compliant;
- acute postoperative atelectasis, sputum retention, pneumonia or depression of respiration caused by analgesic, sedative or neuromuscular blocking drugs.

Frailty and malnutrition contribute.

2   Acute fall in FRC with pulmonary vascular dysfunction. This includes left ventricular failure, fluid overload, pulmonary hypertension, PE, neurogenic pulmonary oedema or adult respiratory distress syndrome (ARDS).

3   Airflow obstruction – including increased lung volume states such as COPD, asthma or other airflow obstruction.

Factors that increase the risk of respiratory problems include:

▨ a history of pre-existing respiratory disease, such as asthma, COPD and obstructive sleep apnoea

▨ obesity

▨ smoking

▨ thoracic surgery

▨ upper abdominal surgery

▨ older age.

## Immediate assessment and management

Although ABG analysis is often the first point at which respiratory failure is diagnosed, the initial assessment and management of the patient with respiratory problems should follow the systematic approach of the CCrISP algorithm.

Remember the ABCDEs. An unconscious patient with no airway must be resuscitated quickly to prevent hypoxic brain damage. Review airway management in Chapters 2 and 3.

Patients with respiratory failure may be easily recognised if they are:

▨ dyspnoeic, tachypnoeic or apnoeic;

▨ unable to speak in complete sentences;

▨ using accessory muscles of respiration;

▨ centrally cyanosed;

▨ sweating and tachycardic;

▨ exhibiting a decreased level of consciousness.

All patients should be given high-flow oxygen via a reservoir bag in the first instance if still spontaneously breathing. During resuscitation, you should not worry about the possibility of depressing ventilation by giving high concentrations of oxygen to a patient with chronic pulmonary disease whose breathing is normally regulated by a hypoxic drive. Hypoxia kills more quickly than hypercarbia.

Apply a pulse oximeter and once the patient has stabilised, the rule is to give the minimum added oxygen to achieve the best oxygenation.

## Pulse oximetry

Pulse oximetry has become a central tool in the monitoring of critically ill surgical patients. It is a method of continuously monitoring oxygen saturations, not absolute oxygen levels or ventilation.

Understanding its working will make you aware of the limitations. Pulse oximetry works by combining two principles based on light transmission and reception through tissue. First, the probe detects pulsatile flow plethysmographically. Second, it differentiates between oxygenated and reduced haemoglobin by their differing light absorption. Signal processing produces a display of heart rate and arterial oxygen saturation ($SaO_2$).

Saturation does not equate to the partial pressure of oxygen (which is responsible for gas exchange). The oxygen dissociation curve in Figure 4.1 links these parameters. Note that $SaO_2$ of 94% often equates to a $PaO_2$ of about 8 kPa so it is advisable to keep the $SaO_2$ above 94% and to set the alarms accordingly. There is a delay of around 20 seconds between actual and displayed values.

If a patient is chronically hypercapnic (identified by a high bicarbonate on ABG analysis) then a target $SaO_2$ of 88–92% is usually appropriate when the patient is stable. The pulse oximeter does not detect hypercarbia or acidosis – only blood gas analysis can do this. Carboxyhaemoglobin can cause a pulse oximeter to give an erroneously high reading. Other factors that can impede accurate pulse oximetry include:

- movement: shivering, rigors, tremor, agitation;
- peripheral vasoconstriction – shock, hypothermia;
- cardiac arrhythmias;
- profound anaemia (rarely seen in UK practice);
- $SaO_2$ below 70% (the device is not accurately calibrated below 75%);
- diathermy;

- bright lights;

- dirty skin, pigmentation including jaundice, or the use of nail varnish (most modern pulse oximeters will work with nail varnish present).

# Full patient assessment

## Chart review

Chart examination may reveal changes in respiratory rate, temperature, pulse rate, blood pressure, level of consciousness, a fall in oxygen saturation or deterioration in ABGs if previously recorded. Fluid balance charts should be assessed and the patient examined for signs of fluid overload. Ask the patient about any changes in the colour or amount of sputum. A deteriorating trend in any of these physiological variables is an essential diagnostic tool and the importance of accurate charting cannot be overemphasised.

## History and systematic examination

You should quickly review the patient's history in an effort to determine any likely source of respiratory difficulty. The patient may be known to suffer from asthma or chronic bronchitis or may recently have received a large dose of opiates. The examination should initially be clinical, based on simple 'Look, Listen and Feel' techniques described in the assessment chapter (Chapter 2) and aimed at detecting the physiological changes of developing respiratory failure.

## Available results

### Full blood count

Correction of anaemia will help to improve oxygen delivery to the tissues if the haemoglobin is less than 80 g/L. An elevated white cell count may indicate concurrent infection that may be pneumonic in origin.

### Urea and electrolytes

The levels of urea and electrolytes in the blood may give some indication of the patient's fluid and renal status.

## ABG analysis

This is the most useful blood test in cases of respiratory failure. You should be familiar with the practical skill of blood sampling and the interpretation of the results. The interpretation of ABGs is outlined in Chapter 5. Treat the patient as a whole and do not act only on the blood gases in isolation from the clinical findings.

## ECG

An ECG will provide information regarding the presence or absence of myocardial ischaemia and rhythm and rate abnormalities that could be responsible for the onset or worsening of respiratory failure. Cardiac and respiratory physiological variables are inseparable when it comes to assessment and treatment of respiratory failure. Further investigation of cardiac function, such as echocardiography or estimations of cardiac output or cardiac index, may be appropriate if the patient is receiving a higher level of care.

## Chest X-ray

Plain chest X-ray remains a valuable diagnostic tool. Radiographic changes often lag behind the clinical changes and it is important to treat the patient, not the X-ray. Interpretation of chest X-rays must follow a systematic approach, as described in Box 4.1. For the acutely deteriorating patient, a portable chest X-ray machine may be helpful.

## Lung function tests

Preoperative lung function tests (peak expiratory flow rate, vital capacity and forced expiratory volume in 1 second ($FEV_1$)) are useful in predicting the patient at risk, although a patient's ability to climb a flight of stairs in one go or to conduct everyday tasks also provides valuable information. Hand-held spirometers are simple and easy to use, and spirometry should be conducted preoperatively in any patient who gives a history of respiratory disease. It is increasingly common for patients undergoing major surgery to undergo formal cardiopulmonary exercise testing (CPET) to determine the dynamic functioning of the lungs and heart as a unit, i.e. measurement of anaerobic threshold. Looking in the notes for this preoperative information may give a valuable clue as to the cause of any current deterioration.

Chest ultrasound is frequently used clinically in critically ill patients to determine the presence of a pleural effusion, and to guide its drainage. CTPA (CT pulmonary angiography) should be used when a patient is hypoxic and there is no clear cause for the deterioration. An alternative investigation in the unstable patient may be to arrange Doppler scanning of the legs and bedside echocardiography to look for evidence of right heart strain. Infection is the most common cause of respiratory failure, and samples of blood for culture should be obtained before commencing antibiotic therapy. Positive blood cultures have been reported in up to 40% of patients with hospital-acquired pneumonia. Sputum samples should be collected at the first opportunity but this should not delay administration of antibiotics. Additional microbiological samples may also be required if there is no clear cause for the respiratory deterioration. Seek advice about further samples, for example the need for flu swabs in a patient recently admitted from home.

## Stable patients – daily management plan

Frequent assessment of all surgical patients, but especially those at high risk, is important.

Routinely assess respiratory rate, $SaO_2$ (along with oxygen requirements), cyanosis, ability to cough and deep breathe and adequacy of analgesia, looking for signs of respiratory distress, sweatiness and tachycardia. Formal examination of the chest should also be carried our regularly. If there any concerns, consider the investigations outlined above.

Prescribe humidified oxygen therapy by mask at an appropriate concentration. Monitor clinical signs (especially respiratory rate), oxygen saturation and ABGs. For patients with lower oxygen requirements, nasal cannulae may be used, but remember that oxygen should be administered to patients to keep their $SaO_2$ above 94%. Communicate with nursing staff and ensure that they are aware of the frequency of observations required and triggers for escalation.

If patients require oxygen by mask for >24 hours, or are likely to have a high sputum load, ensure that appropriate humidification is used. Physiotherapy review should be sought for all patients at risk of, or developing, respiratory problems. Early mobilisation and sitting up are the best ways of preventing later respiratory problems. However, other aspects to be considered are patient positioning, exercises to encourage deep breathing, suction of respiratory secretions using nasopharyngeal airways, techniques such as percussion and use of devices such as incentive spirometry and cough incentive machines.

Ensure that patients' routine prescriptions for any respiratory disease are continued and consider changing inhalers to nebulisers if appropriate. Consider use of nebulised saline to loosen secretions. If a patient develops a wheeze (which can occur in the absence of previous respiratory disease), prescribe nebulised salbutamol and ipratropium. Some patients use home non-invasive ventilation (NIV) or continuous positive airway pressure (CPAP) devices. Ensure that any patient who uses these brings them into hospital and that staff who will be looking after the patients are familiar with their use. Keep interruptions to patients' usual CPAP/NIV regimes to a minimum. Adequate analgesia is important to enable patients to cough and deep breathe. Conversely, overuse of opiates leads to narcotisation and airway and respiratory compromise (see Chapter 14 for advice on analgesia). For most surgical patients, 4-hourly observations are appropriate but, if you are concerned, increase the frequency to hourly. Monitoring consistent with NEWS charts standards is the minimum. Abnormalities in observations should be escalated in accordance with your hospital policy.

## Case scenario 4.1

A 45-year-old man had a laparoscopic gastric bypass 2 days ago. His body mass index (BMI) is 45 kg/m² and he has a history of obstructive sleep apnoea but has refused home CPAP. He has a history of chronic back pain problems and normally takes regular paracetamol and oral morphine as required. You are called to see him because his saturations are 90% and he is complaining of pain.

He is maintaining an airway, and immediate assessment reveals a temperature of 37.3°C, respiratory rate of 24 and $SaO_2$ of 90% on room air. He has not been out of bed since the operation. He also has non-insulin-dependent diabetes mellitus (NIDDM) and hypertension. He is cyanosed but well perfused. You review him in detail and find that he has not been receiving his normal analgesia, oxygen therapy has not been given for 6 hours and that he has not seen the physiotherapist today. He has poor air entry bilaterally, particularly at the right base. Blood gases now show a mild respiratory acidosis and a $PaCO_2$ just above the upper limit of normal. You prescribe humidified oxygen to maintain his oxygen saturation above 95% and start regular nebulised salbutamol as he uses salbutamol as necessary at home. A CXR is requested, which reveals atelectasis at both bases. You arrange for immediate review by the on-call physiotherapist and by the pain team. The physiotherapist obtains a sputum sample for culture but, as this looks clear and the white cell count is normal, you elect not to start antibiotics at present. You review him 1 hour later, confirm that his improved analgesia has allowed him to increase his air entry and clearance of secretions and, thereby, oxygenation. The blood gases have improved. You discuss the case with the nurse and agree the necessary frequency of observations and parameters of saturation, respiratory rate and pain score that would necessitate further urgent medical review. You plan to review in any event at 8am to discuss with (and feed back to) the patient's own team.

## Learning points

- Predict the patient at risk and establish the correct level of care from the outset.
- Ensure early mobilisation – provide good analgesia with regular physiotherapy input.
- Regular nursing observations and medical review vary – once-daily medical review is not enough in some cases.
- Use preventative techniques including chest physiotherapy, nebulised saline, monitored humidified oxygen, adequate analgesia and sputum culture.

## Practice point

The frequency with which early chest problems are encountered cannot be overemphasised, nor can the importance of examining the chest routinely and adopting simple preventative measures.

### Preventing respiratory deterioration following surgery

- Identify those at risk.

- Examine and assess.
- Encourage early mobilisation.
- Provide adequate analgesia.
- Arrange for chest physiotherapy.
- Administer nebulised saline.
- Administer humidified oxygen at a titrated dose.
- Take sputum for culture.
- Reassess regularly.

## Practical skill: interpreting chest radiographs

### Objectives

At the end of this section, participants should:

- be able to view a system for examining chest radiographs in the critically ill;

- be aware of the complementary information provided by clinical and radiographic examination.

The chest radiograph is one of the most frequently ordered investigations in the management of the critically ill. In many cases, abnormal signs will be picked up earlier on clinical examination as radiographic appearances tend to lag behind the clinical findings. The chest X-ray (Figure 4.2) offers valuable confirmatory and complementary diagnostic evidence (or reassurance). The aim here is not to list exhaustively the clinical scenarios and diagnoses in which it may be of help, but rather to revise a system for reviewing chest images.

Always use a system for looking at chest X-rays: you may miss pathology if you don't.

The most useful chest view for assessing the heart is a straight, erect posteroanterior (PA) film, taken at full inspiration. This type of radiograph is more likely to give a true indication of heart size than the portable anteroposterior (AP) film, which may suggest cardiomegaly. Be aware of which type you are looking at and remember to check name, date and time. Compare with previous films.

Your routine should be:

▦   note overall shape of the chest and obvious abnormalities

▦   use a system to assess the CXR fully (Box 4.1).

### Box 4.1  Example system for assessment of CXR

- Soft tissues. Look for air (surgical emphysema), foreign bodies or disruption of contours.
- Bony structures. Use the mnemonic RCS's (ribs, clavicles, scapulae, sternum).
- Lung markings. Do they extend to the chest wall? Is there pneumothorax or haemothorax? Trace around the edge to avoid missing a small pneumothorax. Is the volume of parenchyma increased (chronic obstructive airways disease (COAD), lots of ribs visible) or reduced (poor respiratory effort, abdominal distension)?
- Examine the lung fields for opacities.
- Double check the costophrenic angles for fluid (erect film?).
- Is there air beneath the diaphragm (erect film?) or any obvious intra-abdominal abnormality to investigate specifically, such as distended bowel?
- Note the position of the trachea and heart size. Trace round the mediastinum and check the location of any tubes or lines. The width of the mediastinum should be noted but may be unreliable.

(a)

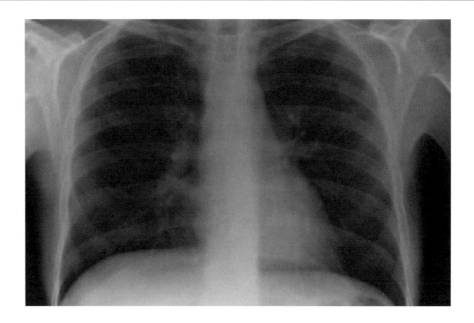

(b)

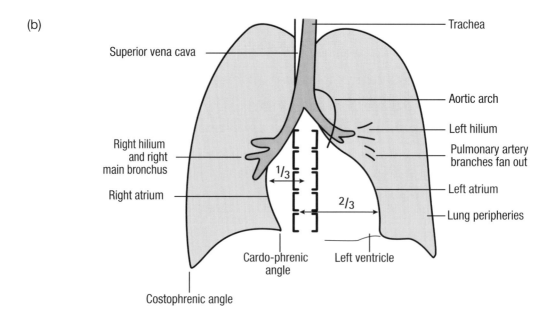

Figure 4.2 Chest X-ray (a) and diagrammatic representation of a chest X-ray (b).

## Air bronchogram

A bronchus is not normally visible if surrounded by aerated lung since both are equally radio-translucent. Anything that causes the normal lung tissue to lose its aerated property will produce a difference in opacity and the bronchus, provided it still contains air, will be visible. The presence of an air bronchogram suggests oedema, infection or other infiltrates in the surrounding lung tissue.

## Kerley B lines

These are horizontal lines that meet the pleural surface at right angles. They tend to be about 1–2 cm long and 1–2 mm thick. They are caused by increased fluid or tissue within the intralobular septa.

## Bronchitis and emphysema

Bronchitis and emphysema can be present even if there are few or no chest X-ray abnormalities. What may be present is increased lucency of the lung and regional or general loss of vascularity in the peripheral lung fields. The lung fields are increased in size.

## Pleural effusion

A small effusion may produce only a blunting of the costophrenic angle. A large effusion will produce evidence of lung compression and is usually associated with clinically apparent respiratory problems. The mediastinum may be displaced to the opposite side and the diaphragm flattened on that side. It is important to be aware that, with an X-ray taken with the patient supine, an effusion may show only as a faint diffuse opacity spread over the lung field. This is because the fluid is spread thinly over a wide area.

Repeat the X-ray after the patient has been sitting up for 15 minutes or obtain an ultrasound scan. An effusion due to a cardiac disorder tends to be bilateral.

## Consolidation

Consolidation will not produce a mediastinal shift unless there is significant collapse, in which case the mediastinum will be drawn over to the side of the lesion.

## *Pericardial effusion*

There are many reasons for an enlarged cardiac silhouette. The most common pathological reasons include ventricular hypertrophy, pericardial effusion and ventricular aneurysm. An effusion may produce an outline that is globular in appearance, but hypertrophy of the left ventricle can do the same. Left atrial enlargement can produce a straightening of the left cardiac border. A significant pericardial effusion is likely to produce evidence of tamponade with poor cardiac function and raised central venous pressure. If in doubt, echocardiography will confirm the diagnosis.

Cardiac failure may give rise to a variety of signs including upper lobe blood diversion, cardiomegaly, pleural effusions, Kerley B lines and parenchymal shadowing (diffuse or hilar 'bat's-wing' shadowing).

## Management of respiratory failure and compromise

The treatment plan for managing respiratory failure follows a stepwise increase/ decrease in support depending on its severity (Figure 4.3).

During initiation of treatment, start at the left of the scale and progress to the right as determined by your assessment of the patient's response.

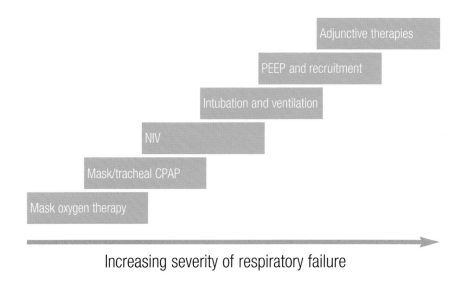

Increasing severity of respiratory failure

Figure 4.3 Treatment plan for managing respiratory failure.

Only conventional mask oxygen therapy is possible on the majority of surgical wards. Fixed-delivery oxygen masks are available up to an inspired oxygen concentration of 60%, ie an $FiO_2$ of 0.6.

All oxygen delivery systems should be humidified. Otherwise the dry, cold gas may contribute towards thickening of the patient's secretions and promote sputum retention. Nebulised 0.9% saline (with bronchodilators if indicated) and regular treatment from a respiratory physiotherapist may prevent worsening of incipient respiratory failure if they are used early.

Devices such as high-flow nasal oxygen therapy (Figure 4.4) are becoming available on the wards although they are not yet in widespread use. They provide higher flows and concentrations of oxygen than conventional facemasks along with gas humidification and are often well tolerated by patients.

The response of the patient is assessed according to the improvement of clinical status, oxygen saturation and ABG analyses. If the patient's condition does not improve with increased inspired oxygen concentration up to 60%, then you have a

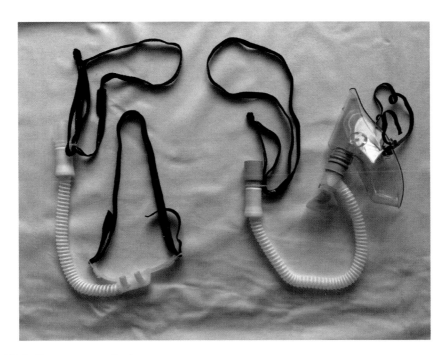

Figure 4.4  High-flow oxygen device.

very unstable patient and further diagnosis and definitive treatment are required. This will require expert help and the safe transfer of the patient to a higher level of care.

Even if the patient responds to supplemental oxygen therapy and the ABGs improve, you must remember that oxygen is only one aspect of treatment – you must treat the underlying cause of the respiratory failure.

### Treat the cause of respiratory failure

Supportive and definitive treatments are needed. Use appropriate antibiotics, physiotherapy, diuretics, bronchodilators and cardiac or other drugs as necessary. Basal signs may indicate continuing abdominal pathology (eg subphrenic abscess). Systemic factors influence respiratory function (eg mobility, nutrition) – it is important to treat these too.

Review the patient's requirement for and response to analgesia; either too little or too much can be a factor in preventing adequate clearance of secretions by inhibiting coughing and by limiting the patient's tolerance of physiotherapy.

Where sputum clearance is the primary problem, a nasopharyngeal airway may be considered, or discuss the use of a cough assist machine with the physiotherapists.

Do not assume that confusion or a depressed level of consciousness is due to the effects of opiate analgesia. Hypoxia may cause an acute confusional state and hypercarbia may lead to obtundation.

### Reassess

Detect failure of improvement or further patient deterioration: persisting or worsening signs and symptoms of respiratory failure require further immediate management and transfer to a higher level of care.

### Detecting respiratory failure

It is essential to be alert to this situation as it is common, can be rapidly fatal and requires a prompt change in management.

Failure of mask oxygen therapy at high $FiO_2$ may be indicated by:

- increasing respiratory rate;

- increasing distress, dyspnoea, exhaustion, sweating and confusion;

- oxygen saturation 80% or less (this may be a late sign);

- $PaO_2$ less than 8 kPa;

- $PaCO_2$ greater than 7 kPa.

## Case scenario 4.2

A 62-year-old woman with chronic bronchitis who underwent right abdominal nephrectomy 4 days ago is now tachypnoeic and pyrexial. Air entry is reduced and examination reveals bronchial breathing and dullness to percussion at the right lung base. Her $FiO_2$ was increased to 0.8 in order to maintain $SaO_2$ above 97%. The physiotherapist obtained a sample of yellow sputum for culture and antibiotics were prescribed for hospital-acquired pneumonia. A CXR showed typical localised changes at the right base. It is now 7pm and the HDU nurse has called you because the patient is again tachypnoeic and hypoxic despite the therapy above. The patient's chest signs are unchanged but she is noticeably sweaty and starting to look tired. She is not in pain and, on detailed review, there does not seem to be anything else you can do to improve matters. Recent blood gases show that the $PaCO_2$ has risen from 4 kPa to 7.3 kPa over the last 10 hours. The HDU nurse is experienced and worried that the patient might suddenly tire and arrest. You accept her advice and ask for an urgent ICU review. The ICU consultant is pleased that you called at this stage. The patient is hypercarbic and it is decided to take her to ICU for intubation and ventilation.

## Learning points

- Use your routine ward rounds to monitor progress systematically but reassess and hand over patients who are not right at the end of the routine day.

- Detect patients who are failing to respond or deteriorating despite reasonable therapy and refer promptly.

- Clinical signs (eg tiredness and sweating) are also important in detecting the patient at risk of respiratory failure and arrest.

The clinical signs and blood gas analysis are the most important factors. Tachypnoeic patients suddenly tire and arrest. You must intervene before this stage by acting on early symptoms and signs, particularly tachypnoea. Transfer the patient to a higher level of care for further therapy to improve gas exchange. An arterial line will probably be inserted if frequent blood gas analysis is to be performed. Anticipate problems in patients with severe chronic lung disease (eg vital capacity less than 15 ml/kg or $FEV_1$ less than 10 ml/kg) and monitor them closely.

## Continuous positive airway pressure

If the primary problem is type 1 respiratory failure, CPAP may help.

A high-flow source of oxygen-enriched air is supplied through a tight-fitting facemask with a range of expiratory valves (Figure 4.5). These valves maintain a set airway pressure, which can range from 2.5 to 10 cmH$_2$O. During ventilation, airway pressure cannot drop below the pressure indicated on the valve. This leads to recruitment of underventilated alveolae, increases FRC, decreases intrapulmonary shunt and the work of breathing and may improve oxygenation.

The masks vary from full face to nasal and may cause nasal pressure sores. If air swallowing occurs, it may result in gastric dilatation and regurgitation. Some patients are unable to tolerate a full-face mask but may tolerate a nasal mask. They must

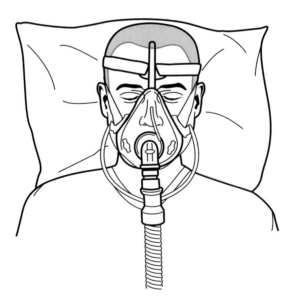

Figure 4.5 Diagrammatic representation of patient receiving CPAP therapy.

keep their mouth closed to prevent loss of pressure. Hood devices are also available; these are noisy and can be claustrophobic to wear, but do not require any patient coordination. After some forms of surgery, eg upper GI surgery, there may be some concerns regarding the effect of CPAP on any high anastomosis.

The CPAP device may also be connected directly via a T-piece to a pre-existing tracheostomy tube. The patient must have a reasonable respiratory rate and tidal volume, be in control of his or her own airway and able to cooperate. Patients who fail to tolerate CPAP are recognised by refractory hypoxaemia, increasing respiratory rate and progressively smaller tidal volumes with subsequent $CO_2$ retention. More obvious clinical signs include intolerance of the CPAP device and agitation or, conversely, obtundation.

Patient selection is key to the success of CPAP. Frequent monitoring of the patient is required, including regular ABGs, within an HDU environment. A plan should be made of how frequently CPAP is to be given, and for what length of time. Generally, to be beneficial, a minimum of 2 hours of continuous CPAP is required. CPAP may also be used as part of the weaning process from formal ventilation or, alternatively, used after major surgery to reduce the risk of respiratory complications, eg following aneurysm surgery.

## Non-invasive ventilation by mask

If type 2 respiratory failure ($CO_2$ retention) develops, NIV support by mask should be considered. Essentially, two different pressures are applied to the patient via a facemask – a higher one during inspiration (around $20\,cmH_2O$) and a lower one in expiration ($5\,cmH_2O$). This may be termed bilevel positive airway pressure mask ventilation (BIPAP). The pressure difference generates gas flow into the lungs during inspiration.

The BIPAP machine detects the initial drop in airway pressure that occurs during inspiration. It then automatically raises the pressure to that set on the machine for inspiration and then changes back to the lower level on expiration. The tidal volume delivered is determined by the lung compliance, duration of inspiration and the driving pressure. This method of respiratory support may pre-empt the need for intubation and ventilation but requires critical care support. It is not effective in all patients and, as with CPAP, careful selection of patients is required. It is not appropriate for patients who are cardiovascularly unstable or those with a decreased level of consciousness, severe metabolic acidosis or a poor respiratory rate. Patients must be in control of their own airway and able to cooperate and a nasogastric tube is usually required to reduce gastric distension. Patients who fail to tolerate mask ventilation are recognised by refractory hypoxaemia, increasing respiratory rate and progressively smaller tidal volumes with worsening $CO_2$ retention. In general terms, if the patient's $CO_2$ has not improved within 30 minutes, mask ventilation is unlikely to succeed. NIV can be used post extubation in patients in whom the risk of reintubation is thought to be high.

## Ventilation

Intubation and ventilation allows administration of oxygen at concentrations of up to 100% and enables the volume of each breath (tidal volume, $V_T$) and respiratory rate or frequency ($f$) to be adjusted to suit the patient's needs. The minute volume (MV $= V_T \times f$) may be varied by altering the frequency or tidal volume. The greater the MV, the greater the removal of carbon dioxide, but if the tidal volume is too high lung damage may result. Use of a low tidal volume approach improves outcome for ICU patients. Target $V_T$ should be 6 ml per kilogram of predicted body weight. Controlling $V_T$ may improve outcome in patients undergoing intrabdominal procedures. Use of sedatives, paralytic agents and permissive hypercapnia may enable these targets to be achieved.

### High-flow nasal oxygen

High flow nasal oxygen can deliver up to 100% $O_2$ with high flows and high humidity. This benefits patients with a high sputum load or those who cannot clear secretions. As the flow is so high, a pressure equivalent to CPAP 5 cmH$_2$O is delivered to the patient, and can help improve the work of breathing. High-flow nasal oxygen is generally well tolerated by patients and, importantly, allows communication and oral nutrition without interruption. However, as with all these methods of respiratory support it is important to ensure that treatment is targeted at the cause of hypoxaemia, and that the patient's response is observed carefully. Unless patients improve rapidly, intubation may be required. The main use of high-flow nasal oxygen in the surgical patient is in treatment of type 1 respiratory failure.

A form of synchronised intermittent mandatory ventilation (SIMV) is used to try and preserve some of the patient's respiratory muscle activity by synchronising ventilation around the patient's own respiratory effort. 'Controlled mandatory ventilation' requires the patient to be fully sedated to tolerate the presence of the tracheal tube and the compulsory positive-pressure breaths from the ventilator. This mode of ventilation allows the patient to play no part in breathing and is rarely used.

Ventilators are increasingly sophisticated and offer different forms of ventilation, which may be used in combination (Figure 4.6). With modern modes of ventilation, such as combining SIMV with pressure-controlled ventilation (PCV), pressure support ventilation (PSV) and positive end-expiratory pressure (PEEP), there is much less need for heavy sedation and paralysis.

PSV, alongside PEEP, may be used once the patient has achieved a good respiratory rate and pattern. Generally, paralysis is necessary only in the most difficult to ventilate patients, and then only for short periods until control is achieved.

With PEEP, pressure is administered during expiration to prevent airway collapse and recruit underventilated alveoli (just like CPAP). Normally 5 cmH$_2$O PEEP is used; however, in very hypoxic patients high PEEP can improve oxygenation rapidly by recruiting alveoli. Once oxygenation is improved, PEEP pressure should generally be brought down. Lung compliance, tidal volume and how fast the tidal volume is 'pushed' into the patient determine the pressure reached within the airways at the end of each breath from the ventilator.

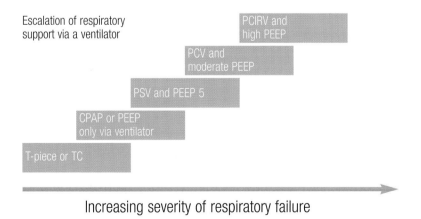

Figure 4.6  There are numerous modes of ventilatory support. A balance needs to be reached between adequate gas exchange and prevention of complications associated with artificial ventilation.

A high peak airway pressure can have adverse consequences. The intrathoracic pressure is always positive on inspiration during ventilation. This causes decreased venous return and a fall in cardiac output, which may be very severe if the patient is hypovolaemic. PEEP can exacerbate this problem. High values of peak airway pressure and PEEP predispose to barotrauma, which can result in tension pneumothorax.

High pressures plus high oxygen concentrations may also promote the toxic effects of oxygen; consequently, concentrations of oxygen greater than 80% are rarely used, and then only for the shortest time possible.

The process of volutrauma promotes alveolar and vascular damage, resulting in fluid leak and worsening of lung compliance. This, in turn, predisposes to even higher airway pressures. Pressure control modes of ventilation allow a breath to be administered to a set pressure, kept below $26\,cmH_2O$; the tidal volume then depends on the patient's lung compliance. By preventing high peak pressures, the risk of barotrauma is reduced. With pressure support, the ventilator senses that the patient has taken an inspiration and administers pressure to provide a higher tidal volume. The aim is not to achieve a normal ABG but to provide adequate ventilation without causing barotrauma. Usual tidal volume is 10–12 ml/kg, but much lower volumes (6 ml/kg predicted body weight) are used during mechanical ventilation. This leads to a higher $PaCO_2$, termed permissive hypercapnia. The $CO_2$ is allowed to rise as long as the pH is above 7.2. This reduces 'ventilator-induced lung injury' and is associated with improved survival (termed 'lung-protective ventilatory strategy'). If lung compliance is very poor, the $CO_2$ may rise too high.

Lung recruitment strategies such as PEEP must be combined with regular physiotherapy, suction and turning the patient to prevent alveolar collapse. CXR, ultrasonography or fibre-optic bronchoscopy should be used to identify any lung collapse amenable to bronchoscopic reinflation, pleural effusions or undiagnosed pneumothoraces.

Normally, the ventilator is set to provide less time for inspiration than for expiration. If the lungs are very poorly compliant and 'stiff', the inspiratory time may be increased to be equal to or even longer than the expiratory time. This process is known as adjusting the inspiratory to expiratory (I/E) ratio. The I/E ratio may thus be normal (1:2 or 1:3), equal (1:1) or inverse (2:1). Applying a limited pressure for a prolonged period of time aims to improve gas exchange by opening the poorly compliant alveoli, holding them open for as long as possible to maximise gas exchange at pressures that will not cause barotrauma or volutrauma or decrease cardiac output.

A patient receiving pressure-controlled inverse ratio ventilation (PCIRV), a high $FiO_2$ of $>0.8$, PEEP $>10\,cm\,H_2O$ and with permissive hypercarbia who fails to achieve oxygen saturation of greater than 85% is at high risk of death. Death will occur from multiple organ failure as tissue oxygen delivery fails to meet demand. At this point, the use of an $FiO_2$ of 1.0 is justified and other adjuncts to ventilation can be considered. The most commonly used is to turn the patient from the supine to prone position. Redistribution of blood flow to the less consolidated or collapsed, more easily ventilated, anterior portions of the lung may result in improved oxygenation and outcome. Finally, extracorporal life support with veno-venous cardiopulmonary bypass could be considered although this is available in only a few centres.

Survival depends on treating the underlying cause of respiratory failure, but all these techniques allow time for interventions such as antibiotics and pleural drainage to work.

## Weaning from ventilatory support

Whatever the method of mechanical ventilatory support used, if treatment of the underlying cause of respiratory failure has been successful, then the patient must be 'weaned' from the ventilator (ie returned to spontaneous respiration in a safe, controlled manner). As soon as patients are able to participate in ventilation, they should be encouraged to do so as prolonged ventilation will lead to atrophy of the respiratory muscles. Various modes of ventilation can be used to allow a gradual reduction in the amount of work performed by the ventilator and an increase in the respiratory effort of the patient.

In general, it is unwise to attempt weaning until:

- The original cause of respiratory failure has been treated successfully.

- Sedative drugs have been reduced to a level at which they will not depress respiration. Daily sedation holds alongside spontaneous breathing trials have been shown to improve survival.

- A low inspired oxygen concentration (40%) maintains a normal $PaO_2$.

- $CO_2$ elimination is no longer a problem.

- Sputum production is minimal.

- Nutritional status, minerals, trace elements are normal.

- Neuromuscular function of the diaphragm and intercostals is adequate.

- The patient is reasonably cooperative.

However, not all of these goals may be achievable, and baseline function must be considered. The most commonly used 'step-down' ventilation modes are SIMV, assisted spontaneous breathing (ASB) and PSV, again often in combination. Alternatively, a simple T-piece, requiring the patient to do all the work of breathing, may be used for periods of time, with mechanical ventilation being resumed when the patient shows objective signs of diminished respiratory effort. The ventilator can be set to simply compensate for the presence of the tube (tube compensation). The periods of time spent breathing spontaneously are increased until extubation is possible. In the majority of critical care units, a combined approach is used with PCV → SIMV → ASB/PSV → CPAP and T-piece followed by extubation. Patients may fail to tolerate extubation as a result of poor airway control, laryngeal oedema, poor cough, sputum retention or simple fatigue. If patients require reintubation or have a decreased consciousness level (eg after head injury) then a tracheostomy may be used as part of the weaning process.

## Discharge from ICU

The period following ICU discharge is critical. When transfer occurs to a general ward without a period in HDU, the patient has to adapt to reduced levels of nursing care, physiotherapy and monitoring. A discharge summary and suggested treatment plan will usually accompany patients as they leave ICU, but it is important that this is understood by the ward staff and is implemented immediately. This does not happen automatically. This period of care exemplifies the importance of good personal communication and organisation – communication between ICU and surgical staff, and between surgical and ward staff, of clear written instructions and repeated assessment of the patient. Apart from clinical reassessment, ensure that medications have been changed to ward format and started, arrange out-of-hours physiotherapy as needed, check the oxygen concentration needed and ensure that any monitoring (such as pulse oximetry) is available on the ward. ITU follow-up by critical care outreach teams should improve communication, and allow monitoring by critical care.

Speak to the on-call team and ask for formal review of the patient. If the patient does deteriorate, contact critical care staff at an early stage; usually, attention to the details of care and ensuring they actually happen will prevent this.

## Common surgical respiratory problems

### Atelectasis

Atelectasis is defined as an absence of gas from all or part of the lung. It is commonly seen in surgical patients, particularly following abdominal and thoracic procedures. Reduced lung expansion from pain and splinting leads to retention of secretions and distal airway collapse. This is exacerbated in the elderly, the overweight, smokers and those with pre-existing lung disease.

It should be anticipated in these patient groups and prevented by preoperative breathing exercises to improve expansion, intraoperative care with humidification, ensuring good tidal volumes and avoiding unnecessarily high $FiO_2$. If unrecognised, it can rapidly deteriorate to respiratory failure.

The symptoms of atelectasis are cough, chest pain or breathing difficulty, low oxygen saturations, pleural effusion (transudate) and cyanosis (late sign) or tachycardia. Diagnosis is by CXR. Generally, the white cell count (WCC) and C-reactive protein (CRP) levels remain in the normal range, though they may be increased if there is superimposed pneumonia. The mainstay of treatment is physiotherapy, focusing on deep breathing, encouraging coughing, and effective analgesia. An incentive spirometer is often used as part of the breathing exercises. Mobilisation should also be encouraged to improve lung inflation. There may be benefit in early use of high-flow nasal oxygen therapy if available.

### Pneumonia

Pneumonia causes parenchymal or alveolar inflammation and abnormal filling of the alveoli with fluid (consolidation and exudation). In surgical patients, pneumonia is usually bacterial or chemical secondary to aspiration. Large-volume aspiration leading to pneumonia is associated with a high mortality rate but can be prevented in patients with gastric dilatation or vomiting by insertion of a large-bore nasogastric tube. Symptoms of pneumonia include cough, chest pain, fever and difficulty in breathing.

Physical examination of the lungs may be normal but often shows decreased expansion of the chest on the affected side, bronchial breathing or crackles. Percussion may be dulled over the affected lung. CXR, WCC, CRP and sputum and blood cultures all help in diagnosis.

Hospital-acquired pneumonia is more likely to be due to resistant bacteria such as methicillin-resistant *Staphylococcus aureus* (MRSA), *Pseudomonas* spp., *Enterobacter* spp. and *Serratia* spp. Ventilator-associated pneumonia is a subset of hospital-acquired pneumonia and occurs after 48 hours of mechanical ventilation.

Aspiration pneumonia is caused by aspirating oral or gastric contents and can occur at any time. Material aspirated may contain anaerobic bacteria, leading to a secondary infective pneumonia. Treatment depends on the clinical classification of pneumonia and also the known bacterial resistances within each hospital. Antibiotic guidelines should be consulted, and if unsure microbiological advice should be sought.

Patients with pneumonia have a high risk of developing respiratory failure and may trigger ARDS, which results from a combination of infection and inflammatory response. The lungs quickly fill with fluid and become very stiff. This stiffness, combined with severe difficulties extracting oxygen due to the alveolar fluid, creates a requirement for mechanical ventilation.

The CURB 65 score, developed for assessment of community-acquired pneumonia, is frequently used when looking at severity of pneumonia: **C**onfusion; **U**rea >7 mmol/L; **R**espiratory rate >30 per minute; **B**lood pressure (SBP <90 mmHg or DBP <60 mmHg); age >**65** years. Although not designed for surgical patients and patients with hospital-acquired pneumonia, it can be a useful tool in flagging up the severity of the condition and likely need for additional critical care support.

### *Pulmonary embolism*

PE comprises embolic obstruction of a vascular branch beyond the right ventricular outflow tract, usually from an associated deep vein thrombosis (DVT). PEs are still relatively common in surgical practice, though thromboprophylactic measures reduce the risk substantially.

Common symptoms include dyspnoea, pleuritic chest pain, cough, haemoptysis and palpitations, while signs include hypoxia, tachypnoea and tachycardia. Diagnosis

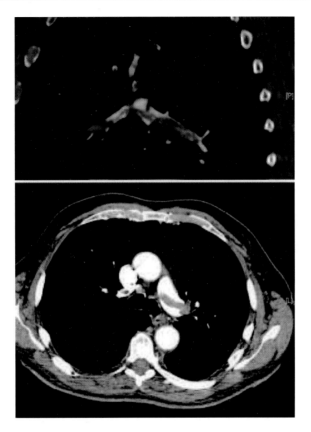

Figure 4.7  CT pulmonary angiogram showing a saddle embolus and substantial thrombus burden in the lobar branches of both main pulmonary arteries.

is based on these clinical findings in combination with laboratory tests and imaging studies. CT pulmonary angiography is commonly used to make the diagnosis (Figure 4.7).

CXR may be helpful in excluding other causes of deterioration. ABG analysis may show hypoxia and hypocarbia. The most common ECG change, apart from sinus tachycardia, is T-wave inversion in the anterior leads and echocardiography may be very useful in the unstable patient to look for right heart dysfunction.

## Treatment

In most cases, anticoagulant therapy is the mainstay of treatment. Usually, low-molecular-weight heparin (LMWH) is administered initially, prior to administration of warfarin or other novel oral anticoagulants (NOACs). In the perioperative patient, treatment is complicated by the risk of bleeding. If the risk of bleeding is moderate, unfractionated heparin by infusion may be used with close monitoring of the activated partial thromboplastin time (APTT).

If there is a concern regarding bleeding, stopping heparin will result in reversal of its effect within 3 hours. Alternatively, it can be reversed with protamine if a more immediate effect is required. The effect of LMWH cannot be fully reversed.

On some occasions it may still be appropriate, in a very high-risk patient, to insert an inferior vena caval filter.

Decisions regarding anticoagulation for PE and DVT in perioperative patients can be complex and should involve discussion with the responsible surgeon and the haematology and critical care departments as required.

## Practical skill: chest drains

Chest drains are inserted either for pneumothorax or for drainage of pleural fluid. There are two main types of drain in common use. Seldinger-type chest drains are mostly used for drainage of pleural effusions and small pneumothoraces, while more traditional drains are inserted for larger pneumothoraces (Figure 4.8). The size of the chest drain used depends on the indication: a large-bore tube (28–30F) should be used for haemothorax, large and/or tension pneumothorax and a smaller calibre tube (10–14F) for pleural effusions. Maintenance of patency of chest drains is important for

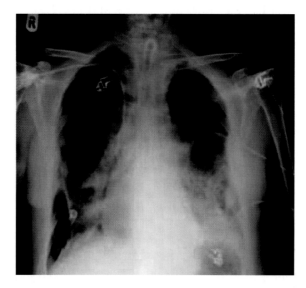

Figure 4.8 Chest X-ray showing chest drain in area of partially resolved right-sided pneumothorax.

safety; frequently, larger tubes are inserted if there is any doubt. However, larger chest drains are associated with increased pain.

The technique of chest drain insertion is not taught on the CCrISP course, however, surgical trainees should be able to state the indications, methods and complications associated with chest drainage.

All chest drains should be monitored for swinging, draining and bubbling and should have an underwater seal. Chest drains should be removed as soon as they are no longer required, ie a pleural effusion drained to dryness (remember that about 100–150 ml of pleural fluid is normally produced per day) or the pneumothorax is fully inflated. Caution must be used when patients are ventilated (including CPAP and NIV) as recurrence of pneumothorax is common and these may well be tension pneumothoraces. If a patient has a pneumothorax, generally any central line required should be put in that side to prevent the occurrence of bilateral pneumothorax.

## Summary

- Assess respiratory function in all ward patients who have undergone major surgery and use simple measures to prevent major respiratory compromise.

- Routine assessment is predominantly clinical and aims to identify the patient who is deteriorating.

- Use the CCrISP system of assessment to identify those patients with respiratory failure.

- Instigate the level of treatment appropriate to the severity of failure.

- Treat the cause of the failure as well as hypoxia/hypercarbia.

- Reassess clinical signs, oximetry and, most importantly, ABGs.

- Arrange transfer to higher level of care for those who do not respond.

# Arterial blood gases and acid–base balance

# 5

## Learning outcomes

This chapter will help you to:

- describe the rationale for blood gas analysis;

- evaluate blood gas analysis in the surgical patient;

- describe how to manage acid–base disturbance using the CCrISP system of assessment.

## Introduction

Blood gas measurements are very useful in the assessment and management of critically ill surgical patients and are probably underused in routine practice. Arterial blood gases (ABGs) can provide a guide to acid–base status, ventilation and global tissue perfusion, as well as showing how well compensatory mechanisms are working. Acid–base status affects blood pH, ventilation (through the partial pressures of oxygen and carbon dioxide) and tissue perfusion through base excess/ base deficit and lactate level. Examining the trends in these values in the critically ill allows clinicians to analyse the severity of patient deterioration and the effectiveness of management plans. Abnormalities in ABGs may arise before a patient becomes obviously unwell and provide clinicians with the opportunity for early intervention: the importance of this in the assessment of the severity of sepsis is reinforced in Chapter 12. Blood gas analysers give rapid results and also provide considerable useful additional information, eg lactate, Hb, $K^+$, $Na^+$, $Ca^{2+}$ and glucose levels. A venous sample may be taken either initially, when taking blood for other tests, or if an arterial sample cannot be obtained, but the results need to be interpreted with caution. A normal venous lactate may be reassuring but an elevated value may or may not indicate significant physiological disturbance and an arterial sample should then be obtained. It is important to ensure that venous blood is not taken from an arm where an IV infusion is running as this may lead to erroneous results.

ABG samples are obtained either by arterial puncture (usually the radial artery) or from an arterial line (a-line; see Chapter 8). The complication rates of such a procedure are low but include bleeding and haematoma formation (particularly in coagulopathic patients), distal ischaemia and pseudo-aneurysm formation (the last usually as a consequence of infected in-dwelling catheters).

The arterial partial pressure of oxygen ($PaO_2$) is a reflection of the amount of oxygen dissolved in the blood. Its relationship with the oxygen saturation of haemoglobin ($SaO_2$) is affected by factors such as temperature, partial pressure of carbon dioxide ($PaCO_2$) and pH, which is reflected by the oxygen dissociation curve (Figure 5.1). The $PaO_2$ can be used as an indicator of the pressure gradient that has the potential to drive oxygen into the tissues. A normal (or supranormal) value does not necessarily ensure effective oxygen utilisation by the tissue but it does reflect adequate management of oxygen delivery by the respiratory and cardiovascular systems.

Regardless of what other ABG values show, hypoxia should be treated with oxygen therapy. A small group of patients with severe COPD rely on hypoxaemia to drive their ventilation, and high inspired oxygen concentrations ($FiO_2$) may suppress ventilation and cause hypercapnia. However, in the acute phase of critical illness, oxygenation is imperative and patients should not be denied oxygen for fear of loss of their respiratory drive. Clinical progress and serial ABG measurement can assist in the management of these patients; trainees should always seek appropriate advice and help if unsure about the potential for causing hypercapnia.

## Practice point

While hypercapnia can kill slowly, **hypoxaemia will kill quickly**. When interpreting the $PaO_2$, any ventilatory support used and the $FiO_2$ should be noted and clinicians should be aware of relative hypoxaemia, ie an absolute $PaO_2$ may be within 'normal limits' (10–14 kPa) but the amount of supplementary oxygen and ventilatory support may be high. A more effective means of assessing for relative hypoxaemia is the $PaO_2/FiO_2$ ratio, with a ratio of <40 kPa deemed hypoxic. Remember that, as the $FiO_2$ increases towards 1.0 (100% oxygen), the $PaO_2$ should increase. An oxygen saturation of 100% and $PaO_2$ of 13 kPa indicates good oxygenation for an individual breathing air ($FiO_2$ 0.21, $PaO_2/FiO_2$ ratio 61.9 kPa) but not necessarily for a patient on supplemental oxygen (ratio 13 if the inspired oxygen is 100%). Note also that pulse oximetry does not measure $CO_2$ so reflects effective oxygenation rather than effective ventilation. ABGs provide a better overall picture of the ventilatory process (see below).

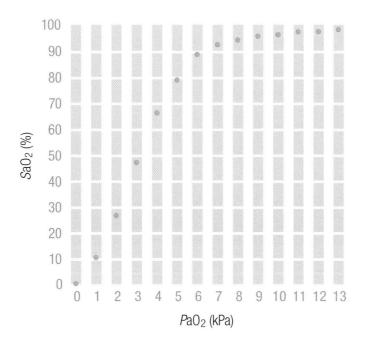

Figure 5.1  The oxygen dissociation curve.

Metabolic activity in body tissue produces energy (heat), carbon dioxide and acid, which reduces the affinity of oxygen for haemoglobin; thus, for a given $PaO_2$, oxygen is less tightly bound to haemoglobin enhancing its off-loading into cells. As this occurs, 2,3-diphosphoglycerate (2,3-DPG) present in red blood cells further loosens the bonds between haemoglobin and oxygen. The reverse is the case in the lungs, resulting in increased binding between haemoglobin and oxygen.

## Interpreting arterial blood gas values

A simple sequential approach to interpreting ABGs can allow you to detect abnormalities, basic pathophysiological processes (metabolic versus respiratory) and compensatory mechanisms of any acid–base disturbance. Approximate normal ranges for ABG components are outlined overleaf.

## Acid–base balance

The concentration of hydrogen ions within the body is normally tightly controlled at 40 nmol/L, which is 7.42 pH units ($pH = -\log_{10}[H^+]$).

## Normal ranges for ABG components

**pH.** Normal range 7.35–7.45. Shows whether a pathophysiological process has resulted in acidaemia or alkalaemia.

***PaCO$_2$.*** Normal range 4.5–6.0 kPa. This provides information about the absolute ventilatory state of a patient and possible respiratory compensatory mechanisms.

**HCO$_3$⁻.** Normal range 24–28 mmol/L. Bicarbonate is the main plasma buffer; a low value suggests consumption, often due to increased acid load (usually lactic acid in surgical patients), and a high value suggests retention of base to compensate for hypoventilation causing an acidaemia (see below).

**Base deficit/base excess.** Normal range +2 to –2 mmol/L. This describes whether the body's buffers are being consumed (deficit) or retained (excess).

***PaO$_2$.*** Normal range 10–14 kPa. Outlines the level of oxygenation (taking into account the $FiO_2$).

**Serum lactate.** Normal range <1.2 mmol/L. This is primarily a reflection of the extent of anaerobic metabolism occurring within the body and secondarily a reflection of the liver's ability to metabolise lactate and regenerate bicarbonate anions.

**Anion gap.** Normal range 10–15 mmol/L. Plasma exists in electrochemical neutrality, ie the numbers of cations and anions balance; however, the majority of laboratory assays measure approximately 95% of cations and 85% of anions, creating a differential described as the anion gap or AG.

$$AG = ([Na^+] + [K^+]) - ([Cl^-] + [HCO^-])$$

The majority of 'unmeasured anions' are plasma proteins but also small concentrations of phosphate, sulphate and organic acids. An acidaemia with an increase in the anion gap indicates an increase in the concentration of these unmeasured anions (eg lactate and ketones). An acidaemia with a normal anion gap equates to the total concentration of measured anions being unchanged usually as a consequence of hyperchloraemic acidaemia. This is most frequently seen following vigorous resuscitation with 0.9% saline but is also associated with bladder surgery and ileal conduit formation.

Over 1000 mmol of hydrogen ion is produced per day, primarily as a result of the production of carbon dioxide. This is excreted by the lung and is dependent upon the minute ventilation as controlled by chemoreceptors in the medulla. A smaller quantity of hydrogen ion is also produced as non-volatile acid products of metabolism of non-carbohydrate substrate, such as phosphates and sulphates. This amounts to approximately 1 mmol $H^+$/kg/day and must be excreted by the distal nephron. There are, therefore, two control mechanisms maintaining hydrogen ion homeostasis – respiratory and renal.

The respiratory mechanism is a rapid response system that requires normal CNS function (central pH chemoreceptors) and lung function to allow carbon dioxide to be transferred from pulmonary venous blood to alveolar gas and excreted in expired gas. Any dysfunction of the mechanics or control of respiration will cause retention of $CO_2$ and a rise in hydrogen ion concentration ($[H^+]$) (respiratory acidosis) or overexcretion and a fall in hydrogen ion concentration (respiratory alkalosis).

The renal mechanism is a slower responding system that depends upon the excretion of hydrogen ions in the urine by the distal nephron. Conditions that impair renal function and, in particular, distal nephron function (eg obstructive uropathy, circulating volume depletion) will prevent non-volatile hydrogen ion excretion resulting in a metabolic acidosis.

The body's homeostatic mechanisms with regard to the maintenance of acid–base balance are powerful, and a patient can have a normal pH in the face of marked physiological disturbance.

The pH scale is a log-based scale, so small changes in pH represent major physiological disturbances. Proteins are the primary buffer of retained hydrogen ion; however, because of the importance of the carbon dioxide/bicarbonate system in the elimination of hydrogen ions, the acid–base status of the body is best reflected by the measurement of carbon dioxide tension and bicarbonate level in the blood. This measures both the volatile and non-volatile arms of the system.

$$(H^+) + HCO_3^- \rightleftharpoons H_2CO_3 \rightarrow H_2O + CO_2$$

Non-volatile                    Volatile
(Renal)                           (Respiratory)

## Respiratory acidosis

The retention of carbon dioxide will cause a rise in [H⁺] by driving the acid–base equation to the left. The kidney will respond slowly over approximately 48 hours to compensate by increasing $H^+$ excretion in the distal nephron, thus returning [H⁺] towards normal, although complete normality will not be achieved.

## Metabolic acidosis

The inability of the kidney to excrete non-volatile hydrogen ion or a sudden increase in non-volatile acid load (such as in sepsis) will drive the equation to the right and respiratory function will rapidly respond by increasing minute volume, reducing $CO_2$ and cause [H⁺] to return towards normal.

## Respiratory alkalosis

Respiratory alkalosis results when the minute ventilation is higher than that required to maintain the $PaCO_2$ appropriate for a [H⁺] of 40 nmol/L. The $PaCO_2$ is driven down and the [H⁺] falls (pH rises). This is usually caused by an increased central respiratory drive commonly caused by fever, hepatic disease, aspirin toxicity or CNS dysfunction.

## Metabolic alkalosis

Metabolic alkalosis occurs when the level of bicarbonate in the blood is increased due to either abnormal retention or administration of bicarbonate or the loss of non-volatile acid from the body (gastric outlet obstruction or chronic nasogastric aspiration). Abnormal retention of bicarbonate can occur in association with chloride depletion due to loop diuretics and is also seen in chronic hypokalaemia.

Knowing the [H⁺]/pH, $PaCO_2$ and bicarbonate allows the patient's acid–base status to be determined, and thus the type of abnormality and degree of compensation to be estimated.

The most useful bicarbonate measure is the standardised value, which corrects the measured bicarbonate to the value that would be present if the $PaCO_2$ was normal (40 mmHg or 5.4 kPa). The non-volatile acid–base state is also summarised by the calculated base excess, which gives a value of the difference between the standardised bicarbonate and the normal value. This is otherwise considered as the amount of acid or alkali needed to return blood *in vivo* to normal pH under standard conditions.

## Management of acid–base disturbance

The first step is to manage the patient in accordance with CCrISP principles and then investigate the nature of the disturbance using ABG samples and other investigations relevant to the patient's history. The importance of determining the underlying primary disturbance is that it can point you towards definitive treatment of an underlying problem. While this is achieved, measures may be required for temporary correction of the pH by other means.

### Aetiology of common acid–base disturbances

#### Metabolic acidosis

- Impaired tissue perfusion – deal with the cause, improve circulation/perfusion.

- Renal failure – deal with the cause; possible treatments include bicarbonate, renal replacement therapy.

- Hepatic failure – ?suitable for transplant.

#### Respiratory acidosis

- Head or spinal injury – ventilation.

- Drug overdose – specific antidote (eg naloxone) and/or ventilation if indicated.

- Chest wall deformity or injury – ventilation if indicated, surgery for flail chest/ multiple rib fractures.

- Myopathy or peripheral neuropathy – ventilation if indicated.

- Pulmonary disease – treat the disease, respiratory support and ventilation if indicated.

- Massive pulmonary embolus – re-establish perfusion of ventilated lung.

## Quick guide to interpreting blood gases

Look at the pH. Is the patient acidotic or alkalotic or is the pH normal?

Then, bearing the pH in mind, look at the $PaCO_2$. If the $PaCO_2$ is high, there is a respiratory acidosis; if it is low, there is a respiratory alkalosis or a compensated(ing) metabolic acidosis.

Then look at the standard $HCO_3$. If the $HCO_3$ is low, there is a metabolic acidosis or a compensated(ing) respiratory alkalosis; if the $HCO_3$ is high, there is a metabolic alkalosis or a compensated(ing) respiratory acidosis.

The primary abnormality is often indicated by the direction of $H^+$ change. The nature of the primary abnormality is determined by considering the clinical context.

Look at the lactate: the higher the lactate, the greater your concern should be.

Look at other variables such as $K^+$, $Ca^{2+}$ and Hb.

## Examples of acid–base disturbance in clinical practice

### Case 1

A 54-year-old man, 14 hours after a laparoscopic hemicolectomy, is receiving oxygen at 4 L/min via a facemask and using a morphine PCA. His respiratory rate is 8/min and his ABGs are as follows:

| | |
|---|---|
| pH | 7.24 |
| $PaCO_2$ | 9.8 kPa |
| $PaO_2$ | 15.1 kPa |
| $HCO_3^-$ | 24.2 mmol/L |
| Lactate | 0.9 mmol/L |
| BE | +0.2 mmol/L |

What is the nature of the blood gas abnormality and how should you manage the situation?

The patient has an uncompensated respiratory acidosis, most probably caused by hypoventilation as a result of excess opiate. Oxygenation remains good; however, in time, the patient will become hypoxaemic without intervention. Assess using the CCrISP system with early administration of supplemental oxygen. The diagnosis may be suspected in 'B' with the slow respiratory rate and in the assessment of 'D' as there may be pinpoint pupils, or at the point of full patient assessment when the observation and drug charts are assessed.

Treatment should include removal of his PCA initially. Analgesia should be ensured by maximising non-opioid analgesia. If the patient has a decreased consciousness level, naloxone should be given. A 400-µg ampoule should be diluted to 10 ml with normal saline and then given in 2-ml aliquots. It is important to remember that giving naloxone rapidly can lead to poor analgesia, and also that naloxone is a short-acting drug in comparison with morphine, so the patient may become drowsy again. Ensure that they are monitored regularly.

## Case 2

An 85-year-old man who has undergone a Hartmann's procedure is shocked and hypotensive with a respiratory rate of 24/min. His ABGs on air are:

| | |
|---|---|
| pH | 7.29 |
| $PaCO_2$ | 2.2 kPa |
| $PaO_2$ | 10.6 kPa |
| $HCO_3^-$ | 10.5 mmol/L |
| BE | −18 mmol/L |
| Hb | 55 g/L |
| $Na^+$ | 140 mmol/L |

| | |
|---|---|
| K⁺ | 6.0 mmol/L |
| Cl⁻ | 111 mmol/L |
| Ca²⁺ | 1.2 mmol/L |
| Glucose | 7.8 mmol/L |
| Lactate | 12.5 mmol/L |

**What is the nature of the abnormality and how should you manage the situation?**

This patient has a partially compensated metabolic acidosis and is hypoxic. He is likely to have either intra-abdominal blood loss or sepsis with increased acid load secondary to organ hypoperfusion, and this has led to a high serum lactate.

The tachypnoea is a consequence of an attempted compensation for the acidosis and also the likely consequence of pain, which in turn can cause diaphragmatic splinting, atelectasis and hypoxia. If ineffectively managed, this will eventually lead to hypercapnia and a mixed metabolic and respiratory acidosis. This patient needs aggressive volume resuscitation, blood transfusion and adequate analgesia. The underlying problem needs to be brought under control. The high K⁺ may be secondary to inadequate renal perfusion and should come down with aggressive fluid resuscitation.

## Practice point

Be aware that blood gases give other vital information, such as Hb level, which can aid early treatment.

## Case 3

A 48-year-old man presents with Crohn's disease, an ileostomy and large stoma losses. He is tachypnoeic and breathing room air. His ABGs are as follows:

| pH | 7.25 |
| --- | --- |
| $PaCO_2$ | 3.2 kPa |
| $PaO_2$ | 17.1 kPa |
| $HCO_3^-$ | 14.2 mmol/L |
| BE | −9.9 mmol/L |
| Lactate | 1.0 mmol/L |

**What is the nature of the blood gas abnormality and how should you manage the situation?**

The patient has a metabolic acidosis with attempts at compensation, but these are not effective enough to prevent a low pH. There is likely to have been large losses of bicarbonate from the stoma. In addition to CCrISP assessment, investigation and treatment of the cause, fluid replacement with a crystalloid such as Hartmann's solution is appropriate to replace many of the electrolytes being lost. If the patient's liver function is normal, the lactate anions can be utilised to generate bicarbonate, help replace losses and correct the acidosis.

## Case 4

A 78-year-old man presents to surgical admissions with abdominal distension and pain, nausea, vomiting and diarrhoea. He has received opiate analgesia. An ABG analysis on air is performed:

| pH | 7.51 |
| --- | --- |
| $PaCO_2$ | 8.0 kPa |
| $PaO_2$ | 8.0 kPa |
| $HCO_3^-$ | 45.5 mmol/L |
| BE | +21 mmol/L |
| Hb | 91 g/L |

| | |
|---|---|
| Na+ | 150 mmol/L |
| K+ | 1.8 mmol/L |
| Glucose | 4.5 mmol/L |
| Lactate | 1.3 mmol/L |

### What is the nature of the blood gas abnormality?

The patient has a partially compensated metabolic alkalosis; his $PaCO_2$ is further raised secondary to excessive opiate administration as hypoventilation as a compensatory mechanism is limited. Important extra information is the presence of hypokalaemia and hypernatraemia. Fluid resuscitation is necessary, as is replacement of K+ losses. As the patient's K+ level is so low, this will most likely need to take place in a critical care unit via a central venous catheter. Careful monitoring will be required.

## Summary

The interpretation of blood gases is an essential part of caring for surgical patients.

- pH indicates whether there is acidosis or alkalosis.

- Base excess indicates whether acidosis is metabolic (negative base excess) or respiratory.

- Low $PaO_2$ indicates the presence of hypoxia and should be interpreted with the $FiO_2$.

- High $PaCO_2$ and acidosis (plus high $HCO_3^-$ and positive base excess) indicates respiratory acidosis.

- Further information, such as the concentrations of lactate, Hb, Na+, K+ and glucose, may be helpful in emergencies.

- Initial management of any acid–base disturbance begins with the CCrISP algorithm.

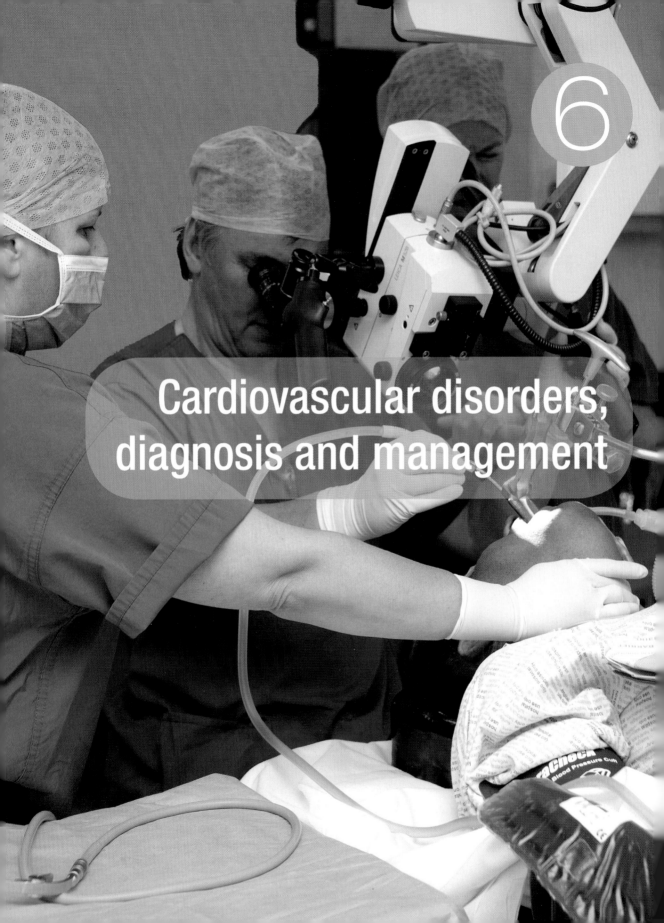

# Cardiovascular disorders, diagnosis and management

6

## Learning outcomes

This chapter will help you to:

- assess if a patient's cardiovascular system is functioning adequately;

- determine if a patient is unwell because of a cardiovascular problem;

- decide where and how the patient should be appropriately treated;

- initiate safe and appropriate management of common cardiac pathophysiologies;

- involve and communicate effectively with other specialists as required.

This chapter and the next two chapters deal with aspects of cardiovascular disorders, shock (Chapter 7) and monitoring (Chapter 8) and should be considered together. This chapter will focus on clinical assessment and the diagnosis and management of cardiac disorders. This first section will introduce a basic pattern of thinking that should enable the early detection of an impending or actual cardiovascular problem. Preventative measures, simple treatments or referral to a specialist unit can then be initiated appropriately.

Disorders of the cardiovascular system (CVS) are very common in the unwell surgical patient with pre-existing comorbidities or may appear as a new disorder following surgery. Despite the presence of an intact airway and adequate ventilation, any problem causing decreased efficiency of the CVS can result in delivery of oxygen to the tissues being inadequate for the patient's metabolic needs. This will initiate a cascade of adverse events that will lead to the development of organ failure. The range of pathologies that cause CVS disturbance is broad, and includes inadequate circulating volume (eg haemorrhage), primary 'pump' problems (eg myocardial ischaemia or arrhythmias) and increased or reduced afterload (eg sepsis). Detecting problems before the development of overt organ failures can be difficult: early signs may be subtle and gradual, i.e. slightly deranged pulse rate and blood pressure. Early recognition of an impending problem and initiation of treatment will increase your patient's chances of survival and help to prevent further complications. Prediction and prevention are vital, hence the role of National Early Warning Scores (NEWS) as a means of detecting these derangements and prompting a trigger for medical review and/or planning of subsequent patient care.

The approach to the examination of the CVS must be systematic, accurately documented and repeated frequently. The effect of any intervention, such as fluid administration, must be reassessed to ensure its efficacy and durability. It is also vital to consider a patient's concurrent cardiac medications and other organ pathologies as managing these can be complex in the perioperative period. It is important to decide what medications to continue and the route of administration should the patient be nil by mouth following surgery.

## Patient assessment and management

### Immediate assessment and resuscitation

Establish that the patient does not need immediate cardiopulmonary resuscitation by making your immediate 'ABCDE' assessment, then progress using the CCrISP algorithm. Keep an open mind and do not try and make the findings fit any preconceived diagnosis, whilst giving immediate and appropriate resuscitation during the assessment. Potential causes of cardiac disturbance are numerous and include hypovolaemia due to haemorrhage or unreplaced fluid losses, sepsis, cardiac dysfunction or PE. Jumping to conclusions can be catastrophic for the patient as the treatments required vary considerably between these conditions.

The presence of dyspnoea increases the likelihood of a cardiac and/or respiratory problem. Respiratory and cardiovascular function are inextricably linked; a disorder of the respiratory system (eg tension pneumothorax) may produce CVS signs and, similarly, a CVS disorder (eg left ventricular failure) may produce respiratory signs. All other organ systems are dependent on the effectiveness of the circulation. This is particularly true of the renal and the central nervous systems, and the integrity of these end organs can give valuable information about the function of the CVS. If the patient is obtunded or too confused to respond coherently, then cerebral hypoperfusion or hypoxia is likely and prompt action will be needed.

Life-threatening CVS disorders are recognisable if you examine the patient appropriately:

- **Look for** pallor, signs of poor peripheral perfusion, underfilled or overfilled central veins, obvious blood loss from wounds, drains or stomas, swelling of soft tissues or other evidence of concealed haemorrhage into the chest, abdomen or pelvis.

- **Listen to the patient:** confusion might be due to poor cerebral perfusion; if the patient complains of feeling faint on sitting up or is thirsty, consider hypovolaemia. A complaint of breathlessness on lying flat may point to pulmonary oedema. Complaints of chest pain and feeling feverish or cold are all helpful in indicating potentially serious underlying pathology and should not be ignored. New-onset pain in the operated cavity may suggest a surgical complication that may need investigation. Listen to the chest and heart and compare what you hear now with what has been recorded previously.

## Practice point

Listen to the heart – are there normal heart sounds or a gallop rhythm? Is there a new murmur?

- **Feel for** carotid and femoral pulses if peripheral radial pulses are not present. Assess rate, quality (weak/thready/strong), regularity and equality. Examine the patient for swelling, distension or painful areas that may indicate internal bleeding or ischaemia.

- **Feel for** changes in skin temperature and always assess capillary refill time.

## Practice point

Unwell surgical patients will benefit from 15 L/min oxygen and consideration of a fluid challenge whilst you are performing your assessment.

# Full patient assessment

## Chart review

The notes and charts contain a lot of data; a systematic approach minimises the chance of missing important facts. It can be useful to complete your note and chart review before speaking in detail to the ward nurses and doctors. This provides you with a factual base for discussing the patient in more detail. The notes will provide basic clinical information on the patient's premorbid status, comorbidities and any procedures performed. On the charts, look at both the absolute values and the trends. Absolute values need to be considered, but trends and, if possible, a comparison with the patient's known observations when well, eg in preassessment clinic, are also important. The charts should indicate the progress of the patient and important parameters include:

- respiratory rate, administered oxygen and measured saturation

- heart rate and rhythm

- blood pressure – systolic/diastolic

- CVP (if measured)

- temperature

- urinary output

- IV lines – position and date of insertion

- fluid therapy – prescribed versus given

- drainage of all types.

Review drug chart for drugs with cardiovascular effects (are they being given or omitted) and the most recent blood results including near-patient testing.

## Respiratory rate

This is the most sensitive marker of the 'ill' patient and often the first parameter to change as the patient deteriorates. Accurate observation and recording is essential. Low rates may be due to opiate/sedative overdose or other causes of CNS depression, including low cardiac output states, whereas a high respiratory rate is an early sign of many kinds of shock, as well as respiratory disease or cardiac failure. An increased respiratory rate may also be found as part of the response to hypoxia and/or metabolic acidosis. If a full patient assessment fails to reveal an obvious cause of a high respiratory rate, check the blood gases to establish if acidosis is a contributory factor.

### Heart rate and rhythm

- Heart rates rise as the body attempts to maintain cardiac output and delivery of oxygen to the tissues. This is supply attempting to match demand. Not all patients will be able to mount a response to an increasing demand, eg if they are on ⎕-blockers or are in receipt of mechanical pacing. The cause may also be autonomically driven; pain, anxiety and pyrexia can all increase heart rate. How a patient responds to a circulatory insult depends on his or her cardiovascular reserve and reactivity. Patients with little reserve will show obvious signs of dysfunction in response to a relatively small insult whilst fitter patients will tolerate a larger insult for longer but will eventually collapse dramatically. These patients will show signs of cardiovascular stress if carefully assessed, eg prolonged capillary refill time. It is important to understand this interpatient variability to successfully manage an unstable patient.

- Tachycardia along with increased respiratory rate and altered mental state can be an early sign of shock, and acute dysrhythmia can be an important sign of biochemical derangement, sepsis or myocardial failure/ischaemia. The rhythm may also change as the heart attempts to maintain supply. This can indicate myocardial ischaemia or biochemical abnormalities that should be investigated further. Myocardial perfusion occurs in ventricular diastole and tachycardia or tachyarrhythmia may precipitate an ischaemic cardiac event that may not be symptomatic.

### Blood pressure

Changes in both systolic and diastolic pressure are often late signs but, when present, should flag up the severity of the underlying problem. It is more useful to think of organ perfusion rather than blood pressure: a high or normal blood pressure with poor perfusion is of little benefit to the patient. Look at the blood pressure and the urine output together. Is there a blood pressure that is associated with a better urine output? Urine output responds less quickly than capillary refill time when cardiac output is improved.

In the elderly, hypertensive patient who usually has a blood pressure of 180/100 mmHg, a pressure of 110/70 mmHg represents significant hypotension and potentially impaired organ perfusion.

---

**Learning point**

- Clinical signs may be unreliable; normal values do not exclude significant abnormality. Abnormal values should be assessed and acted upon.

---

### Jugular venous pressure/central venous pressure

It is unusual for CVP to be monitored in a ward environment, and a more practical and clinically useful assessment of filling can be made by measuring the capillary refill time. Capillary refill time is the time in seconds it takes for perfusion to return and is measured by pressing on a distal nail bed or over the sternum for 5 seconds until blanching occur.

Jugular venous distension is measured with the patient inclined at 45° and will give a clinical indication of the CVP. Collapsed neck veins with the patient at 45° indicates a likely low CVP. An internal jugular vein that is not visible with the patient lying flat is always abnormal.

The response to a fluid bolus is a better guide to fluid status than absolute values. A change in capillary refill time is a very valuable tool in assessing on-going fluid status and response to a fluid challenge.

Formal CVP monitoring may be needed to manage patients where further fluid management is becoming problematic eg the patient whose blood pressure is not responding to several fluid challenges and who is not bleeding. However, if you are considering the need for a CVP line you should probably be asking for expert advice and assistance from critical care.

Abnormalities relating to capillary refill time are detailed in Box 6.1.

## Box 6.1 Abnormalities of capillary refill time and central venous pressure

- A prolonged capillary refill time may be:
  - due to inadequate fluid therapy
  - an indication of continued bleeding
  - due to vasodilatation in response to sepsis
  - associated with a low cardiac output state, eg cardiogenic shock.

  A prolonged capillary refill time must not be tolerated if the patient is hypotensive.

- A high CVP may be:
  - temporary following a rapid fluid bolus
  - a result of fluid overload
  - due to right ventricular failure as a result of MI or PE
  - due to cardiac failure
  - due to chronic respiratory disease
  - caused by pericardial effusion with tamponade.

If in any doubt as to the cause or treatment required, seek expert help.

### Temperature

Low-grade pyrexia may occur after an MI, in bacterial endocarditis (look out for a cardiac murmur and anaemia) or with diurnal variation in a warm environment (highest in the early evening).

### Fluid balance

Assess the losses (urine, drains, stomas and nasogastric aspirates) against the inputs (nasogastric feed, oral fluids, IV fluids and IV nutrition). Urine output is frequently used as a surrogate marker of cardiac output and tissue perfusion as it is relatively easy to monitor on the ward. However it is not an immediate and acute measurement of organ perfusion. Look out for a steady decline in hourly urine output to indicate a problem rather than sudden complete anuria, which is more often due to a blocked catheter.

It is the trend that is most useful and comparing what the other charted vital signs were just before the urine output trended down can provide a timeline for the patient's deterioration.

## Intravenous lines, intracavitary drains and tubes

Large-bore IV access is required to deliver an appropriate rapid fluid bolus and you should aim to insert the largest cannula that will fit into the vein. Tissued lines cause morbidity both locally owing to the effect of extravasated fluids and drugs and systemically as a result of the failure of the fluid and drugs to reach the circulation.

Careful aseptic insertion and management of IV lines is essential, as cannula site cellulitis and sepsis is a significant cause of hospital-acquired morbidity.

Look for the drain that is no longer draining; blocked chest drains (the fluid in the tube should 'swing' and the drain may bubble if there is an on-going air leak) can cause a tension pneumothorax while blocked abdominal drains can conceal blood loss and pus, both of which may result in cardiovascular instability. Examine the colour and possibly the smell of drain contents. Brown or green fluid in an abdominal drain may represent a significant complication. It is much more common for unwell surgical patients to be hypovolaemic than to be fluid overloaded. Pulmonary oedema may be iatrogenic, particularly in the elderly patient who develops a new pathology, eg perioperative MI with associated heart failure. In these patients, fluid should be given in small repeated boluses to correct hypovolaemia and invasive monitoring in an HDU/ICU environment may be necessary. All patients are different and not everyone responds in the same way to apparently similar fluid regimens.

Assess the type and quantity of fluids given, review the fluid balance for the current 24 hours and for the preceding days and link this to the rest of the full patient assessment.

## Drug chart review

Omission of regular cardiac medication while the patient was 'nil by mouth' contributes to perioperative morbidity, eg hypertension and dysrhythmia. Alternatively, the patient may have been given drugs that have produced adverse cardiovascular effects as a result of overdosage, accumulation or interaction with other medication, especially in the presence of renal dysfunction (eg digoxin can accumulate if the patient develops a new acute kidney injury).

## Case notes

### History

Taking a careful and detailed history from the patient and from the notes will help to identify cardiac problems. Remember that nursing colleagues and relatives can be useful additional sources of information. Specific points worth remembering include:

- speed of onset and duration of any symptoms;

- pain, its nature, severity, site and radiation;

- presence of dyspnoea;

- functional exercise tolerance.

The preadmission cardiac status, functional capacity and medication should be identified from the notes when making an assessment of the patient's CVS, both when complications are occurring and when the daily management plan is being formulated.

### Examination

Use all the available clinical information and think about perfusion. Concentrate on the CVS as part of the full patient assessment (Box 6.2).

### Look

- Overview – is the patient alert now that oxygen has been administered? A reduced level of consciousness is often a clear sign of reduced cardiac output.
- Colour – look for peripheral or central cyanosis or obvious pallor.
- Peripheries – assess for peripheral perfusion and the presence of oedema.
- Neck veins – can you see them?

## Listen

### Breath sounds

- Assess for the presence of basal crepitations, which may be indicative of left-sided heart failure.
- In early, left-sided heart failure, bronchial wheeze (cardiac asthma) may be caused by small airway narrowing as a result of interstitial pulmonary oedema.

### Heart sounds

- Assess for the presence of added sounds or murmurs (?new).
- Time the murmur with the carotid pulse: remember that a diastolic murmur is never 'physiological'.

## Feel

- Assess limb temperature. The skin may feel clammy and capillary refill time may be poor in patients with cardiogenic shock. Alternatively, the skin may feel warm and capillary refill may be good in patients with sepsis.
- Liver – assess for presence of hepatomegaly or ascites, which may be an indication of right heart failure. Heart failure can cause abdominal pain as a result of acute distension of the liver capsule.

## Box 6.2 Indicators of a low cardiac output

- Cool, clammy skin with poor capillary refill time
- Rapid, thready pulse
- Peripheral cyanosis
- Oliguria or anuria
- Confusion
- Metabolic acidaemia

## Available results

Include the available results and previous investigations in your assessment. Remember that ward care is different to HDU/ICU care and it is unlikely that the complete range of cardiovascular tests will have been performed. Be realistic; look at what is available and use the findings of your clinical examination and note and chart review to determine if any further specific tests are required. Demanding unnecessary tests is time-consuming and costly and inflicts further discomfort on the patient.

As a minimum to aid your assessment, look at the most recent results of haemoglobin, white cell count, platelet count and electrolytes (potassium and magnesium especially) and compare them with those taken when the patient was well. If no contemporary results are available since the patient's deterioration, these will need to be ordered. Additional tests will be necessary if you suspect particular problems (eg cardiac enzymes for MI).

## Haemoglobin

Anaemia may well precipitate heart failure in patients with critical ischaemia. Transfusions should be used to maintain a haemoglobin level around 80 g/L in the stable patient as this reduces the number of units a patient is exposed to without increasing cardiac morbidity. If the patient is actively bleeding, or has new acute cardiac pathology, a higher haemoglobin and further blood transfusion will be required.

## Electrolytes

Potassium and magnesium are particularly important for cardiac function (see Chapter 11). If infarction/ischaemia is suspected, serial troponin levels should be measured from 6 hours after the onset of symptoms, bearing in mind the problems of measurement in the perioperative period. Troponin levels (either troponin I or troponin T) are the most frequent measure of cardiac ischaemia. An absolute level 6 hours after an index event or a change in the level from baseline is often considered diagnostic; however, troponin levels can be raised in patients with sepsis or other cardiorespiratory pathologies, eg acute heart failure or pneumonia, and levels may be raised several days after an event if the patient has other organ dysfunctions, eg chronic renal failure (CRF). Interpretation can be difficult without integrating the results with the rest of the full patient assessment.

Brain natriuretic peptide (BNP) levels (if available) may help in assessing heart failure.

## Chest radiography

This can help differentiate respiratory conditions from cardiovascular and aids in the positive identification of heart failure. Check previous films and decide if the current clinical picture suggests something different. Refer to the system for looking at radiographs in Chapter 4.

Departmental chest X-rays take time and should not delay treatment. Unwell patients should not be sent to the radiology department unless they can be monitored and receive the appropriate level of care. Portable films are frequently preferable in unwell patients.

## Electrocardiography

As with other investigations, ECGs should never be looked at in isolation but should be interpreted in light of the clinical findings and compared with any previous ECGs. An ECG may show nothing significantly new, even in the failing heart, but it is important to be able to recognise common patterns. Most bedside monitors do not show a trace adequate for accurate diagnosis so a formal 12-lead ECG is essential.

## Interpreting the ECG

Work to a routine when looking at an ECG (Table 6.1). Check the patient name/date/time and compare with previous ECGs.

Table 6.1  The routine for looking at an ECG

| | | |
|---|---|---|
| Axis | Use deflection in bipolar leads | |
| Rhythm | Use the R wave (lead II) | ?Regular |
| Rate | Use the R wave | ?Normal |
| P wave | Presence and morphology | ?Sinus rhythm |
| PR interval | Short or Long | Pre-excitation (eg Wolff–Parkinson–White syndrome, heart block) |
| QRS complex | Height, width, presence Q waves | ?MI, ?bundle branch block |
| ST segment | Depressed or elevated | ?MI, ?ischaemia, ?digitalis toxicity |
| T wave | Height, shape | ?Ischaemia, ?biochemical abnormalities |
| U wave | Presence | ?Hypokalaemia |

## Rotation of the heart and morphology of the precordial QRS complexes

The rotation of the heart determines the appearance of the QRS complexes in the different leads (Figure 6.1). The size of the R wave increases progressively from V1 to V6 because the underlying myocardium becomes progressively thicker over the left ventricle. This reflects myocardial thickness as depolarisation spreads from endocardium to epicardium. Occasionally, the R wave in V6 may be smaller than that in V5 and that in V5 may be smaller than that in V4 – this can occur if the electrodes in these leads are further away from the myocardium.

The size of the S wave (the first negative deflection after the R wave) tends to decrease towards V6.

The direction of the first part of the QRS complex is upwards, ie positive, in V1 to V3 (an R wave) but becomes negative as it progresses to V6 (Q wave). This is not pathological and is due to rotation of the heart about a near-vertical axis (left hip to right shoulder), thus producing a variation in the relative positions of the two ventricles. This rotation causing the variations in QRS complexes is not clinically significant and is dependent on the individual.

Since the height of the R wave and depth of the S wave are influenced by the thickness of the underlying myocardium, these deflections will be abnormally large in conditions producing hypertrophy, for example left ventricular hypertrophy secondary to hypertension or aortic valve disease. However, in thin patients the R wave may be 'abnormally' high over V4 to V6.

## The electrical axis of the heart

The spread of depolarisation across the myocardium produces 'vector loops' of electrical activity. When the depolarisation wave moves towards an electrode, an upwards or positive deflection will be recorded. Conversely, moving away from an electrode will produce a downwards or negative deflection. The angle at which this electrical wave moves in relationship to a particular electrode will determine the degree of upward or downward deflection recorded by it. Each lead of the ECG 'looks' at the heart from a different aspect, or angle. These 'angles' can be displayed using the hexaxial reference system.

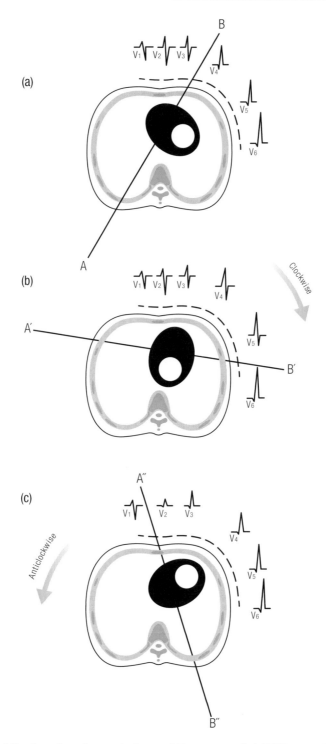

Figure 6.1 Rotation of the heart and morphology of the precordial QRS complexes. The cross-section through the thorax is viewed from below. (a) Intermediate position; (b) clockwise rotation; (c) anticlockwise rotation.

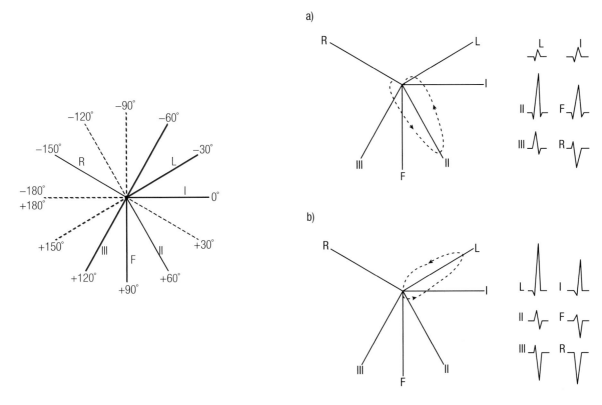

Figure 6.2  Electrical axes of the heart.

Figure 6.2 shows the 'angle' at which each bipolar lead 'sees' the heart. By comparing the relative heights of the R wave and depth of the S wave, the electrical axis or sum of the depolarisation vectors can be determined. Basically, the more the electrical axis points towards an electrode, the greater the deflection produced by that electrode. See leads II and F in Figure 6.2a and leads L and I in Figure 6.2b.

This description is simplified and is only intended to give you an outline of the subject.

Look at the example provided in Figure 6.3. Using the theory above, can you determine the electrical axis?

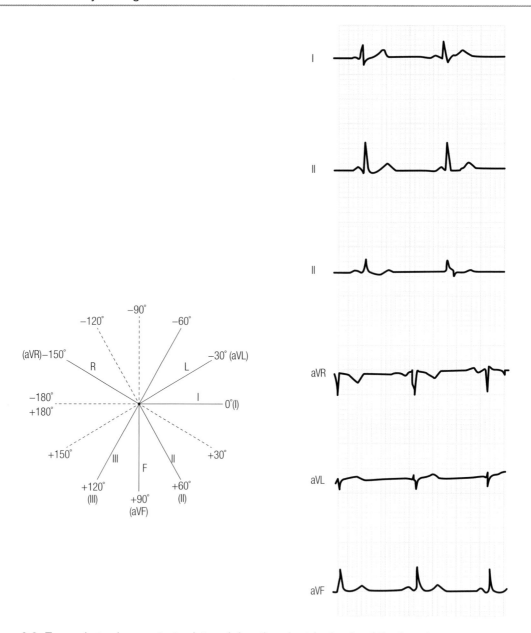

Figure 6.3 Example to demonstrate determining the electrical axis of the heart.

## Normal ranges in ECG interpretation

The normal ranges in ECG interpretation are shown in Table 6.2 and in Figures 6.4 and 6.5.

Table 6.2 Normal ECG ranges

| | |
|---|---|
| At 25 mm/s | Large square = 0.2 seconds, small square = 0.04 seconds |
| QRS width | Normal < 0.12 seconds, wide > 0.12 seconds |
| Tachycardia | Is a ventricular rate > 100 bpm |
| Bradycardia | Is a ventricular rate < 60 bpm |
| Electrical axis | +90° to −30°<br>Vertical +60° to +90° (tall individuals)<br>Intermediate +30° to +60°<br>Horizontal +30° to −30° (stocky, squat individuals)<br>Axis shifts towards the left in the elderly |
| T wave | Normally upright, except in aVR lead. Inversion can also occur in leads III, V1 and V2 |
| P wave | Normally upright<br>Inversion can occur in retrograde P waves in atrioventricular nodal rhythm<br>Tall, peaked waves in pulmonary hypertension ('pulmonary P')<br>Biphasic in mitral valve disease ('mitral P') |
| PR interval | Measured from the start of the P wave to the first deflection of the QRS complex, whether it is upright or inverted<br>Range = 0.12–0.2 seconds |
| QT interval | Variable, depends on rate |
| Q wave | The first downward (negative) deflection after the P wave<br>Normal in lead III and aVR and sometimes in V4, V5, V6<br>Width no more than 0.04 seconds' duration<br>Depth no more than one-quarter the height of the following R wave |
| U wave | Normal when T wave is normal, but in hypokalaemia it may become more prominent as the T wave flattens |

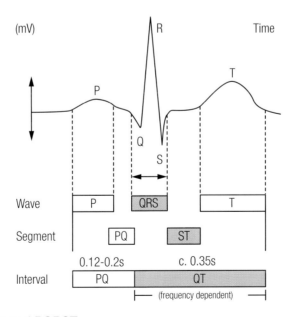

Figure 6.4 Normal annotated PQRST.

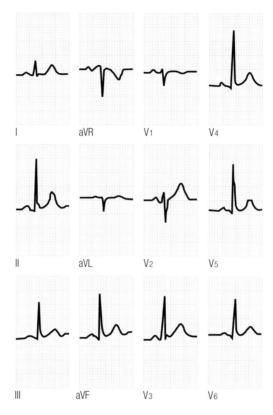

| I | aVR | V1 | V4 |
| II | aVL | V2 | V5 |
| III | aVF | V3 | V6 |

Figure 6.5 Normal ECG trace.

## Decide, plan and treat

The clinical assessment and investigations described above should lead to a diagnosis that explains the patient's deterioration. The next task is to reach a decision based on the findings and, if needs be, arrange further appropriate investigations or specialist opinions. Make a management plan to treat the problem and prevent recurrence.

Conditions that do not rapidly resolve with relatively simple measures will require expert help and a higher level of care. After any intervention you will need to reassess and modify the management plan.

Remember the CVS has considerable reserve and, by the time dysfunction is evident, the problems are marked. Do not leave patients with obviously compromised cardiovascular systems.

## Specific management problems

### Diagnosis and management of hypotension

Hypotension is the commonest cardiovascular problem seen in unwell surgical patients.

### Diagnosis and management of tachyarrythmias

A frequent trigger for NEWS scoring and need for review is the patient with a tachycardia (Table 6.3). A patient with unstable vital signs needs prompt assessment and treatment. At the other end of the spectrum, long-standing, asymptomatic AF is common in the elderly and might simply need attention to fluid balance and electrolytes and reinstitution of routine digoxin treatment. Usually, some action will be required. If any doubt exists, ask for senior help.

■ Rule out/correct hypovolaemia, hypoxia, hypokalaemia, hypomagnesaemia.

■ Check routine medications have been given.

Table 6.3  Causes of tachycardia (the type of tachycardia will only be evident from the ECG)

| | |
|---|---|
| Trauma | Hypovolaemia, anaemia, contused myocardium |
| Inflammatory | Pyrexia, pericarditis, sepsis |
| Metabolic | Acidosis |
| Haematological | Anaemia |
| Circulatory | Shock, from any cause |
| Arrhythmias, PE, MI | |
| Endocrine | Thyrotoxicosis |
| Drugs | Aminophylline, digitalis toxicity, beta-agonists |
| Anxiety and pain | |

#### Autonomic manoeuvres

Valsalva manoeuvres may correct a supraventricular tachycardia as described below, but this is unlikely to be permanent.

#### Drugs

Care must be taken with all drugs, particularly in patients with poor ventricular function or hypotension. Only use/prescribe a drug if you are familiar with its actions and its side effects: if there is any doubt about a drug, it should not be given and advice should be sought.

In the longer term, if atrial fibrillation or atrial flutter persists, anticoagulation may be necessary in order to prevent emboli, but it is rarely required in the acute phase and may have significant risks for the acutely unwell surgical patient. It is not the role of the surgical trainee to decide on long-term anticoagulation for a surgical patient.

### DC cardioversion

Cardioversion can be considered when there is a very rapid rate or evidence of compromise, particularly in the case of ventricular tachyarrythmias. It is less effective in cases of long-standing atrial arrhythmias. Help from the critical care team and/or cardiology must be sought at an early stage.

### Pacing and surgical ablation

The use of these treatments is beyond the scope of this course. They should be used under the guidance of a cardiologist.

## Ventricular tachyarrythmias

### Ventricular tachycardias

Safe and effective management of even the most common arrythmias (Box 6.3) may require cardiology input. Ventricular tachycardias (VTs) are potentially very serious and require prompt specialist referral. They should be distinguished from supraventricular tachycardia (SVT) by the appearance of the ECG (Figures 6.6 and 6.7 and Table 6.4). Cardioversion is often required for VT and is particularly urgent if the patient has evidence of compromised cardiac output. SVT may respond, although sometimes only temporarily, to intense vagal stimulation, eg a Valsalva manoeuvre. Alternatively, adenosine can be administered (6 mg bolus first dose, 12 mg bolus second dose if given via a peripheral cannula). Adenosine has a powerful blocking effect on the atrioventricular (AV) node, thus slowing ventricular rate if the dysrhythmia is atrial in origin. It acts for only 15–20 s and is relatively safe in inexperienced hands. Its use should be avoided in the asthmatic patient and in the presence of dipyridamole, which greatly prolongs its action.

## Case scenario 6.1

A 73-year-old man with hypertension who usually takes amlodipine underwent anterior resection for carcinoma of the rectum this morning. You review him at 8 pm on the HDU on the evening of surgery and find him to be in AF with a rate of 90 bpm. This developed about 30 minutes previously. On your immediate assessment you find that he appears quite well and he tells you that he feels comfortable (he has an epidural infusion in progress). His respiratory rate is 18 breaths/min and his oxygen saturation is 97% with facemask oxygen at 40%. You examine him and find that his peripheries are well perfused. His blood pressure is unchanged from preoperatively at 150/80 mmHg. Your initial assessment reveals no other findings. You review his charts and notes and find that his urine output has only been 40 ml over the last 2 hours. His CVP has been gradually decreasing since return from theatre and is now reading 2 mmHg. He was prescribed two units of blood to run over 3 hours each, followed by 1000 ml of saline 8-hourly. The first litre of saline has just been started. You ask the nurse to give him the 500 ml of saline over 20 minutes, and check a full blood count and his urea and electrolytes. His haemoglobin is satisfactory at 110 g/L. His serum potassium is 3.2 mmol/L. All other electrolytes, including magnesium, are within normal limits. You prescribe 20 mmol of potassium to be given in 100 ml of saline via the central line over the next hour and arrange with the ward nurse in charge of HDU to review him in an hour. When you review him, he is in sinus rhythm with a rate of 75 bpm, his CVP has risen to 6 mmHg and he has passed 30 ml of urine over the past 30 minutes. You change the fluid prescription to 1000 ml saline with 20 mmol KCl at 100 ml/h and arrange to review the patient again later that evening.

## Learning points

- Use the CCrISP system of assessment to review all patients.
- Regular review of patients at risk will lead to early detection of potential problems.
- Correction of hypovolaemia, hypoxia and electrolyte disturbances is simple but is often very effective.

## Box 6.3 Common causes of arrhythmia

- Ischaemic heart disease
- Oxygen, fluid and electrolyte disturbances
- Drugs
- Rheumatic heart disease
- Cardiomyopathy
- Thyrotoxicosis

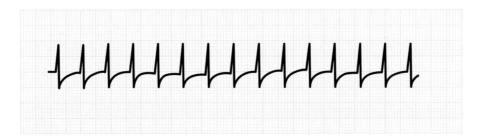

Figure 6.6 Supraventricular tachycardia.

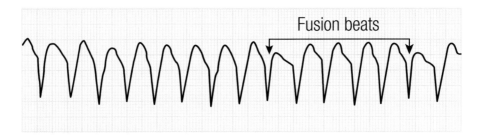

Figure 6.7 Ventricular tachycardia.

Table 6.4 Differentiating SVT and VT

| Supraventricular (SVT) | Ventricular (VT) |
| --- | --- |
| QRS narrow complex | Often broad complex |
| Often no P waves | P waves dissociated rhythm |
| Usually regular | May be irregular |
| QRS right way up | QRS inverted |
| Slowed with adenosine | No response to adenosine |

## Ventricular ectopics

Ventricular ectopics (VEs) may be unifocal (each ectopic will have the same shape) or multifocal (different shapes). The pulse will be irregular.

ECG is the only certain way to distinguish VEs from other causes of an irregular pulse. The danger lies in the fact that an ectopic arising on the apex of a T wave (R on T phenomenon) may produce ventricular fibrillation. Clearly, the more ectopics there are, the greater is the probability of this happening. Treatment should be considered if the ratio of VE to normal QRS is greater than 1:6 or if VEs are multifocal.

Development of new VEs may also indicate another significant underlying problem: sepsis. Although VEs can occur in healthy people without evidence of any disease, they can also occur after MI and in patients with electrolyte disturbance (eg hypokalaemia and hypomagnesaemia), valvular heart disease, cardiomyopathies, hypoxia or digitalis toxicity.

## Common types of atrial tachycardia

### Sinus tachycardia (Figure 6.8)

- The heart is regular: up to 160 bpm or so in young patients.

- The maximum rate is lower in older patients.

- The P wave and morphology are normal.

- Onset is gradual.

- Treat the cause – hypovolaemia, anaemia, PE, sepsis, etc.

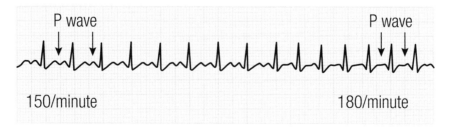

Figure 6.8  Sinus tachycardia.

## Paroxysmal supraventricular tachycardia (Figure 6.9)

■ This term describes any tachycardia originating in the AV node, atria or sinoatrial (SA) node.

■ P waves can be of abnormal shape and may or may not be seen.

■ QRS width is usually normal but may be wide if there is associated bundle branch block (BBB).

■ Paroxysmal SVT may be associated with ST depression, suggesting ischaemia.

■ The heart rate is regular: 150–250 bpm.

■ Paroxysmal SVT can be abolished/slowed by adenosine.

■ Treat with verapamil, digoxin or beta-blockade (avoid ?-blockers in conjunction with verapamil).

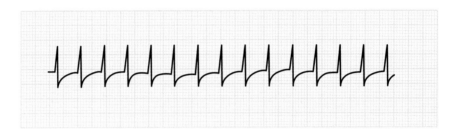

Figure 6.9 Paroxysmal SVT.

## Atrial fibrillation (Figure 6.10)

■ The heart rate is irregularly irregular and ventricular rate variable, but often 100–180 bpm.

■ AF is very common postoperatively in surgical patients.

■ It is associated with hypovolaemia, hypoxia and electrolyte disorders.

■ AF is also associated with cardiopulmonary disease (eg ischaemic or rheumatic heart disease).

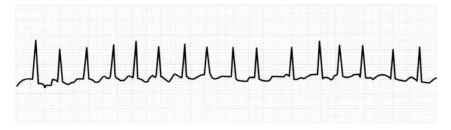

Figure 6.10 Atrial fibrillation.

The management of AF depends on the cause and effects. Many new cases occur after surgery, caused by hypovolaemia, hypoxia or electrolyte imbalance, particularly hypokalaemia and hypomagnesaemia. These episodes can be rapidly treated by correcting the causal factors alone. Identify and treat any underlying problems that would cause these predisposing factors to recur.

When new AF causes serious adverse signs (particularly hypotension, shock, chest pain, heart failure, decreased conscious level or marked tachycardia > 140 bpm), urgent treatment is needed with either DC cardioversion or intravenous amiodarone. Seek expert help immediately.

New AF that does not cause serious adverse signs and which does not respond to the correction of the factors listed above is usually treated with digoxin or amiodarone. Again, if problems persist or recur, or you are unsure, get expert help.

Long-standing AF can worsen after surgery if a patient's usual drugs have been omitted.

## Atrial flutter (Figure 6.11)

- There are regular flutter P waves at 300/min.

- The QRS is normal with variable AV block.

- Atrial flutter is usually associated with cardiac disease.

- It may respond to adenosine or the adenosine may reveal flutter waves.

- Atrial flutter and fibrillation may be present in the same patient.

- Treatment is cardioversion, digoxin or verapamil.

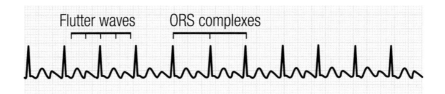

Figure 6.11 Atrial flutter.

**Learning point**

* In all the above cases, investigate the underlying cause.

## Left ventricular hypertrophy (Figure 6.12)

A hypertrophied left ventricle has a greater influence on the electrical axis of the heart and causes left-axis deviation. This gives the picture of tall R waves in I and aVL with S waves in III and aVF. Most noticeably, the increase in the left ventricular muscle mass also produces tall R waves in leads over the left ventricle (V4 to V6), and deep S waves in leads over the right ventricle (V1 to V3).

### Clinical associations

Left ventricular hypertrophy is associated with conditions causing an increase in afterload or work on the left ventricle, for example aortic valve disease and systemic hypertension.

## Right ventricular hypertrophy (Figure 6.13)

When the electrical activity of the hypertrophied right ventricle predominates over the left, there is right-axis deviation (leads I, II, III) with a tall R wave in V1 and deep S wave in V6. A tall pulmonary P wave suggests right atrial hypertrophy.

### Clinical associations

Right ventricular hypertrophy is associated with conditions causing increased right ventricular afterload, for example pulmonary hypertension, cor pulmonale and pulmonary stenosis.

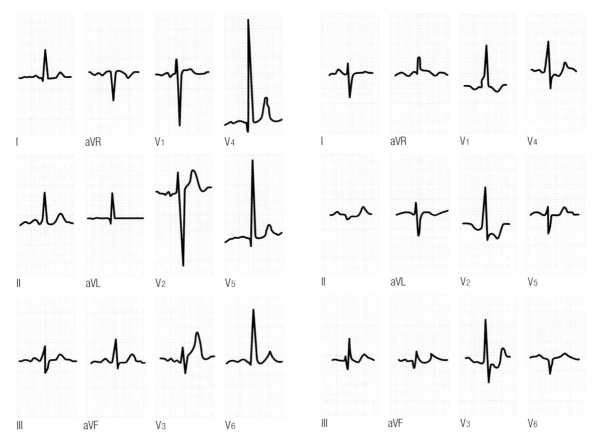

Figure 6.12  Left ventricular hypertrophy.      Figure 6.13  Right ventricular hypertrophy.

## Left bundle branch block (Figure 6.14)

Electrical activity in the left ventricle is delayed because conduction to it must take place via the right ventricle. The resultant delay in left ventricular depolarisation produces the 'M'-shaped QRS wave, typically in V5, V6, I and aVL, and a 'W'-shaped QRS in some of the reciprocal leads, typically leads III and aVF.

## Right bundle branch block (Figure 6.15)

Conversely, in right BBB, right ventricular depolarisation occurs via the left ventricle.

In right BBB the 'M'-shaped QRS would typically be in leads V1, V2 and V3. Right BBB with left axis deviation suggests bifascicular block.

This condition will often necessitate pacing – seek help early.

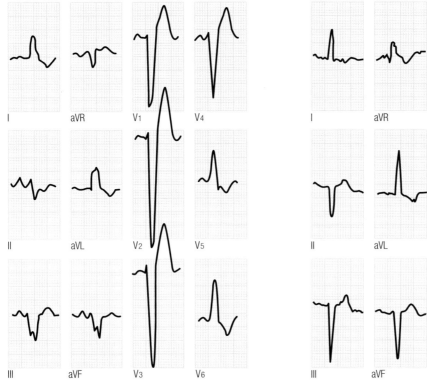

Figure 6.14  Left bundle branch block.

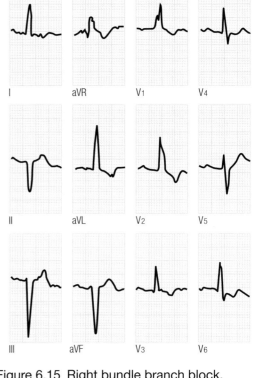

Figure 6.15  Right bundle branch block.

## Clinical associations

Right BBB is associated with coronary artery disease, valvular heart disease, ventricular hypertrophy and fibrosis, and cardiomyopathies.

## Bradyarrythmias

Slow heart rates are problematic if associated with hypoperfusion or hypotension (Box 6.4). They are common in the elderly and should not be taken as evidence that the patient is 'fit'.

### Practice point

The treatment options for a tachyarrhythmia or bradyarrhythmias will be found within your hospital's advanced life support protocols.

## Box 6.4 Conditions associated with bradycardia

### Autonomic

- Pain, especially visceral (may also be associated with tachycardia)
- Raised intracranial pressure
- Drugs: β-blockers
- Epidural

### Non-autonomic

- Myocardial infarction (particularly inferior MI)
- Sepsis
- Hypoxia
- Drugs – digitalis toxicity
- Hypothyroidism
- Hypothermia

Patients likely to develop troublesome heart block (eg those with bifascicular block) should be detected preoperatively and considered for elective pacing and referred for cardiology opinion. In patients with symptomatic bradycardia, atropine (0.6–1.2 mg) may help but pacing may be needed. Isoprenaline infusion may be used under guidance of an intensivist or cardiologist.

## Myocardial infarction

Pre-existing ischaemic heart disease is very common and often occult in patients with poor exercise tolerance for other reasons. This is particularly true of elderly patients or patients with peripheral or cerebrovascular disease or diabetes mellitus. Perioperative MI is associated with a higher mortality rate than MI occurring unrelated to surgery. A recent MI (within the previous 6 months) significantly increases the risk of morbidity resulting from surgery and is a valid reason to delay elective surgery if possible, since the incidence of perioperative MI is higher during this period in this group. Cardiac drugs should be continued up to and including the day of operation and recommenced at the earliest opportunity postoperatively, although care and planning may be needed, and antiplatelet medication may need to be instituted, especially if the patient has had a coronary vessel stent inserted. Patients on the newer antiplatelet drugs with stents require complex multidisciplinary planning and discussion between surgeon, anaesthetist, cardiologist and possibly also the haematologist.

Perioperative MI is often silent, but may present with shortness of breath, hypotension, evidence of decreased organ function (including confusion) secondary to cardiogenic shock, acute dysrhythmias, sudden pulmonary oedema or cardiac arrest. It should also enter the differential diagnosis of acute upper abdominal pain. A high index of suspicion is required, particularly in high-risk groups.

The ECG may show typical changes of anterior, anterolateral or inferior MI with ST-segment elevation of >1 mm in the relevant leads overlying the infarct (primary changes) and inversion in the leads opposite to it (reciprocal changes). T waves flatten and invert within hours to days of MI and Q waves develop over 1–2 days. Changes may be masked by a pre-existing left BBB and new BBB should make you suspicious.

The ECG may be normal after an MI, certainly for the first hour or so. A normal ECG does therefore not exclude MI. If an MI is a potential diagnosis then the ECG should be repeated.

### Practice point

Recognition of patterns of ECG changes in MI:

- anterior infarct – primary changes V1, V2, V3, V4;
- inferior infarct – primary changes II, III, aVF;
- posterior infarct – isolated ST depression V1, V2.

Treatment:

- oxygen, analgesia – refer and transfer to high-care area;
- involvement of cardiologist and senior staff for consideration and planning of percutaneous coronary interventions.

Early treatment influences the outcome significantly and many patients are given percutaneous coronary interventions in the acute phase (see below). If you suspect the presence of an MI, then seek urgent advice from a cardiologist, who will be best placed to arrange the appropriate pathway of treatment for this patient: percutaneous coronary intervention or clot thrombolysis. Inform your surgical seniors as a decision may need to be made regarding the type of intervention required in a patient who has recently undergone surgery, as will decisions regarding on-going anticoagulant or antiplatelet therapy.

In the meantime:

- Check and correct the ABCDEs.

- Make the patient comfortable with a suitable opiate analgesic. Morphine (or diamorphine) is best, titrated to response intravenously (1–2 mg boluses every 2 minutes). Ondansetron 4 mg or cyclizine 50 mg intravenously can be used to prevent or treat nausea.

- Give high-flow oxygen to reduce hypoxia (monitor $SaO_2$).

- Give glyceryl trinitrate (sublingual or spray) to reduce coronary artery spasm. Nitrates also have a synergistic effect with thrombolysis.

- Consider aspirin 300 mg, orally or rectally.

- Commence treating conditions that can exaccerbate myocardial hypoperfusion: anaemia, fluid overload, extreme hypertension.

- Arrange appropriate investigations: (i) ECG (serial ECGs are required); and (ii) blood tests to exclude anaemia and electrolyte disturbances, and for troponin levels.

ECG changes of MI are localised to ischaemic or infarcted areas whereas generalised changes are seen in, for example, hyperkalaemia (peaked T waves) or pericarditis (ST elevation). The timing of changes is shown in Table 6.5.

*Anterior myocardial infarction*

ECG shows raised ST segments in V1–V4 (Figure 6.16).

Table 6.5 Timing of ECG changes after MI

| Change | Onset/duration |
| --- | --- |
| Peaked T waves | Seconds |
| ST changes (usually elevation) | Hours |
| Q waves | Hours to days |
| T-wave inversion | Hours to days |

## *Inferior myocardial infarction*

Raised ST segments and Q waves can be seen in leads II, III and aVF (with reciprocal ST depression in leads I, aVL and V2–V4). Non-pathological Q waves can be present in leads II and III (Figure 6.17). Compare this with the example of the anterior infarction above.

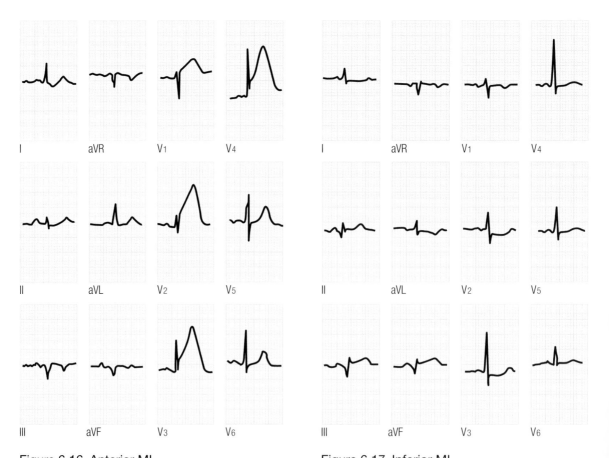

Figure 6.16  Anterior MI.

Figure 6.17  Inferior MI.

## Acute treatment of proven myocardial infarction with ST segment elevation

This should be determined by the cardiology team and will depend on local resources but will require close liaison with the surgical team: there will need to be discussion regarding risks of bleeding versus the benefits of intervention, anticoagulation and anti-platelet treatment. Always inform your seniors if intervention is planned.

Acute treatment (NICE Guideline CG167) involves (i) aspirin; (ii) primary percutaneous intervention followed by anticoagulation with heparin or low-molecular-weight heparin or thrombolysis depending on local arrangements; (iii) glycoprotein IIb/3a inhibitors; (iv) glycaemic control, particularly in diabetic patients (blood glucose <11 mmol/L); and (v) ?-blockers (providing there is no evidence of cardiac failure, bradycardia or hypotension, ?-blockers have been shown to improve survival).
If primary percutaneous intervention is not available, fibrinolytics, eg alteplase (a recombinant tissue plasminogen activator, rTPA) can be used, particularly if there is persistent chest pain and gross ECG changes, though not in the immediate (<2 weeks) postoperative period because of the risk of bleeding. Other contraindications to fibrinolytics include:

- active peptic ulcer;

- previous haemorrhagic stroke;

- recent head injury, however minor;

- prolonged traumatic cardiopulmonary resuscitation (CPR).

NICE Guideline CG167 discusses the management of acute myocardial infarction. Secondary therapy with an angiotensin-converting enzyme (ACE) inhibitor and a statin should also be considered as soon as the patient is haemodynamically stable.

## Acute coronary syndromes

'Acute coronary syndrome' is an all-encompassing term that refers to a variety of myocardial conditions and includes acute MI (both Q wave and non-Q wave) and unstable angina. The full range of conditions included is listed in Box 6.5.

## Box 6.5 The acute coronary syndromes

### Acute myocardial infarction

- Transmural myocardial infarction
- Q-wave myocardial infarction
- ST elevation myocardial infarction (STEMI)

### Non-Q-wave myocardial infarction

- Sub-endocardial infarction
- Non-ST elevation myocardial infarction (non-STEMI)

### Unstable angina

In most of these patients, the development of an acute coronary syndrome is due to rupture or erosion of an atherosclerotic plaque within the walls of a coronary artery, leading to thrombus formation. This is then followed by platelet aggregation and vasoconstriction of the associated vessels. Less commonly, an acute coronary syndrome is the result of emboli or coronary spasm. It is often impossible to distinguish between the different causes clinically.

### Treatment strategies

Again, this will need to be instituted by the cardiology team following surgical discussion regarding risk of bleeding versus benefit of anticoagulation and anti-platelet treatment.

Measure serial troponin levels.

Consider

- aspirin;
- other antiplatelets, eg clopidogrel;

■ anticoagulation;

■ glycaemic control (blood glucose <11 mmol/L);

■ ☐-blockade.

It is likely that patients with acute coronary syndromes will require further cardiology review and investigation prior to discharge.

## Cardiac failure

Cardiac failure varies in severity from mild dyspnoea, which is easily treated, to cardiogenic shock. Demands on the heart are increased by surgical illness and this may unmask or worsen cardiac failure. Signs of heart failure prior to surgery are a significant risk factor for increased morbidity and mortality.

Cardiac function depends on preload, intrinsic myocardial function and afterload. This concept can be simplified in the following way. If the heart is thought of as a simple pump, the preload is analogous to the priming of the pump; it will work well only if it has something (and not too much) to pump. Ensuring adequate cardiac filling is essential. Any condition that disturbs 'pump filling' will affect preload and, therefore, cardiac function (Box 6.6a).

Intrinsic myocardial function is analogous to the function of the pump itself; if the pump fails in any way, it will not be able to cope with the demands made on it. Any condition that directly affects the function of cardiac muscle will affect intrinsic myocardial function (Box 6.6b). Afterload can be thought of as the work that is demanded of the pump to overcome the resistance to forward flow. If the resistance to flow is low, less work will be required of the pump; if it is high, the pump will have to work harder to produce the same output. Conditions that alter circulatory resistance (systemic or pulmonary vascular resistance) or cause an obstruction to flow will affect afterload (Box 6.6c). Increases in afterload raise the cardiac oxygen demand, yet there is decreased supply to the subendocardial areas as the contracting muscle squeezes the subendocardial capillaries. If there is a simultaneous tachycardia, the diastolic time interval is reduced and the coronary artery blood flow is reduced, decreasing myocardial oxygen delivery even further.

## Box 6.6 Causes of cardiac failure in surgical critical care

### (a) Conditions affecting preload

- Hypovolaemia (bleeding, inadequate volume replacement, etc)
- Fluid overload
- Pneumothorax/cardiac tamponade (see (b) and (c))

### (b) Conditions affecting intrinsic myocardial function

- Ischaemia
- Infarction
- Dysrhythmias
- Chronic heart failure + 'operative stress'
- Hypocalcaemia and other electrolyte disturbances
- Myocardial depressant factors (eg in sepsis)
- Pneumothorax/cardiac tamponade (see (a) and (c))

### (c) Conditions affecting afterload

- Aortic/pulmonary valvular stenosis
- PE
- Pneumothorax/cardiac tamponade (see (a) and (b))
- Aortic dissection

After surgery, a patient may develop heart failure as a result of any of the conditions listed in Box 6.6. Sometimes, multiple factors apply in a single patient and the range of specific disease processes that may produce these problems is wide. Most commonly, it is a result of fluid overload. The cause of fluid overload may be obvious (eg giving blood or parenteral nutrition simultaneously with maintenance fluids to a patient with borderline cardiac function). Fluid balance can also become positive insidiously – perhaps as a result of several days of giving slightly too much maintenance fluid to a small, elderly patient, who may also have had routine diuretics omitted or developed AF.

The pathophysiology of heart failure is such that patients enter a downward spiral of increasingly inefficient cardiac function. The physiological response to the failing heart (as it is to surgical pathology) is to increase catecholamine release in an attempt to stimulate cardiac output. Unfortunately, the failing heart has a 'flat Frank–Starling curve': one shifted down and to the right compared with the curve in Figure 6.18. It is unable to respond and maintain cardiac output by increasing its stroke volume and tends to rely on an increase in rate. This is inefficient in that diastole is short, which reduces the time available for diastolic filling (affecting preload) and for perfusion of the coronary arteries, leading to development of relative or absolute ischaemia (and further affecting intrinsic myocardial function).

Cardiogenic pulmonary oedema occurs with acute left ventricular failure or during an exacerbation of congestive cardiac failure. Such patients usually have hypertension and ischaemic heart disease and are often elderly. They may develop symptoms as a result of MI or acute ischaemia precipitated by pain from non-cardiac sources. Sudden withdrawal of epidural analgesia may cause acute afterload increases in susceptible patients while increasing preload as the sympathetic block wears off. The

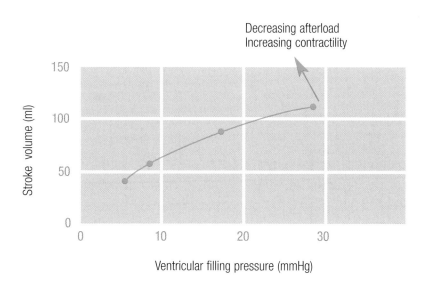

Figure 6.18 Cardiac function: Frank–Starling curve.

commonest causes are iatrogenic fluid overload, dysrhythmia and MI. Patients become acutely dyspnoeic, orthopnoeic and tachypnoeic. They are tachycardic, sweaty and often hypertensive, and a gallop rhythm may be present with a high jugular venous pressure. They become hypoxic with increased work of breathing, which further aggravates myocardial ischaemia. Chest auscultation reveals crepitations basally, possibly with some wheeze (cardiac asthma) and, if oedema is very severe, pink, frothy sputum may be produced. The CXR may show fluid in the horizontal fissure, peribronchial cuffing, upper lobe diversion, a perihilar 'bat's-wing' appearance and, rarely, Kerley B lines.

## Practice point

Treatment follows ABCDE principles:

- Administer oxygen: sit the patient up, and administer CPAP if practicable.
- Administer diuretics and small doses of opiate intravenously to aid vasodilation.
- Reduce afterload as well as decreasing anxiety and dyspnoea, with drugs if necessary.
- If intravenous vasodilators/inotropes are being considered, transfer to a high-care area.

## Case scenario 6.2

A 65-year-old woman with long-standing ischaemic heart disease had a right mastectomy 2 days ago. You are asked to see her on the third postoperative day because she has become acutely short of breath following an episode of severe central chest pain that lasted about 10 minutes but has since settled. When you arrive on the ward, the patient is obviously dyspnoeic and is unable to speak in complete sentences. She looks very unwell, and her skin feels cool and clammy. The staff nurse who is with her reports that her pulse is 110 bpm and her blood pressure is 170/95 mmHg. You ask the nurse to give the patient high-flow oxygen, using a mask with a reservoir bag. You examine the patient's chest and find that she has a respiratory rate of 28 breaths/min and fine crepitations up to the mid-zones on both sides. It is difficult to hear her heart easily but you do not think you can hear any murmurs, although you think she has a gallop rhythm. Her blood pressure is now 140/90 mmHg. You ask the nurse to help you sit the patient up and establish intravenous access. An examination of the patient's ward charts shows that she was progressing well until this episode. The case notes reveal that she is hypertensive, has occasional angina (about one attack every 2 weeks associated with exercise or cold weather) and usually takes bendroflumethiazide 2.5 mg and atenolol 50 mg each morning. From the prescription, it seems that she has not had these since her operation as she has felt nauseous as a result of the morphine PCA she has been using until recently.

Although she seems slightly better with the oxygen and repositioning, you decide to give her 40 mg of furosemide IV. You ask for an ECG to be carried out and order a CXR. The ECG shows a sinus tachycardia of 100 bpm but is otherwise unchanged from the one obtained preoperatively. The CXR confirms pulmonary oedema. You arrange for the patient to be transferred to the HDU, where she can have continuous ECG, oxygen saturation and blood pressure monitoring and be considered for CPAP as well as review from the cardiology team. In the meantime, you arrange for routine blood tests and cardiac enzymes to be sent.

## Learning points

- Treat the ABCDEs first.
- Give high-flow oxygen to all patients during initial assessment.
- Transfer patients to a higher level of care if closer monitoring is required.
- Seek expert help early.

The acute management of heart failure is as follows:

- Assess and treat ABCDEs.
- Give oxygen and monitor $SaO_2$.
- Stop IV infusions (may be only a temporary measure).
- Drugs: consider diuretics (eg furosemide 80 mg IV), nitrates (patch, sublingual, buccal or IV), diamorphine 2.5–5 mg IV.

- Carry out 12-lead ECG.

- Treat any underlying cause such as dysrhythmia, pulmonary embolus or tamponade.

- Consider CPAP if the patient is not improving.

- Montor CVP.

- Consider early specialist referral.

Cardiogenic shock is defined as severe impairment of cardiac function with hypotension of less than 90 mmHg or 30 mmHg less than the patient's 'normal' systolic pressure. The patient may be tachycardic or bradycardic. Among the causes, the commonest is severe myocardial ischaemia or infarction. The cardiac output falls, systemic hypotension occurs and there is a progressive fall in organ perfusion.

Left ventricular end-diastolic pressure rises and pulmonary venous pressure increases, which leads to pulmonary oedema formation. The patient becomes dyspnoeic and hypoxic and a downward spiral develops as low $SaO_2$ and low diastolic pressure further compromises myocardial perfusion.

The acutely failing heart is very sensitive to too much or too little fluid. The patient normally has pulmonary oedema so increasing preload with IV fluid is often detrimental. Occasionally, the failing heart can have a high preload requirement and reducing preload by diuresis may worsen cardiac output. If the afterload is high, reducing it by using vasodilators may be beneficial, but subsequent worsening hypotension may be detrimental to myocardial perfusion.

Accurate individualised treatment requires the measurement of cardiac output, preload and afterload so invasive cardiac monitoring is required to optimise fluid loading, inotropic support and/or vasodilator therapy. Senior critical care input and monitoring are urgently needed.

## Risks of surgery

It is very important to be aware of the risks of surgery in the patient with ischaemic heart disease with recent myocardial infarction and, particularly, of the risk of reinfarction (Table 6.6). It should be clear that delaying surgery, if at all possible, will have a marked effect on the outcome.

Table 6.6  Risk of cardiac disease in non-cardiac surgery

| Higher | Lower |
| --- | --- |
| Recent MI | MI > 6 months |
| Unstable angina | Stable angina |
| Severe aortic stenosis | Abnormal ECG |
| Decompensated heart failure | Compensated heart failure |
| Severe hypertension | Compensated valvular lesions |
| Cardiac arrhythmias | Cardiomegaly |

The risk of perioperative MI is greater with abdominal and thoracic surgery and is related to the duration of operation. The chance of re-infarction has been estimated as:

- 60% if within 3 weeks of MI

- 27% if MI within 3 months of procedure

- 11% if MI within 3–6 months of procedure.

The presence of cardiac failure pre-operatively indicates a significant anaesthetic risk.

Measurement of cardiorespiratory function and reserve, eg by means of echocardiography and cardiopulmonary exercise testing can help quantify this.

## Hypertension

In patients with chronic hypertension, avoid stopping long-term antihypertensive medication suddenly unless the patient is hypotensive. Remember to review the prescription chart of patients on cardiac drugs on a daily basis. As with almost all cardiac medication, antihypertensive drugs (with the exception of ACE inhibitors and angiotensin receptor antagonists) should be given on the morning of surgery and reinstituted as quickly as possible afterwards. Many antihypertensive drugs have side-effects including hypokalaemia (diuretics), hyperkalaemia (ACE inhibitors) and impaired responses to hypovolaemia (vasodilators and ▯-blockers).

Acute, life-threatening hypertension is rare. If the blood pressure remains at 220/120 mmHg or above with signs of organ dysfunction, involve cardiology immediately.

## Pacemakers

Patients who have pacemakers frequently require surgery. Pacemakers can vary between the simple fixed-rate type (rarely used) to the complex demand type with or without internal defibrillators. They can be bipolar or unipolar, the casing acting as the return earth in the latter. It is vital to be aware that your patient has a pacemaker because the use of diathermy can inhibit the demand type, though this is less likely to cause problems with a standard fixed-rate type. The important points are:

- Any patient who has a pacemaker and requires surgery should have had a recent cardiology review to ensure that the pacemaker is functioning optimally. This may mean switching off the internal defibrillator function on the day of surgery.

- The diathermy earthing pad should be placed as far from the pacemaker as possible (eg on the thigh or under the buttocks). Never place the pad on the back of the patient behind the pacemaker.

- Use short bursts of diathermy rather than long bursts.

- Bipolar diathermy is safer than unipolar.

- Avoid using diathermy near the pacemaker if possible.

- Always monitor the ECG during any procedure. Pacemaker types are classified using a three- or four-letter code. Classification is based on which chambers are paced, the response of the pacemaker to a sensed beat and programmability. Recognition of the codes and details of pacemaker function are beyond the scope of this manual and the CCrISP course. If you have any doubts or worries consult a cardiologist.

## Summary

- The detection and treatment of early clinical signs can prevent major deterioration.

- Abnormal signs must be acted on quickly – patients deteriorate rapidly from cardiovascular problems and abnormalities need to be corrected as quickly as possible.

- Normal clinical findings do not always exclude significant abnormality – further investigations and monitoring can help.

- New and long-standing cardiac disorders occur frequently in surgical patients – be aware of common management strategies.

- Impaired perfusion, hypotension, end-organ dysfunction and poor response to treatment suggest severe problems.

- Patients with acute abnormalities of cardiovascular function should have a clear management plan including appropriate treatment and a timely reassessment

- Higher levels of care are often required – either pre-emptively if the patient has long-standing problems preoperatively, or in response to acute events.

- Seek specialist help (anaesthetic/cardiology/critical care) as appropriate at an early stage.

## Further reading

National Institute for Health and Care Excellence (NICE) produce the following guidelines:

- Acute Coronary Syndromes (QS68);

- MI with ST Segment Elevation (CG167);

- Acute Heart Failure (CG187);

- Atrial Fibrillation (CG180).

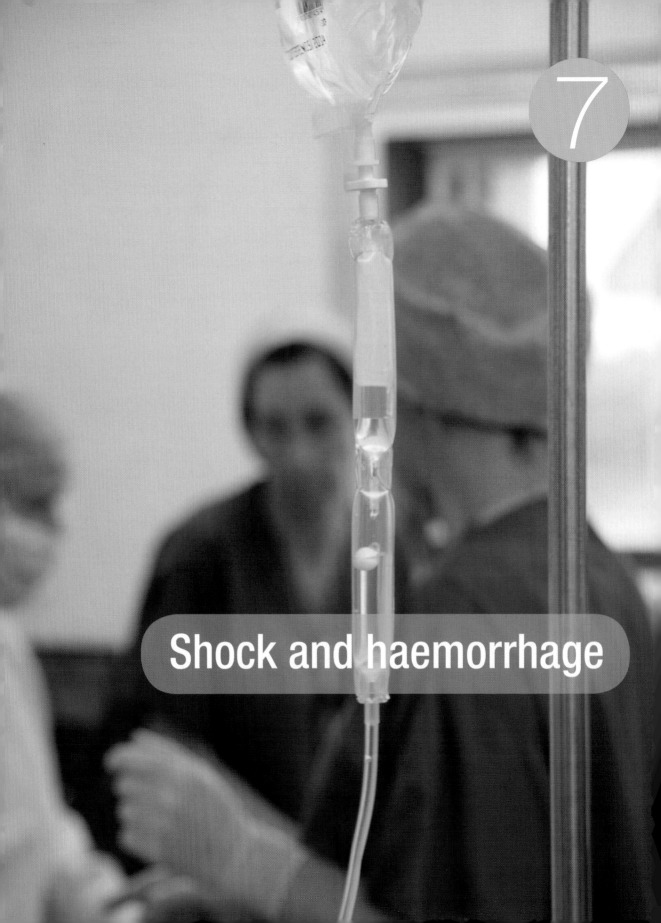

7

Shock and haemorrhage

## Learning outcomes

This chapter will help you to:

- define shock;

- understand the various aetiologies of shock;

- recognise the clinical features of a patient with shock;

- initiate early treatment of the shocked patient;

- Decide on an appropriate level of care based on the history, clinical condition and response to treatment.

## Definition

Shock is acute circulatory failure, with inadequate tissue perfusion causing cellular hypoxia.

Regardless of the underlying cause, shock is characterised by an acute alteration of the circulation in which inadequate perfusion leads to cellular damage, dysfunction and failure of major organ systems.

The clinical features of shock are so variable that they cannot be used to define the shocked state. Although the terms 'hypotension' and 'shock' are often considered synonymous, cellular perfusion may be inadequate despite a normal blood pressure. Perfusion includes blood flow but also the supply of substrates (including glucose and oxygen) and the removal of waste products. Use of phrases such as 'inadequate tissue perfusion' rather than 'reduced perfusion' is important since blood flow and substrate supply may be increased in hypercatabolic states (eg trauma and sepsis) and yet inadequate for the demands of the tissues due to increased metabolism and failure to extract substrates from the circulation. In the shocked state, the distribution of blood flow is also important. While some organs preserve flow through autoregulation (eg brain, heart, kidney), others cannot (eg gut, skin) and may be hypoperfused preferentially to maintain the integrity of perfusion of the other organs. Intestinal hypoperfusion may occur in the face of a normal blood pressure and pulse and, following a brief hypotensive episode, a prolonged period of intestinal hypoxia may occur, with generation of cytokines. This mechanism is the commonest pathway for the initiation of a mediator response that results in the onset of systemic inflammation. Systemic inflammatory mediators can, in turn, lead to further deterioration in organ function and begin the decline to multiple organ dysfunctions and refractory shock. This is why it is so important to detect the early more subtle signs of shock and initiate treatment straightaway: predict and prevent.

## Learning point

- Patients may be in shock despite a normal systolic blood pressure.

## Aetiology of shock

Failure of end organ perfusion can occur through several mechanisms (Table 7.1), which can be grouped into four principal categories:

- hypovolaemic

- cardiogenic

- obstructive

- vasodilatory or (apparent hypovolaemia).

It is helpful within this classification to consider the underlying problem as one of either reduced preload, pump failure (including obstructive causes) or reduction in afterload (Figure 7.1).

Rapid assessment of the patient may give an early indication of the cause of shock, but the classification system is helpful to avoid the risk of a given diagnosis being overlooked. This is especially the case when more than one factor may be contributing to the shocked state, eg when a patient presents with shock secondary to abdominal sepsis, in which case the primary problem is vasodilatation but hypovolaemia due to ileus also contributes.

Table 7.1  Common mechanisms of shock

| Type of Shock | Aetiology |
| --- | --- |
| Hypovolaemia | Haemorrhage |
| | Fluid loss |
| | Dehydration |
| Cardiogenic | MI |
| | Heart failure |
| | Arrhythmia |
| Obstructive | PE |
| | Cardiac tamponade |
| | Pneumothorax |
| Vasodilatory | Sepsis |
| | Neurogenic |
| | Anaphylaxis |
| | Adrenal insufficiency |

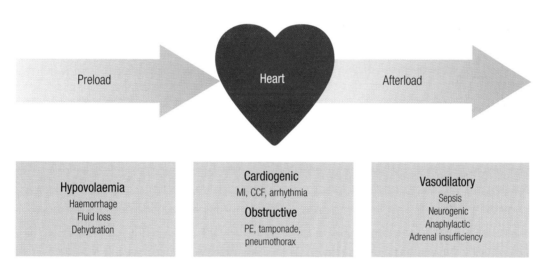

Figure 7.1  Classification of shock in relation to the effect on the circulation.

## Hypovolaemic shock

Stroke volume dictates cardiac output, and is directly linked to ventricular filling pressure by the Frank–Starling curve (Figure 7.2). The curve can be shifted up and to the left (ie improved cardiac contractility for the same degree of filling) by the use of inotropic drugs and sympathetic stimulation. It is important to consider the Starling curve when thinking about the clinical manifestation of shock, but also the rationale for and response to treatment.

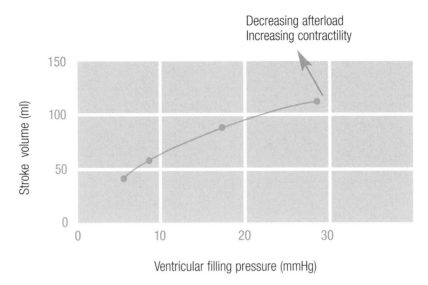

Figure 7.2 Frank–Starling curve plotting ventricular filling pressure (venous return) against stroke volume (cardiac output). The curve is shifted up and to the left by sympathetic stimulation or inotropic agents.

Hypovolaemia is the commonest cause of shock in a surgical patient. The low cardiac output is a direct reflection of reduced venous return (preload). It may result from any of the following causes:

◻ Haemorrhage is a common cause of hypovolaemia. Its effects vary with the duration and severity of blood loss, the patient's age and myocardial condition, and the speed and adequacy of resuscitation. It has been classified, according to the degree of blood loss, into four stages: stage 1, <750 ml; stage 2, 750–1500 ml; stage 3, 1500–2000 ml; and stage 4, >2000 ml. In practice this classification serves little useful purpose as the clinical signs of haemorrhagic shock are not directly correlated with the degree of shock and the physiological response to a given amount of volume loss in an individual patient is determined by the patient's cardiovascular responsiveness, physiological reserve and any concurrent cardiac medication.

◻ Loss of gastrointestinal fluid may be due to vomiting and diarrhoea, fistulae or sequestration of fluid in the bowel lumen in intestinal obstruction.

◻ Trauma and infection increase capillary permeability with local sequestration of fluid and oedema. In addition to causing hypovolaemia, trauma and infection may lead to sepsis.

- Burns lead to direct loss of fluid from the burned surface and tissue fluid sequestration.

- Renal loss of water and electrolytes (eg in sodium-losing chronic nephritis, diabetic ketoacidosis or Addisonian crisis) is an occasional cause of shock.

- Iatrogenic surgical factors often contribute to hypovolaemia (eg poor fluid prescription, slow or tissued intravenous infusion, inappropriate use of diuretics, mechanical bowel preparation, fasting prior to anaesthesia, and insensible fluid losses during prolonged operations and on-going fluid loss from dissected areas for some hours after surgery).

## Cardiogenic shock

Primary impairment of cardiac function may result from myocardial infarction or ischaemia, acute arrhythmias, acute cardiomyopathy, acute valvular lesions (caused by aortic dissection or trauma) or myocardial contusion.

## Obstructive shock

Secondary impairment to cardiac function can result from obstruction to cardiac output. Causes include cardiac tamponade producing constriction of the heart, pressure on the heart from a tension pneumothorax or major PE with obstruction to right ventricular outflow.

In all shock states, myocardial performance is affected adversely by reduced coronary arterial perfusion and, in some cases, by circulating myocardial depressant substances (particularly in septic shock).

## Vasodilatory or distributive shock

### Neurogenic factors

True neurogenic shock follows spinal transection or brainstem injury with loss of sympathetic outflow beneath the level of injury and consequent vasodilation. The rapid increase in size of the vascular bed, including venous capacitance vessels, leads to reduced venous return and reduced cardiac output. There is often a relative bradycardia. An analogous condition may be seen during epidural analgesia, although, in this case, the block is seldom high enough to cause a bradycardia unless it involves the higher thoracic segments.

## Anaphylaxis

Anaphylactic reactions are mediated by IgE antibodies, which results in massive degranulation of mast cells in sensitised individuals. Activation of mast cells releases histamine and serotonin and, with systemic kinin activation, this leads to rapid vasodilation, a fall in systemic vascular resistance (SVR), hypotension, severe bronchospasm with hypoxia and hypercarbia. In contrast to sepsis, the fall in SVR is so sudden and profound that blood pressure falls markedly. Prompt treatment with oxygen, fluids, adrenaline, hydrocortisone and an antihistamine is required, plus removal and subsequent avoidance of the trigger substance.

## Endocrine factors

Although adrenal failure is in itself a potent cause of shock due to the sudden withdrawal of circulating cortisol and aldosterone, the role of the adrenal cortex in the production of shock by other causes is debatable. Acute adrenal failure may occur in severe sepsis (Waterhouse-Friderichsen syndrome), usually meningoccal in origin. Adrenal insufficiency (often subacute) is also seen in patients in whom necessary perioperative steroid cover has been omitted or in cases of severe sepsis requiring high levels of pressor and inotropic support. In these cases, patients may need additional doses of steroids, eg 50 mg hydrocortisone QDS.

## Septic shock

Sepsis and septic shock are complex and are covered in more detail elsewhere. In septic shock, the patient becomes hypotensive and the tissues are inadequately perfused as a result of organisms, toxins or inflammatory mediators. Common sources include the abdomen, chest, soft tissues, wounds, urine and intravascular lines (central or peripheral) or other medical implants.

## Case scenario 7.1

You receive a trauma team call to the emergency department – the paramedics have advised that they will be arriving in 4 minutes with a 34-year-old patient who has a BP of 80 mmHg systolic and a stab wound to the back between the shoulder blades.

### What form of shock might this patient be suffering from?

Haemorrhagic shock? 'Pump failure' due to pericardial tamponade? 'Pump failure' due to tension pneumothorax? Neurogenic shock due to spinal cord transection? All are possible.

### What action may be necessary?

This depends on the cause, but immediate attention to an ABCDE assessment with administration of oxygen and consideration of a fluid challenge, along with diagnosis and definitive treatment, are the mainstays of treatment.

## Clinical features of shock

### Assessment

The early signs of shock can be subtle and the CCrISP system of assessment allows a logical approach to assessment and management with simultaneous resuscitation where appropriate in the initial assessment stage. Provided that there is some response to these manoeuvres it is important to proceed with a full patient assessment, including chart review, history, examination, review of the notes and gathering the results of available recent investigations. The whole picture will then inform the decision regarding the patient's progress. A shocked patient is generally unstable and may require special investigations. It is important to discuss the patient with the consultant in charge, to obtain the opinions of other specialists and consider an intervention or an operation. This will all require careful planning and coordination.

## Case scenario 7.2

The nurses ask you to see a 75-year-old patient 5 days following a right hemiarthroplasty for a subcapital fracture of the head of femur sustained when tripping over a carpet at home 24 hours before the operation. She has become agitated and uncooperative. Her response to your initial questions is in short phrases but the words are confused. The respiratory rate is 18 breaths/minute, the trachea is central and chest expansion equal with a resonant percussion note and basal crepitations. You ask for an oxygen saturation probe, which records 90%, and arrange for supplementary oxygen at 15 L/min via a non-rebreathe mask (which she repeatedly tries to take off). Her peripheries feel cold, the capillary refill is 4–5 seconds and her pulse is 90 bpm with dropped beats and BP 130/95 mmHg. You place a wide-bore cannula, taking bloods for FBC, chemistry profile and serum to be stored in the blood bank: the blood glucose level is 4.8 mmol/L. A bolus of 500 ml of compound Ringer's lactate is started through the cannula (the patient's body weight is 60 kg). The pupils are equal and react to light normally and her Glasgow Coma Scale (GCS) score is 14. On exposure, the chest findings are the same, the abdomen mildly distended and non-tender with bowel sounds present and there are faecal rocks in the rectum (bowels have not been open since the operation). Her hip wound is mildly bruised, but with no obvious collection or leakage. There is no drain in place.

Charts show that the pulse has been around 75 bpm and BP 140/90 mmHg for the last few days. Over the same time period, her temperature has been <37°C, but was 37.3°C this morning. Oral intake has been poor and the last recorded urine output was early the previous evening: her 24-hour urine output over the preceding 3 days has been 550 ml, 610 ml and 590 ml. Her GCS score has not been formally recorded for the past 3 days, but the nurses report that she was progressing well and being cooperative with her early mobilisation. The drug chart reveals daily administration of prophylactic subcutaneous (SC) low molecular weight heparin (LMWH), a single shot of antibiotic at the time of her surgery, bendroflumethiazide and amlodipine daily, glyceryl trinitrate (GTN) spray, Gaviscon and oral analgesia all prescribed prn, none of which has been required. The notes reveal a trip over the edge of a carpet at home (where she normally lives alone, independently), sustaining the fracture. She has treated hypertension, hiatus hernia with oesophagitis and underwent laparoscopic cholecystectomy

5 years ago, when she was a current smoker of 20 cigarettes per day and developed a DVT. Recent investigations (on the third postoperative day) show a Hb level 90 g/L, WCC $10.1 \times 10^9$/L, platelets $150 \times 10^9$/L , Na$^+$ 131 mmol/L, K$^+$ 3.1 mmol/L, HCO$_3^-$ 20 mmol/L, urea 9.9 mmol/L, creatinine 129 μmol/L (compared to admission values of Hb 115 g/L, WCC $8.8 \times 10^9$/L, platelets $120 \times 10^9$/L, Na$^+$ 138 mmol/L, K$^+$ 4.0 mmol/L, HCO$_3^-$ 25 mmol/L, urea 7.0 mmol/L, creatinine 99 μmol/L). A preoperative ECG showed sinus rhythm with T-wave inversion in the lateral chest leads. A postoperative hip X-ray shows a right hemiarthroplasty prosthesis in good position.

This patient has evidence of shock and a problem which requires further management. Initially it is good practice to reassess the patient and her response to your initial treatment and then consider the possible diagnoses so that your investigations may be targeted to defining the problem. This patient has deteriorated postoperatively and is showing subtle signs of shock associated with hypoxia, which may be due to cardiac disease, PE, infection or hypovolaemia.

## Important features to note

- Is there an obvious cause that requires immediate treatment?

- Does the age or previous history of a patient suggest a possible myocardial component?

- Has the patient recently received medication that may have an effect on the cardiovascular or respiratory systems?

- Does the fluid balance chart of the patient show a gradually deteriorating urine output or likelihood of a significantly abnormal fluid balance? Remember that trends in the charted observations may be more important than absolute values and that patients with hypovolaemic shock may still have a normal systolic blood pressure.

- Does the patient have a temperature, high WCC or a history of an operative procedure that may make sepsis a more likely diagnosis?

Most patients with shock have a low cardiac output; an exception is septic shock, in which the cardiac output may be increased. The classic appearance of a patient with low-output shock is that seen after haemorrhage. The features are partly due to loss of circulating volume and tissue perfusion and partly to intense sympathetic stimulation. Early diagnosis of shock depends on recognition of the signs of decreased tissue perfusion, particularly of the skin, kidneys and brain.

Signs of decreased tissue perfusion are summarised in Box 7.1. These are accompanied by varying degrees of tachycardia, hypotension and tachypnoea.

Increased respiratory rate is frequently seen before any significant tachycardia, but marked tachypnoea is an important sign of impending deterioration. Confusion may be an early sign of marked cerebral hypoperfusion whilst coma is often a late sign.

In haemorrhagic shock, decreased venous return to the heart results in a low right atrial pressure, low right ventricular end-diastolic volume and reduced right heart output. This usually reduces the left atrial and ventricular end-diastolic volumes and stroke volume (SV) falls. Since cardiac output (CO) = heart rate (HR) × stroke volume (SV), for a fixed SV, an increase in HR is the first compensatory measure available. The only way the body has to increase the SV acutely is to decrease the amount of blood contained in the resistance and capacitance vessels by vasoconstriction, squeezing the periphery to return more blood to the heart. This gives the appearance of cold, shut-down peripheries. The heart rate response to hypovolaemia may be modified in the elderly, in patients with ischaemic heart disease, in patients on β-blockers, in trained athletes and in young adults.

## Box 7.1  Signs of decreased tissue perfusion

- Cool peripheries
- Poor filling of peripheral veins
- Increased respiratory rate
- Increased core–peripheral temperature gradient
- Capillary refill time prolonged (>2 seconds)
- Poor signal on pulse oximeter
- Poor urine output (<0.5 ml/kg body weight/h)
- Anxiety and restlessness
- Decreased consciousness level
- Metabolic acidosis or raised serum lactate levels

The effect of haemorrhage on blood pressure is particularly variable. It depends on the duration and magnitude of blood loss, the patient's age and cardiovascular status, and the speed and adequacy of resuscitation. Initially, the systemic blood pressure is maintained, and may actually increase, particularly in young patients. The pulse pressure may drop (difference between systolic and diastolic pressure) as a result of peripheral vasoconstriction, but this is a subtle sign. It is possible for up to 25% (or even 30%) of circulating volume to be lost without affecting systolic pressure because of the intense vasoconstriction and, to a lesser extent, the shift of fluid from the interstitial to intravascular space.

A small further volume loss can lead to serious cardiovascular collapse, perhaps with bradycardia rather than the expected tachycardia.

## Practice point

Systolic blood pressure may be normal in the presence of significant loss of circulating volume.

### Specific features of cardiogenic shock

Cardiogenic shock is inadequate tissue perfusion resulting directly from myocardial dysfunction. Common causes in surgical patients include myocardial infarction, acute arrhythmias, post-cardiac surgery myocardial 'stunning' and cardiac contusions due to trauma. The clinical features are similar to those of hypovolaemic shock. Although there is no primary loss of circulating volume, cardiac output falls and catecholamine-induced vasoconstriction produces cool clammy peripheries, reduced capillary return, reduced urine output and reduced level of consciousness. The picture is modified, however, by elevation of cardiac filling pressure leading to elevation of the CVP or JVP and pulmonary oedema, but low arterial pressure.

A careful history and examination of the chest, heart sounds (there may be a gallop rhythm or associated murmur) and neck veins, together with assessment of a chest radiograph and ECG, should prevent the possibility of cardiogenic shock being overlooked in a surgical patient. Urgent echocardiography may be valuable in making the diagnosis and should be attempted if the diagnosis is unclear.

## Specific features of obstructive shock

Cardiac tamponade, tension pneumothorax and PE are the principal causes of obstructive shock. Through a variety of mechanisms, each restricts the work of the heart, leading to a drop in the cardiac output. Typically, the JVP can be elevated in each and assessment of the JVP should be routine. Tamponade and tension pneumothorax need prompt intervention to relieve the pressure on the heart, but all can respond temporarily to intravenous fluids and oxygen pending arrival of expert assistance.

## Specific features of septic shock

Sepsis is dealt with and defined elsewhere in this book and further comments here are limited to establishing a diagnosis only. Clearly, haemodynamic instability and pyrexia 5–7 days after a colonic resection with primary anastomosis should raise considerations of anastomotic leak or chest infection as a source of sepsis but, in general, the early features of sepsis (Table 7.2) are subtle. Diagnosis is difficult and a high index of suspicion is essential. The patient may look remarkably well, largely because of the pink, well-perfused extremities. As already stressed, clues may be obtained from the history or the patient's charts; in postoperative patients, blood gas measurements can aid early diagnosis if you are suspicious and are part of the early assessment and response to patient with suspected sepsis (see Chapter 12).

> ### Practice point
>
> - A serious error for inexperienced staff is to treat restlessness (due to hypoxia and hypovolaemia) with sedation rather than appropriate patient assessment and resuscitation.

In septic shock, an early effect of the mediators is to cause a fall in SVR due to vasodilation. The decrease in SVR reduces the afterload on the heart and leads to a reflex increase in cardiac output, provided the patient has a healthy myocardium and adequate volume state. In early sepsis, blood pressure may be well maintained, and often the patient is pink with flushed peripheries and possibly a low diastolic pressure. This is in contrast to cardiogenic or pure hypovolaemic shock, in which the SVR rises in response to the drop in cardiac output.

Table 7.2  Clinical features of sepsis

| Early | Late |
|---|---|
| Restlessness and slight confusion | Decreased consciousness level |
| Tachypnoea | Tachypnoea |
| Tachycardia | Tachycardia |
| Vasodilation | |
| High cardiac output | Low cardiac output |
| Systolic BP normal or slightly decreased | Systolic BP less than 80 mmHg |
| Oliguria | Oliguria |
| Metabolic acidosis, elevated blood lactate | Metabolic acidosis, elevated blood lactate |
| Warm, dry, suffused extremities | Cold extremities |

In the later stages, or if the patient is already hypovolaemic, the heart may be unable to maintain an adequate output in the face of a falling SVR, so that blood pressure falls (BP = CO × SVR). The patient may then become almost indistinguishable from someone suffering from hypovolaemic shock. Hence, the patient may be hypothermic or hyperthermic depending on the phase. As the septic process progresses, fluid loss due to increased capillary permeability may also contribute to hypotension and, in addition, myocardial depressant factors reduce cardiac function directly. Initially, the patient requires oxygen and fluids but it is vital that cultures are taken and the source is identified and treated.

## Principles of monitoring and management

Restoration of adequate perfusion at the cellular level is the essential aim of treatment. In practice, the initial resuscitation of patients with any form of shock is influenced more by the nature of the associated physiological disturbances than by the specific underlying cause. On the other hand, the ultimate success of treatment depends largely on detection and elimination of the underlying cause (such as arrest of bleeding or drainage of a source of sepsis).

The mainstays of early treatment are infusion of fluid and oxygen administration with the aim of improving cardiac output and oxygen transport. If cardiogenic and obstructive forms of shock are not suspected from the details of the clinical presentation, all patients with shock can be initially treated with fluid administration (initial bolus 10 ml/kg body weight of crystalloid if normotensive, 20 ml/kg body weight if hypotensive). Oxygen should initially be given in high flow (12–15 L/min via a non-rebreathe bag) until blood gas analysis or saturation measurements are available.

## Practice point

In monitoring and management, the essential principles are:

- resuscitate
- diagnose
- treat the underlying cause.

You may encounter a patient with major haemorrhage who requires operative resuscitation, eg because of leaking abdominal aortic aneurysm. You will find it very difficult to fully resuscitate a patient with major haemorrhage; prolonged attempts are futile and merely lead to coagulopathy, hypothermia and death.

Exsanguinating patients need immediate definitive treatment – usually by surgery or interventional radiology.

It is the indices of tissue perfusion which are most useful in the early management of hypovolaemia. Do not be misled into thinking that a patient is well perfused simply because the blood pressure and heart rate are normal, a lucid patient with rapid capillary refill, warm dry skin and a good urine output is unlikely to have significant hypovolaemia.

### Monitoring and instrumentation

Successful clinical monitoring depends on the frequent measurement of simple haemodynamic indices and assessment of tissue perfusion. The following guidelines apply to all forms of shock.

### Venous access

Reliable venous access must be obtained early by inserting at least one large-bore (16G) peripheral cannula in a reliable vein. Access is normally obtained in the antecubital fossa or via the cephalic vein at the wrist. If vasoconstriction makes it difficult to gain access, a 'cut-down' can be performed in the antecubital fossa or on the long saphenous vein in front of the medial malleolus. In profoundly shocked patients, it may be necessary to obtain the initial access by cannulating the femoral vein percutaneously in the groin. Draw blood for urgent cross-matching, haematology and biochemistry.

## Bladder catheterisation

A bladder catheter is inserted transurethrally unless there is a possibility of urethral injury (as in severe pelvic fractures), or when dealing with young children. Under these circumstances, a suprapubic catheter is inserted under ultrasound control once the bladder has filled. Urine output must be measured hourly.

## ECG monitoring

ECG monitoring will detect arrhythmias and myocardial ischaemia. It is indicated particularly in primary cardiogenic shock, myocardial dysfunction secondary to ischaemia, direct thoracic injury and sepsis. Arrhythmias are more likely when there is electrolyte or acid–base disturbance. In many hospitals this may require transfer from a general surgical ward to a level 2 area.

## Pulse oximetry

A pulse oximeter attached to a finger or ear lobe allows transcutaneous estimation of oxygen saturation of haemoglobin. The accuracy of such peripheral probes depends on good peripheral perfusion. In poorly perfused patients, good equipment gives a visual or audible warning of a poor signal, giving a useful index of tissue perfusion.

## Central venous catheterisation

A catheter can be inserted percutaneously via the internal jugular or subclavian veins so that it lies in the superior vena cava, thus allowing measurement of the CVP. An aseptic technique is important for this procedure and accurate insertion is now commonly aided by the use of B-mode ultrasound guidance. It is important to obtain a chest X-ray to ensure correct positioning and exclude serious complications such as pneumothorax or haemothorax, which are potentially fatal. The length and bore of central venous catheters makes them less suitable for rapid fluid administration than large-bore short peripheral catheters and the latter should preferably be used in an overtly hypovolaemic patient. However, following initial administration of fluid and oxygen, measurement of CVP can be useful for monitoring the response to shock over time, measuring central venous oxygen saturation or when there is clinical uncertainty as to volume status and cardiovascular function. Patients will generally be in high dependency or intensive care situations when this monitoring is being employed.

In a shocked patient, a low (<5 mmHg) or even negative CVP indicates the need for more fluid. At the other extreme, a very high CVP (>20 mmHg) may indicate right ventricular or biventricular failure and the need for diuretics, vasodilators or inotropic agents, or an obstructive cause. In practice, static measurement of CVP can be misleading. For example, a young patient may have an apparently normal CVP (say 10 mmHg) as a result of vasoconstriction. A 'fluid challenge' can resolve doubt. This is performed by measuring CVP before and after the administration of a small fluid bolus (100–200 ml). If the CVP does not rise and remain elevated after 15 minutes, further fluid can be given safely; a significant rise in CVP to a small fluid challenge suggests myocardial failure or dysfunction and avoids inadvertent fluid overloading (Figure 7.3).

## Core and peripheral temperature measurement

Using your hand to assess skin temperature is useful in shocked patients. If thermistors are used to measure core and peripheral temperatures, the core–

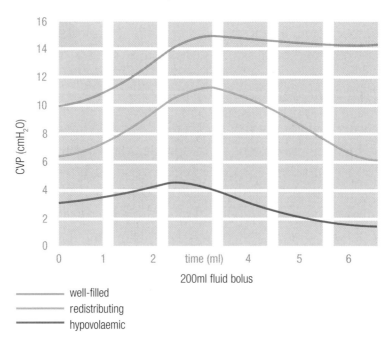

Figure 7.3 CVP response to a 200-ml bolus in different clinical situations.

peripheral gradient provides a useful index of skin perfusion. Core temperature measurement also detects hypothermia, as in injured patients who have been exposed to a cold environment (eg water immersion) or following prolonged open abdominal and chest surgery.

## Fluid administration

In most cases, the type of fluid lost in shock has little influence on the choice of fluid for initial replacement. Successful initial resuscitation depends more on the rapidity and adequacy of fluid replacement. Initial fluid management consists of boluses of warmed crystalloid ( up to 20 ml/kg body weight). Subsequent administration depends on monitoring the response to treatment, and all shocked patients need careful and repeated assessments (Box 7.2).

## Box 7.2  Continuing assessment of the shocked patient

Monitor clinical appearance, noting respiratory rate, state of the peripheral circulation and restlessness or confusion (cerebral hypoxia).

Monitor pulse rate, capillary refill time, systemic blood pressure, hourly urine output and CVP (if appropriate).

Gain valuable additional information by monitoring or periodically checking:

- blood urea and electrolyte concentrations;
- haemoglobin concentration, white cell count and haematocrit;
- ABGs including lactate level;
- pulse oximetry;
- core and peripheral temperature.

Remember to send appropriate samples (eg blood, urine, sputum, drain fluids) for bacteriological examination when sepsis is suspected, and institute cardiac monitoring and perform serial ECG in cases of cardiogenic shock.

Most importantly, diagnose and treat the underlying cause.

For those patients with major blood loss or on going haemorrhage, there are strategies to replace the losses early with red cell concentrate, platelet and fresh-frozen plasma transfusion, and most hospitals have major blood loss and transfusion protocols. This will include early intervention to stop bleeding, either surgically or using interventional radiology, and to provide best haemostasis, prevent coagulopathy, increase organ perfusion and reduce the risk of multiple end-organ dysfunction. Selective use of other blood fractions or synthetic clotting analogues to replace deficient clotting factors will need to be performed with expert haematological advice.

Considerable degrees of coagulopathy can be simply observed and monitored in the absence of active bleeding, but clotting factors are required early if the patient is bleeding or surgery is likely. Hypothermia also contributes to a bleeding diathesis by causing platelet dysfunction and so strategies are required to reduce the risk of this, including warming of resuscitation fluids, particularly when massive transfusion is needed.

## Colloid or crystalloid?

Fluid resuscitation in shock has been subject to extensive research. Normal saline and Ringer's lactate solution are the most commonly used crystalloids. Currently, Ringer's lactate is preferred because it can buffer metabolic acidosis and avoids the hyperchloraemic acidosis associated with large-volume normal saline infusions. In most circumstances either fluid can be used initially but there is a theoretical risk of hyperkalaemia when using Ringer's in patients with an acute kidney injury or chronic kidney disease.

Colloid infusions are theoretically retained in the intravascular space more than crystalloids. In spite of this quality, studies do not show any benefit over crystalloid use in clinical outcomes and there are concerns about the safety of colloid use in patients with sepsis. In a mixed ICU population, colloid administration was associated with a poorer outcome. Colloid infusions, both albumin and those based on synthetic starch polymers, carry risks of anaphylaxis, coagulopathy and acute kidney injury.

Important points:

- In most situations, both colloid and crystalloid are able to replenish blood volume if given in sufficient quantity.

- To replace a given amount of blood loss, the volume of crystalloid required is approximately three times that of colloid.

- When crystalloid resuscitation is used, there is a greater weight gain and probably more tissue oedema than when colloid is used.

- There is no fixed relationship between serum albumin concentration and colloid osmotic pressure until serum albumin falls very low (below 15 g/L).

- In septic shock with increased capillary permeability, both colloids and crystalloids pass through the vascular basement membrane.

- Many experienced practitioners would limit the volume of crystalloid used during resuscitation to <50% of non-blood fluid infusion.

The principal changes in practice that occur with experience are the early identification and rapid treatment of hypovolaemic states, prompt use of blood when haemorrhage is occurring and, most importantly, the surgical treatment of any underlying cause, particularly haemorrhage.

### Assessment of response

One of the most important steps in the management of the shocked patient is the assessment of the response to treatment. For every exsanguination, you will meet many more patients who become critically ill with shock in a less dramatic, but no less important, manner. During resuscitation, and at least every 30 minutes or so, you should reassess the patient's progress. If the patient's signs are not improving, you need to change your plan of action (Box 7.3). The aim is to detect those patients you have initially misjudged or those who are temporary responders. These patients are common and it can be difficult to assess the need for surgery. Involve senior help if you are in doubt.

### Case scenario 7.3

You are called to see a 68-year-old man on the surgical ward. Five days ago he underwent a difficult anterior resection for a colonic tumour. He weighs 125 kg and has NIDDM, and a history of hypertension. He has been spiking a temperature for the last 48 hours but has remained reasonably well until now. It is

8pm, and the nurses on the ward are concerned because he has become cold, clammy and restless. You follow the CCrISP algorithm and establish that the airway is clear. His $SaO_2$ is 92%, respiratory rate 28 per minute, pulse 110 and the urine output has been 20 ml over the last hour. He is restless but cooperative.

### What form of shock might this man have and what would you do?

Hypovolaemic/haemorrhagic shock? Cardiogenic shock? Septic shock? Obstructive shock? All are possible and there may be more than one pathology here. He has been spiking a temperature, so sepsis is possible. This might also have led to a secondary haemorrhage. He has risk factors for cardiac disease, and myocardial infarction or acute arrhythmia, possibly related to sepsis, is possible. He may also have had a PE causing obstructive shock. Following the CCrISP protocol, you should be able to tell which type of shock is most likely. You institute high-flow oxygen, gain intravenous access and send blood samples including cross-match and cultures. The patient's BP is 115/60 mmHg, which, you note from chart review, is lower than before. His urine output has also tailed off. Abdominal examination is difficult but feels tense. There is no acute change on ECG.

### How would you further manage this situation?

This man is clearly shocked and needs simultaneous assessment and resuscitation. The response to a fluid challenge while you wait for available results will give you a much better idea of the problem. You give a fluid challenge of 20 ml/kg body weight and reassess. His BP initially rises to 140/80 mmHg, but then drops again and he remains restless and tachycardic. On a blood gas, his Hb is 70 g/L, and he has a metabolic acidosis with lactate of 5 mmol/L.

### What action may be necessary?

The most likely cause here is secondary haemorrhage, possibly secondary to intra-abdominal sepsis. He has responded temporarily to fluid challenge but further intervention (probably surgery) is necessary to deal with the cause. You must seek senior help at this stage as you have treated the patient appropriately but he remains unstable. As a bare minimum, he needs a higher level of care, with invasive monitoring and further aggressive resuscitation.

## Learning points

- There may be more than one cause of shock – the CCrISP system will help you to decide the correct cause in any particular case.

- Shock may not be amenable to resuscitation alone – surgery may be required to stop the bleeding or deal with the cause.

- Some surgical patients are difficult to assess – if you are not sure, or the patient fails to respond to simple resuscitative measures, get help early.


### Box 7.3  Responses to treatment of shock

- No response, eg exsanguination
- Temporary response, eg continuing slow but steady postoperative haemorrhage
- Full response, eg simple sepsis caused by repeat urinary catheterisation which responds to fluid resuscitation and early administration of antibiotics


### *Refractory shock*

If hypovolaemic shock proves refractory to fluid replacement and oxygen administration, the factors shown in Box 7.4 may be responsible.


### Box 7.4  Refractory shock

- Underestimation of the degree of hypovolaemia
- Failure to arrest haemorrhage
- Presence of cardiac tamponade or tension pneumothorax
- Underlying sepsis with inadequate source control
- Secondary cardiovascular effects due to delay in instituting treatment

Further action is necessary.

## Algorithm of cardiovascular monitoring/support

An algorithm of cardiovascular monitoring/support is given in Box 7.5. Many surgical patients become hypovolaemic and present with oliguria, hypotension, tachycardia, hypoxia or acidosis in isolation or almost any combination. Many do not develop a full picture of shock but require prompt treatment just the same. Most are simply treated with conventional measures including adequate fluid replacement (and other necessary treatments). You need to have a method of management clear in your mind. You should review them later to ensure that normal function has been re-established. Patients who need anything more than simple correction of minor to modest fluid deficit should be managed in a high-dependency environment.

Treat any underlying pathology, particularly haemorrhage (which often needs surgery), in addition to giving intravenous fluids and oxygen.

## Box 7.5 Algorithm of cardiovascular monitoring/support

### Establish and maintain normovolaemia

- Assess with CCrISP system
- Give reasonable intravenous fluid challenge (10–20 ml/kg crystalloid initially; see text)
- Treat any underlying cause (blood loss, sepsis, etc)
- Determine recent fluid balance

### Assess response

- Clinically (skin perfusion, BP, urine output, JVP, pulse)
- By simple investigations (repeat FBC, pulse oximetry, pH, BE, lactate)
- Improving: adjust fluid regimen, treat underlying cause, plan to review shortly
- Deteriorating: resuscitate and involve expert help directly
- No progress, reassess: if different diagnosis, treat and seek help; if still hypovolaemic, continue fluids and find/treat cause
- Not sure if normovolaemic: measure CVP and seek higher level of care

## CVP

- Inadequate: establish normovolaemia

- Adequate: (>8cmH$_2$O), but inadequate circulation: reassess cause (and treat as necessary); consider inotrope in higher level of care; no/poor response, seek help directly

- High: (>15cmH$_2$O), and patient exhibits signs of cardiac failure: simple LVF, treat; suspect cardiogenic shock, call for help

## Invasive monitoring and inotrope treatment

- Transfer to HDU/ICU

Patients who have incipient failure of more than one system need the help of an intensivist directly and you should have a very low threshold for involving help and informing your consultant. All these patients should be receiving monitored oxygen therapy.

Young and fit patients tolerate rapid infusion well and CVP line insertion is indicated when there is doubt about progress, adequacy of filling or likely tolerance of the administered fluid.

Patients who continue with inadequate cardiovascular function and whose good cardiovascular filling has been confirmed by CVP measurement may require inotropic support. In these cases senior help is mandatory and patients should be treated in a critical care environment.

## Metabolic monitoring in refractory shock

Urea and electrolyte levels are required to establish a baseline and monitor progress. Arterial pH and blood gas measurements are essential to assess hypoxia, hypercapnia and acid–base balance. Blood lactate levels are a good index of cellular hypoxia and hepatic function.

Metabolic acidosis associated with inadequate perfusion should correct once cardiac output is improved; its disappearance is a marker of adequate resuscitation. It is rarely necessary to give bicarbonate in a ward setting to treat acidosis, but it may be considered in a higher care area if the patient's pH is very low (<7.1) and myocardial depression from acidosis may be contributing to the shock.

Respiratory acidosis with an increase in arterial $PaCO_2$ usually indicates the need for endotracheal intubation and assisted ventilation.

### Higher levels of care

Shock is an immediate life-threatening condition and should be treated as such. The ability of the cardiovascular system to compensate has been discussed and shock reflects the state that is reached once decompensation is occurring. Although uncomplicated hypovolaemia can often be managed satisfactorily without intensive care facilities, patients with severe trauma, sepsis, cardiogenic shock or shock complicated by secondary myocardial dysfunction will all benefit from the monitoring and support available in a critical care environment.

Consideration should be given to early critical care referral for patients with significant comorbidity. Patients who fail to respond quickly and completely should be discussed with the critical care team and a surgical consultant. Assessment and monitoring of the cardiovascular system is detailed elsewhere (Chapter 8). The basis of critical care is the same as outlined previously, with attention to fluid administration, oxygenation and definitive treatment.

Based on the underlying cause of shock and measurement of cardiovascular parameters (particularly the confirmation of an adequate circulatory volume), some patients require inotropic support. The selection of an inotropic agent is based on the cardiovascular effects of the drug and the underlying pathophysiology. The cardiovascular effects of many agents can be predicted from a knowledge of their particular effect on adrenergic receptors (see Chapter 8).

## Summary

### Definition

- Shock is inadequate tissue perfusion causing cellular hypoxia.

## Diagnosis

- Assess the patient and determine the degree of organ perfusion and not simply blood pressure.

- Identify the different common patterns of presentation of shock.

## Treatment

- Restore perfusion as a matter of urgency.

- A common initial approach is treatment with oxygen and fluid bolus administration.

- Find and treat the underlying cause.

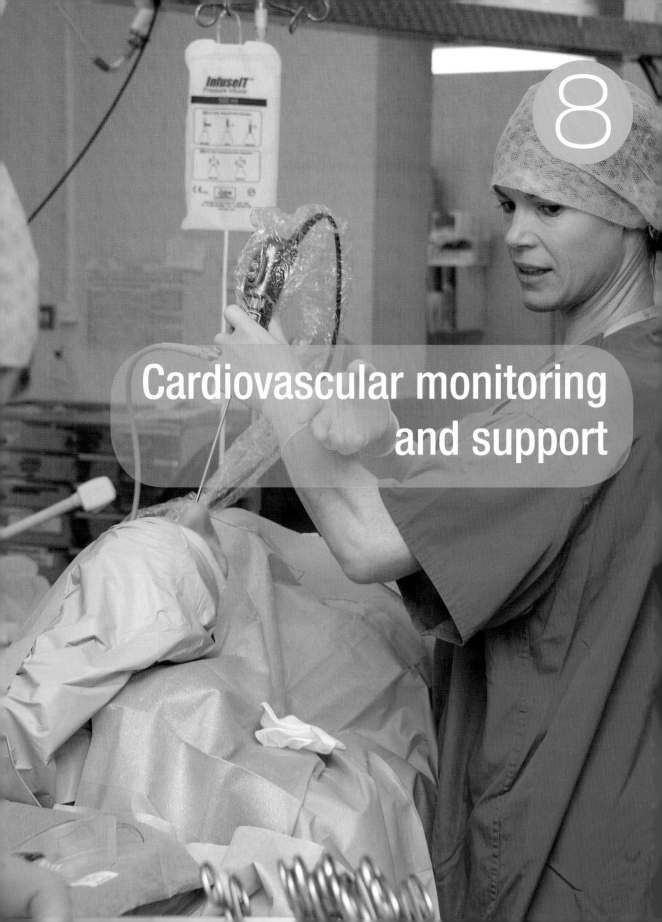

8

Cardiovascular monitoring and support

## Learning outcomes

This chapter will help you to:

- understand the indications for cardiovascular monitoring and support;

- be familiar with the methods used to assess cardiovascular function in a critically unwell or perioperative patient;

- understand how drug and fluid therapies may be used to manipulate cardiovascular function.

## Introduction

Maintaining adequate tissue perfusion and hence oxygen delivery to the cells is one of the primary goals in the management of the critically ill surgical patient.

The main determinant of oxygen delivery is cardiac output; therefore, the monitoring and therapeutic manipulation of cardiac output are essential components of critical care practice. Cardiac output is, in turn, determined by preload, cardiac function and compliance, and afterload (Figure 8.1), all of which can be monitored and manipulated.

In most patients a full clinical assessment, eg RR, HR, BP, capillary refill time and urine output, provides a suitable first step bedside evaluation of cardiovascular functioning. The efficacy of oxygen and nutrient delivery to the tissues, and removal of carbon dioxide and other products of tissue metabolism, depends upon a cardiac output sufficient to meet the demands of tissue metabolism. This is highly variable depending on how ill a patient is. Furthermore, the cardiac output must be regionally matched to the metabolic needs of individual organs.

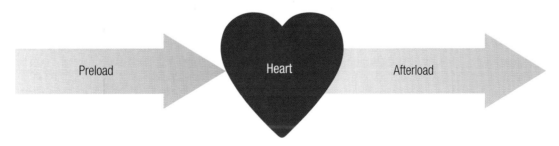

Figure 8.1  The determinants of cardiac output.

In the early stages of deterioration, deviation from the normal ranges of any of these components of cardiac output can occur unexpectedly, rapidly and with only subtle clinical changes. Therefore, reliance on clinical assessment alone may well be inadequate and the accuracy of estimation of volume status compared with more intensive monitoring techniques may be as low as 30%. Objective measurements showing change should be detected as early as possible to allow rapid corrective therapy before vital organ damage occurs. At this stage arterial blood gas measurement can provide additional useful information on the adequacy of tissue metabolism, which is especially helpful in determining whether the patient might need additional monitoring and a higher level of care. Monitoring equipment can provide rapid, accurate and reproducible measurements of cardiovascular performance and the effects of treatment.

Organs vary in their ability to maintain their own perfusion usually through autoregulation. Certain organs, notably the gut, are prone to cellular hypoxia as they cannot autoregulate and hypoxia may continue to drive the inflammatory process (including multiple organ failure) even once the initial causal factors have been dealt with. One approach to overcome this was to try and ensure that the critically ill patient with multiple organ failures has a circulation that provides an oxygen delivery which is, if anything, greater than normal, minimising the chance of occult cellular hypoxia. This is less commonly attempted nowadays but a related approach is to monitor plasma lactate level and/or negative base excess (BE) and central venous oxygen saturations on the grounds that elevated values of these suggest that tissue hypoxia may be present.

An alternative strategy has been to try and measure specific visceral perfusion (eg that of the intestine, brain) by techniques such as tonometry or microdialysis catheters.

There is much to be said for pursuing similar objectives, at an appropriate level, in all unwell patients and particularly in the pre-operative preparation of the critically ill surgical patient.

Indications for intensive monitoring of the cardiovascular system are:

- failure to restore and maintain cardiovascular homeostasis with simple techniques (IV fluids, oxygen, surgery, non-invasive blood pressure, pulse oximetry);

- procedures that may give rise to rapid or profound changes in preload or afterload, eg emergency abdominal aortic repair;

- treatment with vasoactive drugs that influence preload, afterload or myocardial function, to monitor response to treatment and guide management strategies;

- any patient who has, or is at risk of developing, a low perfusion state from any cause, eg the high-risk patient with poor cardiac function.

The parameters that can be monitored include:

- blood pressure

- CVP

- cardiac output or cardiac index (CI).

## Measurement of blood pressure

Non-invasive intermittent measurements of arterial blood pressure can be performed using an automated sphygmomanometer. Non-invasive readings can be erroneous if cuff size or positioning is incorrect. Automated devices are useful to demonstrate trends in blood pressure and are reliable in most stable patients as well as easy to use in a ward setting.

In unstable patients, better accuracy is achieved using invasive techniques. A line can be inserted into an artery and the mechanical energy of blood pressure changes converted to electrical energy using a transducer, allowing continuous monitoring on a screen as well as frequent blood sampling. CVP monitoring utilises the same principles and has the same potential pitfalls as arterial pressure monitoring.

### Transducers

The physical principles of how these individual measurements are made are beyond the scope of this course; however, certain basic scientific principles apply. Changes in any parameter to be measured must be detected accurately with sufficient sensitivity, over the range required, at a suitable frequency response, often from inaccessible sites, and converted by a transducer so that the signals vary in proportion to the changes in the parameters under study. A transducer converts the mechanical energy of pressure changes to electrical energy so that the electrical output of the transducer varies directly with the change in pressure. An example of this kind of system is shown in Figure 8.2.

A pressure wave is transmitted from the vessel (in this case an artery) to the transducer through rigid tubing. The transducer converts the mechanical signal to an electronic one, displayed on the monitor. The three-way tap on the transducer allows zeroing to atmospheric pressure and sampling of arterial blood. Patency of the cannula is maintained by a slow constant flush of saline (up to 3 ml/h) under pressure and most systems incorporate a button for bolus flushing to clear any debris and improve the signal.

The electrical signals must be displayed and processed so that derived results may be calculated. The measurement system must be zeroed and calibrated. If pressure is measured, it should be done with the transducer level relative to the point within the patient at which the pressure is to be measured, eg midaxillary line for the measurement of arterial and central venous pressures in a supine patient, external auditory meatus for intracranial pressure measurement. Care should be taken to minimise the interference and damping of the measurement signal to ensure optimal signal-to-noise ratio. Failure to zero or calibrate will produce erroneous results. This can also happen when the cannula or catheter is kinked, abuts the vessel wall or is partly occluded by clot.

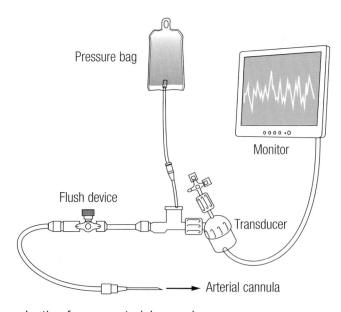

Figure 8.2 Signal transduction from an arterial cannula.

## Safeguards

Certain standards are common to all procedures used during invasive monitoring methods:

▫ The operator should have a sound knowledge of relevant practical anatomy.

▫ The operator should be competent in the technique of insertion of the line.

▫ The procedure should be explained to the patient.

▫ All procedures must be performed using an aseptic technique.

▫ Contraindications and complications of the procedure and monitoring technique must be known.

▫ The benefit accrued must exceed the risks of the procedure.

▫ The patient must be looked after by staff who know how to manage the lines, all of which must be Luer-locked to prevent disconnection.

▫ All lines should be clearly labelled and injections into or sampling from lines performed **only** at designated sites by people trained to do so.

▫ Attendants should be familiar with the monitors to ensure that the data derived from them are accurate.

▫ Lines must be dressed aseptically and other equipment, eg line transducer sets changed at appropriate intervals.

## Arterial pressure monitoring

A peripheral artery can be cannulated either to allow continuous measurement of arterial blood pressure by connecting the cannula to a transducer or to allow for repeated sampling of arterial blood for analysis. The radial artery is the anatomical site most frequently used, followed by the dorsalis pedis artery, and a 20G or 22G cannula is used. The brachial and femoral arteries should be avoided if possible because of lack of collaterals and, in the case of the femoral site, the risk of sepsis.

When using the radial artery, check for ulnar flow supply to the palmar arch using Allen's test prior to cannulation (Figure 8.3). Local sepsis and coagulopathy are the main contraindications, while complications include haematoma, thrombosis, distal ischaemia, intimal damage, false aneurysm formation, disconnection and injection of irritant drugs. Samples from arterial cannulae should be taken aseptically and the line flushed and re-sealed afterwards. After cannulation of the artery, the cannula should be connected to a continuous-flush device containing saline under pressure, which maintains patency and allows blood pressure changes to be conducted without letting blood flow out of the artery into the line.

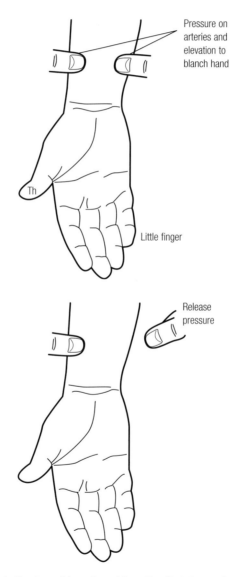

Figure 8.3 Allen's test. Blanch the hand by clenching the fist then simultaneously occlude the radial and ulnar arteries at the wrist. An adequate pink flush of the hand on release of the ulnar pressure confirms an adequate ulnar supply to the palmar arterial arches.

## Technique for radial arterial puncture/cannulation (Figure 8.4)

### Position and palpate

- Position the hand and yourself comfortably, with adequate light and assistance.
- Palpate the artery with two fingers.
- Feel and imagine its course above and below the point of entry.
- Insert at 45°, avoiding the superficial vein which often overlies.

### Puncture

- Advance needle tip in a linear fashion – do **not** wiggle it around.
- If you miss, repalpate and search in a systematic fashion with further straight insertions.
- Let syringe fill and withdraw.
- Pressure haemostasis – 5 minutes.

### Cannulation: the Seldinger technique

This requires strict asepsis:

- Puncture as above.
- Advance guidewire through hollow needle.
- Remove needle.
- Railroad cannula over guidewire.
- Check backflow and secure cannula.
- Connect transducer and flushing set-up.

If the arterial cannula is to be used for pressure monitoring, it is connected via a short length of rigid tubing to a three-way tap, flush device and transducer. Check that the transducer is zeroed and calibrated at the correct level, and that the line does not contain air bubbles, which would cause damping of the signal. The arterial waveform gives real-time information about the blood pressure and heart rate, but can also transform pressure changes into variations in stroke volume or cardiac output using commercial devices, i.e. LIDCO™.

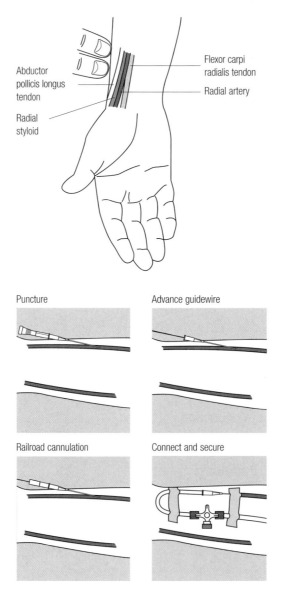

Figure 8.4 Technique for radial arterial puncture/cannulation.

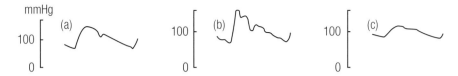

Figure 8.5 Arterial waveforms showing influence of damping. (a) Adequately damped; (b) underdamped; (c) overdamped.

Some devices, such as LIDCO™, need to be calibrated by an independent mechanism in order to compensate for the different levels of vascular compliance seen between and within patients. The shape of the individual waveform can give information about the systemic vascular resistance and cardiac contractility in both normal and pathological conditions. In particular, a sharp peaked up-swing and down-swing with a low dicrotic notch can reflect significant hypovolaemia, but it is dangerous to draw such conclusions unless the system is adequately damped (Figure 8.5).

Changes in the arterial pressure trace with the fluctuations in intrathoracic pressure during artificial mechanical ventilation can be used to determine which patients will respond to a fluid challenge by increasing their stroke volume.

These changes can be characterised by the systolic pressure variation, the pulse pressure variation or when combined with a cardiac output monitor, the stroke volume variation.

## Central venous pressure measurement

CVP measurement is one of the most commonly used monitoring tools in critical care, indicating preloading of the pulmonary circulation and a rough guide to systemic preload given a number of provisos. The CVP is the pressure within the superior vena cava as it enters the right atrium, and reflects the ability of the right heart to accept and deliver circulating volume. The CVP is influenced by various factors, including venous return, right heart compliance, intrathoracic pressure and patient position.

While absolute measurements of CVP are useful (with the normal range 0–8 mmHg or 0–10 cmH$_2$O), often the trend in CVP, and response to fluid challenge or therapeutic manoeuvres is more important. This is particularly useful when trying to find and treat the cause of shock (see Chapter 7).

## Central vein cannulation

### Infraclavicular subclavian route

This technique is rarely used blindly by experienced operators and access is more likely to be achieved using ultrasound guidance.

- Tilt the patient 20° head down, arms by the side and head turned away from the side of entry.
- Make a skin nick and insert the cannula 1–2 cm below the midpoint of the clavicle.
- Advance horizontally towards the suprasternal notch – remember to advance needle tip in a linear fashion – do **not** wiggle it around.
- Try to visualise the anatomy beneath as you do it – think where your needle tip is, particularly in relation to the clavicle and pleura, and the narrow gap between clavicle and first rib, where the subclavian artery and vein run.
- If you miss, search in a systematic fashion with further straight insertions, trying to picture where the vein is most likely to be.
- When venous blood is aspirated freely, remove syringe and insert the guidewire.
- Leave enough guidewire outside to let you railroad the catheter over it without losing the wire inside the patient.
- Advance the catheter to a previously measured point, so the tip lies in the distal superior vena cava (SVC).
- Secure the catheter and check its position by chest X-ray.

### Ultrasound image of the jugular vein and carotid artery

- Using ultrasound, the vein is located at the medial border of sternomastoid, at the level of the thyroid cartilage and anterolateral to the carotid artery.
- Displace the artery medially and, under ultrasound guidance, advance the needle through a skin nick.

- Advance inferiorly at 30° to the skin, parallel to the artery but lateral: this is often towards the ipsilateral nipple.
- Puncture and proceed as above.

## CVP access

The route for access to the central venous circulation depends on the skill and experience of the operator and the presence of site-specific contraindications such as local sepsis, coagulopathy, abnormal anatomy, operative site and previous vein usage. While the techniques are illustrated in Figure 8.6a, the UK National Institute for Health and Care Excellence (NICE) recommends that ultrasound imaging should be used to guide placement of central venous catheters into the internal jugular vein in elective situations. NICE also recommends that those involved in placing central venous catheters should undertake training to achieve competence in the use of ultrasound for this purpose. Ultrasound should also be used in emergency cases, although the anatomical landmark method may still be used for the subclavian route due to poor ultrasonic visualisation of the subclavian vein behind the clavicle.

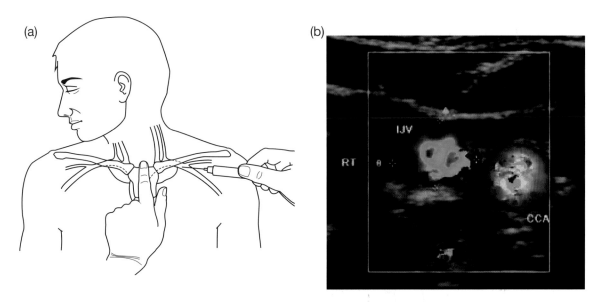

(a)  (b)

Figure 8.6  (a) Infraclavicular subclavian vein cannulation using the Seldinger technique. (b) Ultrasound image of the jugular vein and carotid artery.

The internal jugular site is better in terms of a lower rate of complications, but access at this site is uncomfortable and difficult to dress. The subclavian route has a higher risk profile, in particular the risk of pneumothorax and intrathoracic bleeding, which can be difficult to control.

## Practice point

Central venous catheterisation should only be done by an experienced person.

### CVP measurement

The best zero reference point, which represents the level of the SVC, is the midaxillary line at the fourth intercostal space, with the patient supine. The alternative, the second intercostal space at the sternal edge, represents a point about 5 cm above the atrium. For readings to be comparable at separate times, they should always be taken from the same point (Figure 8.7).

The electronic transducer produces an electronic signal, analysis of which allows the mean pressure to be displayed in mm of mercury. The set up of the transducer is identical to that for arterial pressure measurement.

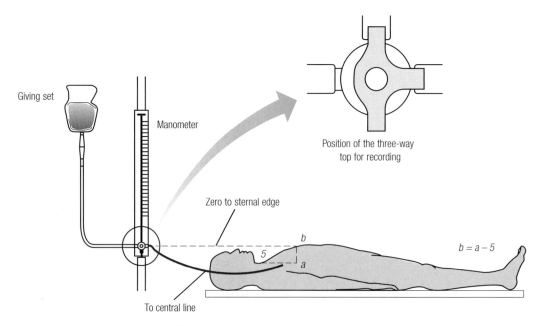

Figure 8.7 Liquid manometer for CVP.

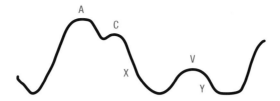

Figure 8.8 The CVP waveform. A wave, atrial contraction; C wave, bulging of the tricuspid valve into the right atrium; X descent, atrial relaxation; V wave; rise in atrial pressure prior to tricuspid valve opening; and Y descent, atrial emptying.

## CVP waveform

The CVP waveform has a characteristic pattern that reflects changes in atrial pressure during the cardiac cycle, as shown in Figure 8.8.

## Indications for CVP measurement

CVP measurement is indicated in the following situations:

- administration of fluid replacement therapy for hypovolaemia when conventional access is not possible, when concern exists about overtransfusion or when there is uncertainty about fluid volume status;

- central vein cannulation is **not** advocated as a primary route of access because of the risk of complications and low flow rates achievable (remember Poiseuille's law);

- to measure the effect of vasoactive drugs on venous capacitance, particularly vasodilators;

- to aid diagnosis of right ventricular failure, when a high pressure will be seen in the presence of poor cardiac output;

- administration of potent drugs, eg inotropes;

- administration of parenteral nutrition, which must be done using a dedicated clean lumen.

### Practice point

CVP as a value does not 'equal' intravascular volume and is not an indicator of left ventricular function.

## Pitfalls in practice

▨ Inaccurate readings can result from failure of zeroing or calibration, placement of the cannula tip in the right ventricle, tricuspid regurgitation and incompetence, AV dissociation and nodal rhythms.

▨ Variations in intravascular volume, sympathetic tone, cardiac output and intrathoracic pressure (particularly during positive pressure ventilation) may lead to a false impression of a much higher right ventricular filling pressure than is actually present (Figure 8.9).

▨ Before using the line and acting on measurements made, always check for easy aspiration of blood and pressure fluctuation with respiration and confirm the position of the line by X-ray.

▨ Complications of central line insertion are numerous and relate to damage to either the veins themselves or adjacent structures. They include rupture of vessel and haemorrhage with local haematoma or haemothorax, tension pneumothorax (particularly if the patient is on positive-pressure ventilation), air embolism, extravascular catheter placement, knotting of catheters, catheter breakage, catheter misplacement, neurapraxia, arterial puncture, lymphatic puncture, tracheobronchial puncture and sepsis. Do not underestimate the potential severity of central line sepsis.

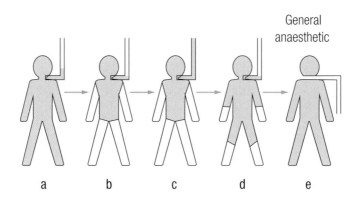

Figure 8.9 CVP and intravascular volume: pitfalls in the shocked surgical patient. (a) Normal. (b) Shocked but compensating (by peripheral vasoconstriction) with low CVP. (c) Rapid refill and (temporarily) high CVP. (d) Redistribution and falling CVP as degree of compensatory vasoconstriction lessens. (e) General anaesthesia with vasodilatation, loss of compensation and very low CVP.

Staff involved in the care of patients with central venous access should ensure compliance with care bundles for central venous catheter care to prevent catheter-associated infections. The care bundle approach considers aspects of line insertion, including aseptic techniques, skin preparation and hand hygiene and on-going care of the line, including regular inspection, aseptic techniques and regular replacement of administration sets.

## Measurements of cardiac output/cardiac index

In shock states, the delivery of oxygen to the tissues is at least as important as the level of systemic arterial pressure. Global oxygen delivery is a product of cardiac output and arterial oxygen content. Cardiac output is a pivotal variable in the management of the critically ill surgical patient.

The understanding of the relationship between cardiac output and other parameters allows an estimate of systemic vascular resistance, using the following equation:

Cardiac output = driving pressure (mean arterial pressure (MAP) − CVP)/systemic vascular resistance

With a measurement of cardiac output, MAP and CVP, an estimate of SVR can be calculated and the combination of variables used to guide rational decisions about volume resuscitation and vasoactive therapies.

The pulmonary artery catheter (PAC or Swan–Ganz catheter) was the gold standard for advanced haemodynamic monitoring. Its use is now limited to cardiac and some vascular surgery. Pulmonary artery pressure and pulmonary artery occlusion (or 'wedge') pressure can be used to monitor right heart function and preload of the systemic circulation. This is achieved using thermodilution techniques and a thermistor on the PAC. The technique is highly invasive and is associated with a significant risk of serious complications. This, combined with ready availability of less invasive cardiac output monitors, has led to reduced use of PAC in general critical care units and in theatre. Cardiac indexing corrects any variable for patient size (Box 8.1).

## Box 8.1 Variables derived from cardiac output measurements

### Systemic vascular resistance (SVR)

- If too high (vasoconstriction), tissue hypoperfusion is likely
- If too low, maintenance of an adequate mean blood pressure will be difficult

### Stroke volume (SV), stroke index (SI)

- A major determinant of cardiac output and governable by preload

### Left ventricular stroke work index (LVSWI)

- An index of the function of the systemic side of the heart

### Oxygen delivery ($DO_2$)

- An index of the oxygen delivered to all tissues

### Oxygen uptake ($VO_2$)

- Index of oxygen consumption

## Non-invasive measurement of cardiac function

There are several less invasive techniques, including trans-oesophageal Doppler (TOD), echocardiography, pulse contour cardiac output with indicator dilution (PiCCO) and the LiDCO™ (lithium dilution cardiac output) system.

### Trans-oesophageal Doppler

TOD uses the Doppler shift principle to make measurements of blood velocity in the descending aorta. A disposable Doppler probe contained at the tip of a $90 \, cm \times 5.5 \, mm$ probe is passed down the oesophagus to lie at the level of the descending aorta (around 35–45 cm) and rotated until the arterial waveform is displayed. This appears as a triangular waveform since the shift signal is displayed as a velocity–time plot. The shape of the waveform provides information on preload,

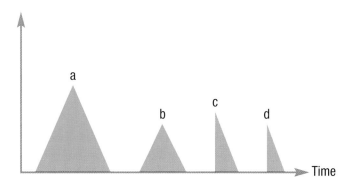

Figure 8.10 Stylised TOD waveforms for vascular abnormality. (a) Best waveform, normal configuration. (b) Failing left ventricle – decreased waveform height and low peak velocity. Giving inotropes increases waveform height and restores velocity. (c) Hypovolaemia – narrow waveform base with decreased FTc (giving volume lengthens flow time and widens waveform base). (d) High systemic vascular resistance/afterload – reduced waveform height and narrow base.

stoke volume and afterload (Figure 8.10). The area under the curve represents the stroke volume flowing through the descending aorta and applying a factor determined from the patient's age, height and weight allows the stroke volume to be calculated. The corrected flow time (FTc) is calculated: it is low in hypovolaemia and may be used to derive SVR. The disadvantage of TOD is that the patient must be anaesthetised and intubated to tolerate the probe. The technique is very position and therefore operator dependent. It cannot be used in patients who have coarctation of the aorta or who are on intra-aortic balloon pumps, or in those undergoing surgery to the oesophagus or in whom insertion of the probe into the oesophagus would carry additional risks, eg patients with known bleeding from oesophageal varices and/or oral surgery patients.

## Trans-thoracic and trans-oesophageal echocardiography

Bedside echocardiography is becoming increasingly available and training in echocardiography image acquisition and interpretation at a basic level is becoming widespread. Its main role in critically unwell patients is the assessment of preload and cardiac contractility before and after an intervention, and the diagnosis of major cardiac structural abnormalities (pericardial tamponade, severe valvular and regional wall motion abnormalities). Some image windows, eg transhepatic views, allow assessment of inferior vena cava size and therefore patient filling. It can be difficult to get good views in ventilated patients or those who have recently undergone abdominal surgery.

## Indicator dilution and pulse contour analysis

Instead of measuring cardiac output by means of temperature changes in the pulmonary artery, which requires a PAC, a thermistor can be placed in the systemic arterial circulation. PiCCO calculates cardiac output from a peripheral arterial cannula providing beat-to-beat information to a computer, which in turn follows the heart rate and pressure waveform and integrates the area under the curve. The accuracy of the method is improved as the cannula contains a sensitive thermistor, allowing thermodilutional calibration. The small drop in the temperature of arterial blood that follows the injection of a bolus of ice-cold saline into a central vein is proportional to cardiac output. The thermodilution measurement is used to calibrate the continuous cardiac output monitoring software, which calculates changes in cardiac output by analysing the pulse contour of the arterial waveform. PiCCO requires recalibration at regular intervals and becomes unreliable when the arterial waveform is suboptimal, for example with a kinked line, air or blood clots in the system or any other cause of a damped trace.

Other indicators can be used to replace thermodilution techniques. For example, lithium chloride can be injected into a central vein and the lithium concentration analysed with an ion-sensitive electrode (LiDCO™). In this case, the blood can be sampled from a normal peripheral arterial line. Several drugs interfere with the lithium analysis, notably some muscle relaxants, eg atracurium, and lithium is contraindicated in some patients, eg pregnant women. As with thermodilution, lithium dilution is combined with continuous pulse contour analysis and similar recalibration requirements and issues with damped arterial traces apply. Some devices provide information on the pulse waveform without calibration; these use the arterial waveform to compute cardiac output continuously by multiplying heart rate by a calculated stroke volume. Although easy to use and providing continuous data, the lack of calibration may make these devices inaccurate, particularly when large cardiac output changes occur, eg during haemodynamic instability due to haemorrhage or sepsis.

## Cardiovascular support using vasoactive drugs

In the normal heart, cardiac output is determined by preload, afterload, heart rate, rhythm, contractility and balance of oxygen demand and supply. If the heart is damaged, for a given preload or afterload, cardiac output will decrease. This can be represented graphically either by pressure–volume loops or by the more familiar Frank–Starling curve (see Figure 7.2).

If the cardiac output remains low after correcting any hypovolaemia with a fluid challenge, inotropic or other vasoactive drugs are used to optimise myocardial contractility by balancing myocardial oxygen supply and demand. Measurements of derived variables can predict the best therapeutic regimens (Table 8.1).

Inotropes are drugs that increase cardiac output and ejection fraction. Ideally, in addition to these properties, they should reduce afterload and preload, resulting in decreased transventricular wall tension, promoting coronary blood flow, increasing myocardial oxygen delivery and reducing oxygen consumption. Regrettably, the ideal inotrope does not exist, but the most commonly used are adrenaline and dobutamine. They all act by providing an upward and left shift in the Frank–Starling curve, as shown in Figure 7.2. Noradrenaline has a specific use in septic shock as a vasopressor: it is used to increase and maintain SVR within the normal range.

Table 8.1 Action of inotropic agents

|  | Receptor | Effect | Clinical use |
| --- | --- | --- | --- |
| Noradrenaline | α-Adrenoreceptor agonist | Arteriolar vasoconstriction | Septic shock with low SVR |
| Adrenaline | α- and β-adrenoreceptor agonist, predominantly β1-adrenoreceptor agonist at low doses | Positive inotropic and chronotropic. Vascoconstricts at high doses | Widespread in conditions of low cardiac output; useful in emergency situations |
| Dopamine | α- and β-adrenoreceptors. Dopamine (DA) 1 and 2 receptors | Low dose: splanchnic vasodilation, increased renal and hepatic blood flow (DA1). High dose: vasoconstriction | Used less frequently |
| Dopexamine | DA1, DA2 and β-adrenoreceptor agonist | Increases splanchnic blood flow | Controversial – in perioperative optimisation |
| Dobutamine | Similar to dopexamine | Reduces SVR and increases cardiac output | Cardiogenic shock |
| Milrinone | Prevents breakdown of cAMP by phosphodiesterase | Inotropic action by increasing intracellular calcium | Heart failure, cardiogenic shock |

Vasodilators such as sodium nitroprusside or nitrates are of use when pulmonary oedema occurs in heart failure, although they can produce a reflex tachycardia if the blood pressure falls. Occasionally, both inotropes and vasodilators are used in combination (eg adrenaline and nitroglycerine in severe LVF) or inotropes and vasoconstrictors are used in combination (eg dobutamine and noradrenaline in severe sepsis).

Inotropes and vasodilators can only be used safely where a full range of monitoring is available. They should never be used on ordinary surgical wards and **never** in the presence of hypovolaemia. Their dose ranges, modes of delivery, etc, are outside the scope of this course, although there should be opportunity to discuss these more during the workshops. Your task as a surgical trainee caring for ward-level patients is to recognise the clinical conditions that mandate their use and refer the patient for the appropriate level of monitoring and care.

## Summary

- Adequate cardiovascular function is a prerequisite for survival.

- To determine cardiovascular function accurately, invasive monitoring is necessary when ward based assessment and therapy is failing to produce a response.

- All techniques of advanced CVS monitoring have complications and limitations to their use.

- The method of monitoring chosen should be appropriate to the specific patient and problems.

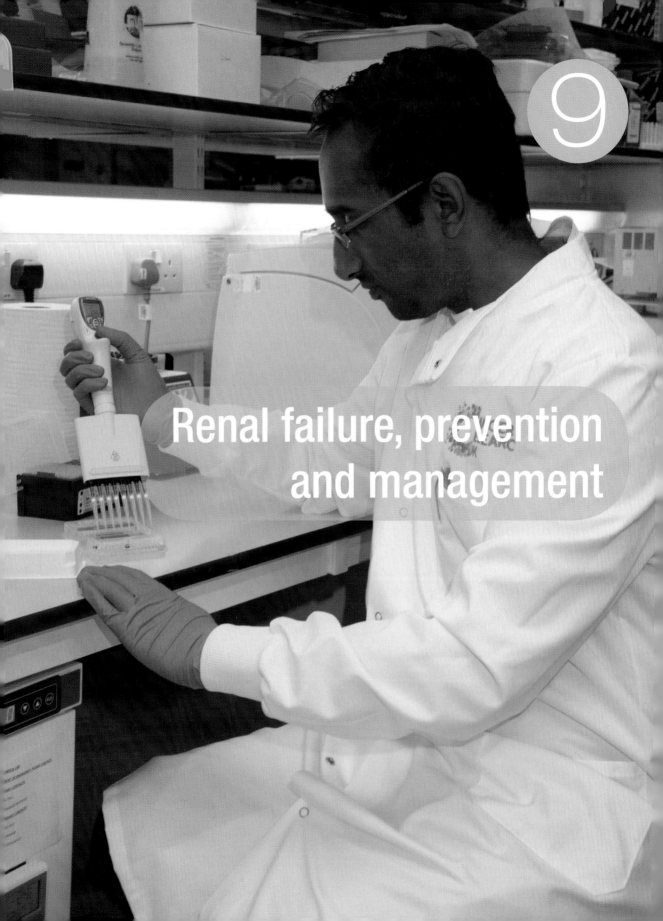

9

Renal failure, prevention and management

## Learning outcomes

This chapter will help you to:

- understand the functions of the kidney;

- anticipate and predict patients at risk of developing acute kidney injury (AKI);

- outline the initial management of a patient with AKI and associated life-threatening emergencies;

- state the common causes of AKI in the critically ill surgical patient;

- be aware of the implications for management of chronic kidney disease in the surgical patient.

Abnormal renal function is not infrequent in surgical patients and poor urine output is one of the most common reasons why you and your team may be called to see a patient. The kidneys have a wide range of functions and play a vital role in homeostasis. In the context of the critically ill patient, they can also be thought of as 'bilateral retroperitoneal indicators of cardiovascular stability'. Abnormal renal function is frequent in surgical patients, and poor urine output is one of the most common reasons for you and your team being called to see a patient. The kidneys have a wide range of functions and play a vital role in homeostasis.

Acute kidney injury (AKI) in critically ill patients is associated with increased mortality and is often preventable, particularly by careful fluid balance management in the perioperative period. It is the responsibility of the surgical team to anticipate and prevent AKI where possible. When it occurs, treatment is essentially supportive, but you must be aware of the associated life-threatening complications of AKI (hyperkalaemia, pulmonary oedema) and know how and when to refer for renal replacement therapy.

## Functions of the kidney

The primary functions of the kidney are:

- elimination of water-soluble waste products of metabolism other than carbon dioxide;

- elimination of water-soluble drugs;

- fluid and electrolyte homeostasis;

- acid–base balance;

- blood pressure control: renin–angiotensin system;

- endocrine function: erythropoietin and vitamin D production.

## Physiology of renal function

The kidney regulates fluid and electrolytes by filtration, secretion and reabsorption. Renal blood flow is approximately 20% of cardiac output (1000 ml/min in an adult) and renal plasma flow (RPF) is approximately 600 ml/min. The glomerulus filters 125 ml/min of renal plasma. This glomerular filtration rate (GFR) is a more accurate marker of renal function than plasma creatinine and can be estimated from the serum creatinine, BMI and gender. Most filtered fluid is reabsorbed, with only 1% passed as urine (0.5–1 ml/kg/h).

Renal blood flow is autoregulated and relatively constant over a wide range of mean arterial pressure (MAP). At low MAP, RPF and GFR become supply dependent and urine output decreases – this is the kidney protecting itself from further reduction in perfusion pressure (Figure 9.1). It is reversible in the short term but the kidney becomes more vulnerable to other insults, particularly the tubular cells deep in the medulla, which is more poorly perfused than the cortex.

The plasma creatinine level and GFR are inversely related. If the plasma creatinine level drifts outside the normal laboratory range, the GFR may already be 50% of normal values. It is important to recognise that a borderline creatinine may pose an increased risk of AKI, particularly in the elderly, as the GFR decreases with age (Figure 9.2).

### Practice points

- Normal adult urine output is 0.5–2.0 ml/kg/h.
- Oliguria is <0.5 ml/kg/h.
- Anuria is <100 ml/day (approximately 0.1 ml/kg/h).

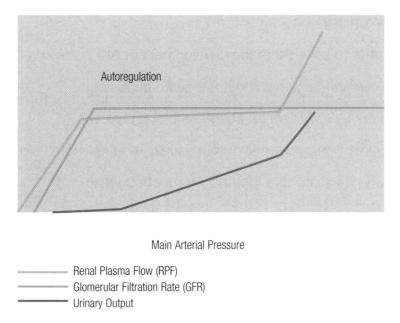

Main Arterial Pressure

———————— Renal Plasma Flow (RPF)
———————— Glomerular Filtration Rate (GFR)
———————— Urinary Output

Figure 9.1 Autoregulation maintains a steady GFR through a wide range of renal perfusion pressures.

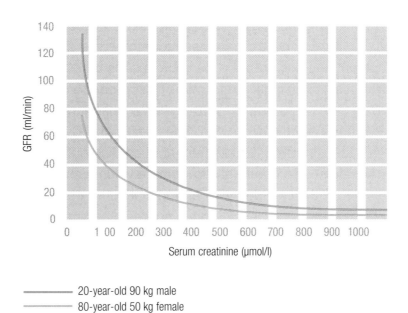

———————— 20-year-old 90 kg male
———————— 80-year-old 50 kg female

Figure 9.2 The GFR steadily decreases with age, but this is not evident in raised creatinine until a relatively low level is reached.

## Acute kidney injury

There are five points to consider in the development of AKI in the surgical patient:

- The kidneys cannot function without adequate perfusion.

- Renal perfusion is dependent on adequate blood pressure.

- A surgical patient with poor urine output usually requires more fluid.

- Absolute anuria is usually due to urinary tract obstruction.

- Poor urine output in a surgical patient is not initially treated with diuretics.

### Case scenario 9.1

Eight hours following an expedited open abdominal aortic aneurysm repair for leak, a 68-year-old man develops oliguria despite receiving 100 ml/h Hartmann's solution with no major change in pulse rate or blood pressure. He is ventilated and there are no signs of major haemorrhage or excess loss from the nasogastric tube. His CVP is 16 mmHg but the critical care nurse feels that the trace is unreliable and 'positional', and suggests that the patient is suboptimally perfused. The patient's Hb is 111 g/L. The junior trainee recommends a dose of furosemide (80 mg IV) to improve the urine output. This improves the urine output to 100 ml for 2 hours, after which it falls again to 20 ml/h. The on-call senior trainee prescribes a further dose of furosemide (40 mg IV) by telephone. This has no effect and the ICU consultant is contacted. She re-sites the CVP line and CVP is found to be very low (2 mmHg). Establishment of cardiac output monitoring (pulse pressure variation) also confirms a low stroke volume and intra-abdominal pressure is measured with no evidence of abdominal compartment syndrome. Immediate circulatory volume expansion does not restore urinary output despite improved stroke volume and a small increase in CVP. By the next day, the plasma creatinine and urea levels have risen rapidly and renal replacement therapy is required. The patient has a long and complicated course and dies of multiple organ failure 3 weeks later.

## Learning points

- Adequate renal perfusion is the critical factor – this is achieved with careful attention to fluid balance and cautious fluid challenges.

- Insensible and tissue fluid losses continue after surgery – postoperative hypovolaemia is common and is not necessarily caused by acute postoperative haemorrhage.

- CVP readings may complement clinical assessment but are influenced by multiple factors, particularly in the context of positive pressure ventilation.

- Consider advice from experienced nursing staff and always perform a three-stage CCrISP assessment of the patient.

- Furosemide will not salvage renal function in a hypovolaemic patient.

- The five points to consider in AKI would have helped in planning management of this patient.

## Definition of AKI

Acute kidney injury is a biochemical diagnosis associated with an acute increase in serum creatinine resulting from injury or an inability to excrete the nitrogenous and other waste products of metabolism.

There have been over 20 different classifications of acute renal failure. The system currently in use is that of Acute Kidney Injury Network (AKIN). The term AKI is preferred to renal failure as the pathophysiology may be reversible. AKI is compatible with the multiple insult hypothesis that a kidney exposed to multiple insults is more likely to be damaged, and so attention should be paid to ensuring other insults are dealt with or prevented. AKI is recognised as one of three clinical scenarios:

- an abrupt (within 48 hours) reduction in kidney function defined as an absolute increase in serum creatinine level of >26.4 µmol/L (0.3 mg/dl); or

- a percentage increase in serum creatinine level of >50% (1.5-fold from baseline); or

- a reduction in urine output (documented oliguria of <0.5 ml/kg/h for >6 hours.

These criteria should be applied in the context of the clinical presentation, following adequate fluid resuscitation and the exclusion of urinary tract obstruction.

There are three stages of AKI based on GFR and urine output, detailed in Table 9.1.

## Epidemiology

The incidence of AKI depends on the population being studied, from 5% of general acute hospital admissions, to 10% of unplanned surgical admissions to ICU and 50% of those with septic shock.

## Aetiology

There are diverse aetiologies to AKI, usually classified as prerenal, intrinsic renal and post-renal (Box 9.1). In surgical patients, prerenal failure is the most common aetiology (75%), followed by intrinsic renal and post-renal (20% and 5%, respectively).

In prerenal aetiologies, the kidney is structurally and functionally intact but blood flow, and GFR is reduced. This is a reversible state if treated urgently, but it can progress to acute tubular necrosis (ATN) in hours.

The renal vasculature, glomerular and tubulo-interstitium may all be affected in intrinsic renal damage. ATN also results from a combination of ischaemic and nephrotoxic injury. Post-renal failure results from obstruction and back-pressure, which disturbs tubular function. Relief of obstruction enables urine to flow, but tubular function may be disturbed during the recovery period.

In some people with certain genotypes, normal renal function may be restored more rapidly because some cells aestivate, ie they effectively shut down with hypoperfusion but maintain their microanatomical architecture throughout the period of AKI.

Table 9.1 Acute kidney injury classification: the AKIN criteria

| Stage | GFR criteria | Urine output criteria |
| --- | --- | --- |
| 1 | Increase in creatinine >26.4 µmol/L or 1.5- to 2.0-fold from baseline | <0.5 ml/kg/h over 6 hours |
| 2 | Increase in creatinine 2- to 3-fold from baseline | <0.5 ml/kg/h over 12 hours |
| 3 | Increase in creatinine 3-fold from baseline or serum creatinine >354 µmol/L | <0.3 ml/kg/h over 24 hours |

## Box 9.1 Common causes of AKI

### Prerenal

- Hypovolaemia
- Sepsis
- Low cardiac output

### Intrinsic renal

- Acute tubular necrosis
- Ischaemic injury – hypoxia, hypoperfusion
- Nephrotoxic injury – endotoxins, drugs, contrast, pigments
- Abdominal compartment syndrome
- Hepatorenal syndrome

### Post-renal

- Bladder outflow obstruction
- Bilateral ureteric obstruction

## Management of renal dysfunction

In surgical patients, there are four common scenarios regarding renal dysfunction:

- an elective patient at risk of AKI (with or without pre-operative chronic renal impairment);
- AKI in a critically ill patient;
- a patient with established AKI;
- a patient with chronic kidney disease (CKD).

*Preoperative management and prevention of renal dysfunction: predict and protect*

It is essential to identify patients at risk of developing perioperative renal dysfunction, particularly those with pre-existing renal impairment. Common causes of CKD include hypertension, diabetes, renal artery stenosis, glomerulonephritis and long-term use of drugs, eg diuretics, ACE inhibitors, non-steroidal anti-inflammatory drug (NSAIDs or aminoglycoside).

In the case of patients scheduled to undergo elective procedures, it is sometimes prudent to delay surgery, investigate the cause of pre-existing renal impairment and look at measures to protect renal function, including a review of drug therapy and considering the effect of nephrotoxins such as contrast media. Relevant investigations may include urinalysis, renal ultrasound and more detailed tests of split renal function, such as a MAG3 scan, although this is usually reserved for patients in whom nephrectomy is being contemplated. It is worth seeking the opinion of a renal physician at an early stage. Ensure optimum perioperative fluid balance and optimise the patient's cardiovascular status, especially in terms of volume, avoiding hypotension and hypovolaemia. Diabetes should also be closely monitored and controlled.

In the emergency setting, strict attention to fluid balance and maintenance of optimum cardiac output is essential, as is further avoidance of renal insults, including nephrotoxic drugs, and aggressive management of any sepsis. It is often a combination of factors that tip a patient into renal dysfunction, in particular the combination of hypovolaemia, nephrotoxic drugs and sepsis, rather than one specific insult. In both the elective and emergency setting, patients at risk should be reviewed regularly.

*Management of acute kidney injury*

Management involves the three-stage CCrISP assessment protocol, with particular attention to:

- recognition and correction of respiratory and circulatory problems;

- immediate identification and management of any life-threatening consequences of renal impairment;

- exclusion of urinary tract obstruction if anuric;

- careful search for, and correction of, the underlying cause;

- help early from appropriate specialists.

## Case scenario 9.2

A 45-year-old previously healthy woman presents with jaundice and cholangitis. She has a pyrexia (38.4°C) and a tachycardia (115 bpm) but is normotensive. She is treated with intravenous antibiotics and fluids and her condition improves. An urgent ultrasound scan suggests stones in the common bile duct. She is scheduled to undergo ERCP later in the week.

ERCP proves difficult and adequate drainage of the common bile duct is not achieved. External biliary drainage (EBD) is scheduled for the following day but, 12 hours after ERCP, the patient becomes hypotensive and pyrexial. The serum amylase and radiography are normal. Treatment is started with oxygen, and intravenous fluid challenges and intravenous antibiotics are continued. She is transferred to the HDU and a CVP line inserted (> 10 mmHg). The blood pressure is restored but the urine output remains poor and by the following morning the urea is 25.7 mmol/L and creatinine 229 μmol/L. The patient is not on any nephrotoxic drugs.

It is clear that definitive treatment in the form of biliary drainage is needed urgently. Emergency EBD is arranged for later the same day. The EBD is performed by a consultant radiologist with an anaesthetist and an HDU nurse in attendance and with appropriate monitoring. Successful biliary drainage is achieved but the patient requires several days of haemofiltration. She eventually makes a slow, but full, recovery, followed by successful ERCP and, subsequently, elective laparoscopic cholecystectomy.

## Learning points

- Multiple factors often contribute to AKI in surgical critical care – biliary obstruction, sepsis and hypovolaemia are a potent combination.

- Patients with obstructive jaundice tend to be hypovolaemic and need adequate fluid therapy and clinical monitoring.

- Procedures such as ERCP and EBD can exacerbate hypovolaemia or sepsis in a number of ways and adequate periprocedural antibiotics and intravenous fluids are needed in such cases – they are easily overlooked.

- Timely, definitive treatment of the underlying cause is usually the key to success.

## Practice point

Complete anuria means lower urinary tract/catheter obstruction until proven otherwise.

## Patient assessment

An accurate history is essential, supplemented by information available from relatives, the patient's GP and the case notes. A note should be made of any factors that predispose the patient to increased risk of renal failure.

Frequently, there are no specific symptoms associated directly with AKI. Uraemic symptoms, commonly seen in CRF (such as anorexia, nausea, vomiting and itching), are rare. Signs caused by the uraemic state, particularly fluid overload and pulmonary oedema, may be attributed to other clinical problems, especially in the patient with multi-organ failure. A thorough systematic examination is essential to identify any subtle signs of underlying disease, such as skin lesions in vasculitis, enlarged prostate and/or bladder and polycystic kidneys.

A thorough and repeated assessment of intravascular volume should be performed. This can be difficult in the critically ill patient, who may have adequate or excessive fluid but in the wrong compartment. The signs of hypovolaemia should be revised, but note that hypovolaemia can exist in the presence of normotension and significant extravascular oedema. Fluid overload may lead to an elevated blood pressure and a raised JVP/CVP. Extravascular fluid overload may manifest as peripheral and pulmonary oedema, ascites and effusions.

## Investigations in acute kidney injury

Dipstick urinalysis is mandatory in renal dysfunction. Marked proteinuria or microscopic haematuria with casts suggests a primary renal insult. Urine biochemistry and microbiology should also be considered, with biochemistry sometimes helping to distinguish between prerenal and intrinsic renal failure (see below). A renal ultrasound scan is also mandatory in any anuric patient. This should be performed immediately in an anuric patient, if an obvious urinary tract obstruction is not detected clinically. Ultrasound will also provide information regarding renal size and blood flow.

Plain abdominal X-ray is rarely useful, but plain chest X-ray can reveal pulmonary oedema. Further radiological investigation should be ordered only after discussion with your seniors, as it will often entail a contrast load and further renal insult for the patient. CT is the most useful investigation, along with radionucleotide studies, in identifying problems with renal blood flow, renal function and obstruction.

Blood tests should be considered to complement routine biochemistry depending on the clinical scenario (Box 9.2).

### Box 9.2 Blood tests to complement routine biochemical analysis

- FBC: to detect anaemia, infection
- Routine biochemistry: urea, creatinine; check potassium
- LFT: to recognise hepatorenal syndrome
- Calcium phosphate: if associated malignancy, rhabdomyolysis or tumour lysis suspected
- Creatine kinase: to detect rhabdomyolysis
- C-reactive protein: as a measure of infection and/or inflammation
- ABG and lactate: to assess hypoxia, acidosis and tissue/organ ischaemia

# Treatment

Look for a reversible cause and act urgently to:

- restore and maintain renal perfusion;
- relieve any obstruction;
- oxygenate the tubules;
- remove/avoid toxins;
- identify and treat any underlying cause.

## Checklist

### Is it prerenal?

Consider the clinical scenario. Surgical patients often become hypovolaemic, for a variety of reasons. Often, oliguria can be corrected by restoring volume.

### Distinguish prerenal from intrinsic renal problems due to ATN

Classically, with prerenal pathology, the concentrating ability of the tubular system is retained, producing urine with high osmolarity, high urea and creatinine and low sodium concentration. ATN results in a low osmolar urine with high sodium and low urea/creatinine is produced (Table 9.2). Note there are many confounding variables and, in clinical practice, the full biochemical analysis is rarely performed as a routine.

Table 9.2  Urine values in prerenal and intrinsic renal failure

| Investigation | Prerenal | Intrinsic renal |
| --- | --- | --- |
| Urinary specific gravity | >1.020 | <1.010 |
| Urinary sodium (mmol/L) | 10–20 | >20 |
| Urinary osmolality (mosmol/L) | >500 | <350 |
| Urine/plasma osmolality ratio | >2 | <1.1 |
| Urine/plasma urea ratio | >20 | <10 |
| Urine/plasma creatinine ratio | >40 | <20 |
| Fractional sodium excretion | <1% | >1% |
| Renal failure index | <1 | >1 |

Note that: fractional sodium excretion = (urine/plasma sodium ratio)/(urine/plasma creatinine ratio) × 100, and renal failure index = (urine sodium)/(urine/plasma creatinine ratio).

### Restore renal perfusion with volume

Aim to restore euvolaemia (using balanced salt solutions) and ensure regular monitoring of cardiovascular parameters, including urine output. Once the patient is euvolaemic, give maintenance fluid to match urine output and any on-going hourly losses. If circulating volume is not rapidly restored, invasive cardiovascular monitoring may be required. This may include central venous access and inotropic/vasoconstrictor support.

There is no significant evidence to support the use of diuretics or 'low-dose' dopamine in the prevention or treatment of renal impairment.

### Exclude post-renal obstruction

Exclude post-renal obstruction with ultrasonography and treat accordingly.

### Distinguish between acute and chronic renal problems

Ultrasound may reveal small kidneys (<9 cm) with echo-bright parenchyma, suggesting chronic damage. The acutely injured but normal kidney will be echo bright due to oedema, but will be of normal size and is more likely to recover. Acute on chronic renal failure is much less likely to recover.

### Oxygenate the tubules

Give oxygen and maintain a saturation of greater than 94%. Also ensure that the Hb level is greater than 70 g/L.

### Exclude toxins

Review the drug chart and avoid nephrotoxins, including contrast medium. Common examples are aminoglycosides, NSAIDs, ACE inhibitors and □-blockers (because of their hypotensive effect). When renal function is impaired, the dose of any drug excreted by the kidney, eg opioids, must be altered to prevent toxic side-effects. This is often overlooked on surgical wards. If in doubt, ask a pharmacist. Test for pigments such as myoglobinuria and haemoglobinuria where appropriate.

Rhabdomyolysis is the breakdown of damaged muscle with release of myoglobin into the circulation. This commonly occurs following crush injuries or acute limb ischaemia and is also recognised after prolonged surgery or immobility. Myoglobinuria manifests as dark-brown urine that tests positive for myoglobin on urinalysis. Treatment includes aggressive volume expansion and sodium bicarbonate to alkalinise the urine, creating a diuresis and limiting the negative effect of acid breakdown products of myoglobin on renal tubules. This is successful only if the condition is recognised early and treated immediately.

## Management of established AKI

### Indications for dialysis

If acute kidney injury fails to respond to the above measures, renal replacement therapy (RRT) will be required. The indications for RRT are summarised in Box 9.3.

### Box 9.3 Indications for renal replacement therapy

#### Absolute

- Refractory hyperkalaemia (>6 mmol/L)
- Refractory pulmonary oedema and fluid overload
- Uraemic encephalopathy

#### Relative

- Acidosis (pH <7.2)
- Uraemia
- Pericarditis
- Toxin removal

### Haemodialysis

Haemodialysis is a process by which low-molecular-weight solute equilibrates between a blood compartment and a dialysate compartment separated by a semipermeable membrane. Solute waste moves across the membrane down a concentration gradient (Figure 9.3a). The dialysate contains normal solutes, including sodium, calcium, magnesium and chloride, in the appropriate concentration to maintain normal levels. Dialysis can be intermittent or continuous. Intermittent dialysis creates rapid changes in plasma osmolality and volume, making continuous methods preferable in critically ill patients.

## Haemofiltration

In haemofiltration, there is a continuous convection of molecules across a permeable membrane (Figure 9.3b). The fluid that is removed is replaced with a buffered physiological solution. This is more effective in removing large quantities of fluid, but not as effective as dialysis at clearing smaller molecules. Filtration is usually performed using a continuous veno-venous method (ie continuous veno-venous haemofiltration, CVVH). This method provides the least risk of significant intravascular fluid shifts and haemodynamic instability and is therefore frequently the method of choice for providing renal support to patients in ICU.

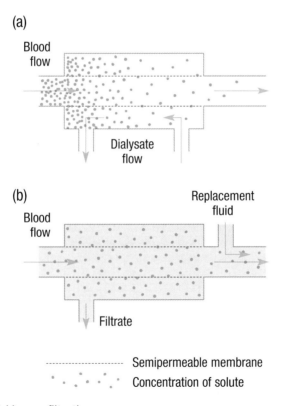

Figure 9.3 (a) Dialysis. (b) Haemofiltration.

The threshold for RRT in uraemia is controversial and relates to the rapidity of rise as well as the absolute level of urea and the presence of symptoms. A rise above 35 mmol/L unresponsive to other therapies is usually an absolute indication. RRT can be performed by dialysis or haemofiltration, depending on the clinical circumstances.

## Management of life-threatening complications

### Hyperkalaemia

Acute hyperkalaemia ($K^+$ above 6.5 mmol/L) requires immediate treatment to prevent life-threatening cardiac dysrhythmia and VF/asystolic arrest. Rate of rise is also important: a rapid rise to 6 mmol/L is equally a cause for concern. There are usually no symptoms specific to a rise in potassium and clinical suspicion in the vulnerable patient is crucial.

Any underlying contributory cause should be identified and stopped, including blood transfusions, drugs that reduce renal potassium excretion (potassium sparing diuretics, ACE inhibitors, etc) or intravenous fluid containing potassium and potassium supplements.

An ECG should be performed. Hyperkalaemia may cause peaked T waves, absent P waves, widened QRS and ventricular arrhythmias. In the presence of ECG changes and a potassium above 6 mmol/L, emergency measures should be instituted to reduce $K^+$ levels temporarily, though this will only shift the potassium into the intracellular space. Immediate measures include (also see Table 9.3):

Table 9.3  Emergency therapy for hyperkalaemia

| Drug | Mechanism of action | Pros and cons |
| --- | --- | --- |
| Calcium gluconate IV (10–30 ml of 10% solution) | Membrane stabilisation | Rapid effect but transient action |
| Insulin/dextrose [insulin (10–20 U of Actrapid) in 100 ml of 20% dextrose IV over 30 minutes] | Drives potassium into cells | Rapid effect, intermediate action but may cause hypoglycaemia |
| Sodium bicarbonate (50 mmol IV over 5–10 minutes followed by IV infusion of 1.26% or 1.4% solution at 100 ml/h) | Transfer of potassium into cells by exchange for hydrogen across membrane | Rapid effect – intermediate action, best with metabolic acidosis; beware sodium overload |
| Salbutamol (5–10 µg/min by IV infusion, or nebulised) | Transfer of potassium into cells | Rapid effect, short action; risk of tachycardia, vasodilator effect, frequent use can raise serum lactate |

- commencing continuous cardiac monitoring;

- insulin (10–20 units of Actrapid) in 100 ml 20% dextrose intravenously over 30 minutes;

- sodium bicarbonate 50 mmol intravenously over 5–10 minutes;

- 10% calcium gluconate intravenously (10–30 ml);

- $\beta_2$-agonist, eg nebulised or IV salbutamol.

If, after emergency treatment, renal function is not improving, treatment should be introduced to reduce total body potassium. This can be achieved by (i) renal replacement therapy (particularly if combined with fluid overload); or (ii) ion exchange resin (in the form of calcium resonium, 15 g 6- to 8-hourly or 30 g rectally (this binds potassium within the gut but is very unpleasant to take and is of limited benefit).

## Pulmonary oedema

Pulmonary oedema presents as acute shortness of breath, associated with anxiety, tachycardia, tachypnoea, cool peripheries, and widespread crepitations/wheeze. If pulmonary oedema is suspected, a chest X-ray should be performed immediately (if safe to do so). Sit the patient upright, stop all intravenous infusions, give high-flow oxygen and monitor saturations with a view to achieve $SaO_2$ of greater than 94%. Further treatment options include:

- intravenous diamorphine 2.5 mg for vasodilatory and anxiolytic effects;

- intravenous GTN infusion, if systolic BP is greater than 100 mmHg: commence infusion at 2 mg/h and titrate upwards every 15 minutes;

- intravenous furosemide, 250 mg in 50 ml saline over 1 hour;

- review regularly;

- discuss higher level of support, particularly in the presence of oligo/anuria, continued tachypnoea (>30/min), signs of fatigue, respiratory failure ($PaO_2$ <8 kPa, $PaCO_2$ >7 kPa), acidosis (pH <7.2).

CPAP can also be helpful in treating pulmonary oedema.

## Checklist when making a nephrology referral

Expect to answer the following:

- Clinical scenario – what do you think is going on?

- What is the patient's premorbid state?

- What are the most recent creatinine, serum potassium and ABG results?

- What is the patient's volume and cardiovascular status?

- What volumes of urine is the patient passing?

- What was the 'pre-insult' renal function?

- What does the ultrasonography show?

- What drugs is the patient on (in particular have they received any nephrotoxins)?

## Prognosis and recovery

As individual nephrons recover, the kidney behaves as in CRF. Because only a proportion of the nephron mass has recovered, each nephron has a much higher solute load to excrete. There is, therefore, a major limitation in the kidneys' ability to conserve sodium, potassium, bicarbonate and water. With modern management of renal dysfunction, it is unusual to see major problems with large fluid and electrolyte losses. The major exception is in postobstructive diuresis, when losses need to be measured and replaced as appropriate. It is important that the recovering kidney is not exposed to further hypotensive or nephrotoxic insults. By 6 months, the kidney will normally have recovered 85–90% of premorbid function, though some 10% of patients may progress to CRF requiring permanent RRT or transplantation.

Prognosis is often determined by the severity of the underlying incident that caused the injury. However, in-hospital AKI due to ATN carries 20–30% mortality, most commonly due to infection or cardiovascular complications.

## Case scenario 9.3

You are asked to see a 75-year-old hypertensive diabetic woman on the ward who had a reversal of Hartmann's procedure 2 days ago. Her observations reveal a BP of 110/70, pulse 100 bpm, temperature 37.8°C, $O_2$ saturations 89% (on air) and urine output of 20 ml for the past 3 hours. Her blood tests this morning are available: Hb 101 g/L, urea 8 mmol/L, creatinine 123 μmol/L, $Na^+$ 130 mmol/L, $K^+$ 5.0 mmol/L.

**What are your priorities and what other information do you want to know?**

- Follow the CCrISP three-stage assessment, in particular with regard to assessing the renal dysfunction. This patient is unstable and careful monitoring is required. She may be developing AKI.

- Oxygenate the tubules by sitting the patient up, administering high-flow oxygen and instituting continuous $O_2$ monitoring.

- To restore renal perfusion, you should prescribe fluid challenges. You do not want the patient to develop pulmonary oedema, so use smaller volumes over short time periods, eg 500 ml of normal saline over 15 minutes, then reassess.

- Review drugs for nephrotoxins. Stop any ACE inhibitors or NSAIDs.

- You need to know the preoperative blood pressure and serum creatinine, weight of the patient, plus fluid balance since surgery on chart review.

- Your plan should include regular observations (every 30 minutes), aiming for a systolic BP of 130–140 mmHg, BP < 100 bpm, $SaO_2$ > 94%, RR 12–15/min, and urine output of 30 ml/h. Set a time for review in 1–2 hours.

After the fluid challenge, you find that the patient's blood pressure has improved and systolic pressure is now 140 mmHg, which is good for renal perfusion, although urine output is still poor at 20 ml in 2 hours. Her $SaO_2$ is 94% on supplemental oxygen and, worryingly, the respiratory rate has risen to 24/min.

How would you manage this situation now?

The findings are compatible with the development of pulmonary oedema and you should reassess the patient. You should consider stopping further fluid challenges, and arranging a chest X-ray and ABGs, re-checking biochemistry.

The chest X-ray shows interstitial oedema, and ABG analysis reveals an acidosis (pH 7.25, $PaO_2$ 9 kPa, $PaCO_2$ 4.5 kPa, BE –5 mmol/L, lactate 2 mmol/L) and the biochemistry is worse (urea 12 mmol/L, creatinine 148 μmol/L, $Na^+$ 129 mmol/L, $K^+$ 5.9 mmol/L).

What is your assessment? What should you do?

It looks as though the patient is developing pulmonary oedema (interstitial oedema, hypoxaemia) and established acute kidney injury (creatinine and $K^+$ rising, metabolic acidosis). She needs a higher level of care than can be provided on the ward. Discuss her organ failure and need for renal and respiratory support with the critical care team.

Learning points

- Predict and prevent renal dysfunction by identifying the surgical patient at risk.

- Immediate management of AKI requires close attention to fluid balance while recognising the risk of developing pulmonary oedema.

- Pulmonary oedema can be life-threatening and often requires a higher level of care with respiratory and renal support.

# Future developments

Creatinine and urine output are relatively insensitive markers of renal function and hence new 'biomarkers' are being sought to identify and predict those at risk of impending AKI. These include neutrophil gelatinase-associated lipocalin and kidney injury marker-1.

## Chronic kidney disease

CKD is defined as chronic irreversible loss of nephron mass resulting in permanent impairment of solute waste excretion. These patients do not necessarily need permanent RRT. When using the Cockcroft–Gault formula to estimate the GFR, 5% of the adult population will be found to have subclinical stage 3 CKD (a GFR 30–60 ml/min). Such patients deserve special attention to detail in the perioperative period due to:

- significant risk of developing AKI;

- multiple medications, especially cardiovascular drugs;

- concomitant silent cardiovascular disease;

- abnormal cardiovascular physiology, eg autonomic dysfunction reducing normal response to volume changes, especially in diabetic patients;

- abnormal gastrointestinal function, delayed transit, impaired absorption;

- abnormal drug handling – impaired excretion requires dose modification; consult a pharmacist.

Patients who have CKD have much less ability to compensate for circulatory stress and the effects of nephrotoxins. A simple example is the patient with significant CKD (creatinine of 300 µmol/L) who is fasted overnight prior to surgery. This will cause mild intravascular volume depletion. As there are far fewer nephrons, each has to carry increased solute, and this acts as an osmotic diuretic that prevents concentration of the urine. This prevents maximum sodium and water retention until there has been a significant fall in GFR secondary to a contracted circulating volume. The patient becomes hypovolaemic and renal function decreases. Depriving patients with CKD of oral fluid for lengths of time greater than 4–6 hours should be avoided unless fluid is given intravenously.

Many patients with severe CKD will be chronically anaemic. Preoperative transfusion will acutely impair renal function by altering the flow characteristics of the blood and is seldom necessary.

Patients with a transplanted kidney must be managed in conjunction with their nephrologist or transplant centre. Skilled assistance will be required to manage their immunosuppression and reduce the likelihood of an acute rejection episode.

## Summary

Predict and prevent acute kidney injury, and remember the five points to consider in the development of AKI:

- The kidneys cannot function without adequate perfusion.

- Renal perfusion is dependent on adequate blood pressure.

- A surgical patient with poor urine output usually requires more fluid.

- Absolute anuria is usually due to urinary tract obstruction.

- Poor urine output in a surgical patient is not treated initially with diuretics.

## Further reading

### Acute kidney injury

Bellomo R, Kellum JA, Ronco C. Acute kidney injury. *Lancet* 2012; **380**: 756–766.

Mehta RL, Kellum JA, Shah SV et al. Acute Kidney Injury Network: report of an initiative to improve outcomes in acute kidney injury. *Crit Care* 2007; **11(20)**: R31.

### Chronic kidney disease

Plantinga C, Tuot DS, Powe NR. Awareness of chronic kidney disease among patients and providers. *Adv Chronic Kidney Dis* 2010; **17**: 223–236.

### Fluid assessment/management

Powell-Tuck J, Gosling P, Lobo DN et al. British Consensus Guidelines on Intravenous Fluid Therapy for Adult Surgical Patients (GIFTASUP). NHS National Library of Health, London. Available at http://www.ics.ac.uk/downloads/ 2008112340_ GIFTASUP%20 FINAL_31-10-08.pdf.

Steddon S, Chesser A, Cunningham J, Ashman N, *Oxford Handbook of Nephrology and Hypertension*, 2nd edn. Oxford University Press, Oxford; 2014.

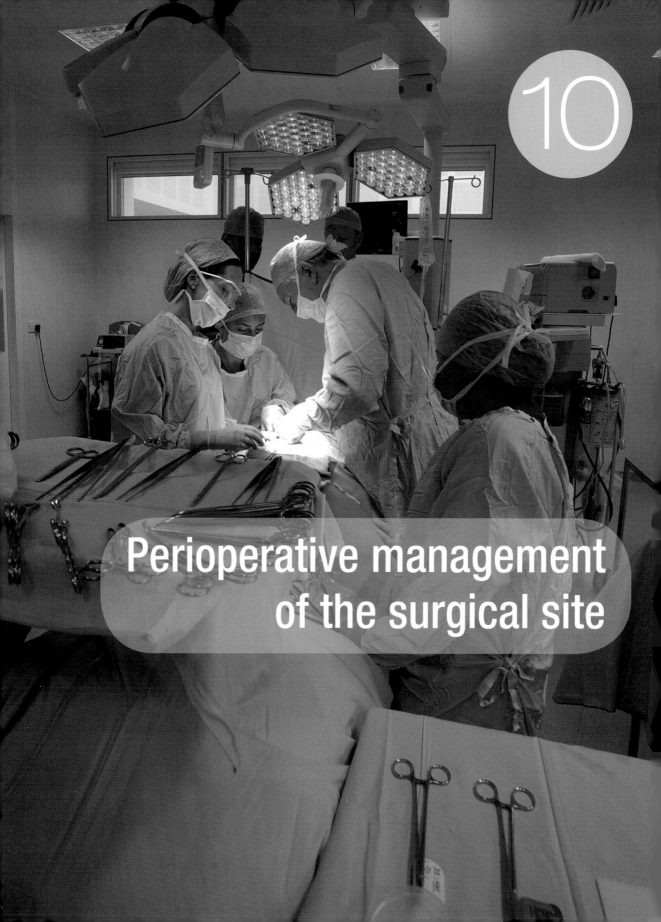

10

Perioperative management of the surgical site

## Learning outcomes

This chapter will help you to:

- utilise the CCrISP system to assess and manage patient problems associated with the surgical site;

- discuss the presentation of common and/or serious complications in surgical patients;

- contribute to planning the management of patients in the HDU or ICU;

- outline the management of surgical wounds, drains and stomas.

## Introduction

Surgery is a significant physiological insult, especially when performed for a life-threatening condition in a patient who is significantly unwell at first presentation. Preoperative patient optimisation balanced against the need to correct the underlying pathology in a timely manner is key to success. Likewise, in the period following the procedure, it is essential to have a plan for on-going resuscitation and recovery, which should be discussed prior to surgery with the relevant multidisciplinary team members, including the anaesthetic consultant, critical care consultant and surgical consultant. This discussion should include whether surgery has a realistic chance of success, management of patient expectation and possible ceilings of care. The patient (and his or her relatives if appropriate) should be involved in these discussions.

Even with all these factors in place there is a risk that complications may arise, including infection, haemorrhage, ischaemia or incomplete resolution of the original pathology. The challenge is to be able to recognise any deterioration early and intervene before the advent of organ failure. In this way it may be possible to avoid some critical care admissions but, if admission is unavoidable, the patients are transferred as early as possible and in the best possible state to enhance the chances of a successful outcome. While recognising physiological deterioration in the immediate management phase, the history of the presentation or the operation notes will give a better guide to a likely cause, and allow successful intervention if events are predicted. The ability to anticipate problems is an important skill to acquire (see Table 10.1), allowing earlier and targeted intervention and decreasing the chance

Table 10.1 Examples of anticipated postoperative complications associated with initial presentation

| Surgical presentation | Potential postoperative complication |
| --- | --- |
| Infarcted bowel from intestinal ischaemia | Further ischaemia causing anastomotic breakdown, abscess/collection, fistula formation |
| Ruptured abdominal aortic aneurysm | Open repair: reactive or secondary haemorrhage/abdominal compartment syndrome/lower limb ischaemia/postoperative ileus Endovascular repair: stent thrombosis and limb ischaemia/abdominal compartment syndrome/renal impairment |
| Diverticular abscess and systemic sepsis | Anastomotic leak and recurrent sepsis. Intraperitoneal abscess Any inotropic support will increase risk of anastomotic leak or end stoma infarction |
| Penetrating abdominal trauma | Increased risk of sepsis/need for laparostomy if regular relook laparotomy required Risk of abdominal compartment syndrome |
| Appendicitis | Wound infection and abscess formation Intraperitoneal pelvic collection |
| Any presentation with comorbid risk factors: age, obesity, smoking and diabetes | Consider these comorbidities and the complications which might occur related to these factors. Then refer to Chapters 16 and 17 for further information |

of deterioration. Operative mortality can be in excess of 50% among patients who develop organ failure.

It is often difficult, when you are time pressed on a routine ward round, to assess the surgical site properly on a ward or critical care area. However, it is the surgical team's responsibility to ensure that there is appropriate monitoring and a management plan in place for all patients. This includes all components of the surgical site, including wound management and plans for drains, stomas or fistulae.

### Practice task

Reflect on your last major operation. Consider what the potential complications were, and how they may have presented. If the patient did experience complications, what could have been done to prevent them?

## Postoperative assessment of the surgical site

The end of an operation is equivalent to the 'decide and plan' component of the CCrISP assessment system. The desired outcome would be for the patient to be stable and progressing safely with a structured management plan in place.

That plan begins with the operation note, which should clearly document the indication for the procedure and the essential findings. The operative procedure and any difficulties encountered should be described, as this may assist others when assessing any subsequent deterioration in the patient. For example, a long dissection for dense adhesions may have resulted in an unrecognised enterotomy, and repairs to serosal tears may give way. An operative diagram is often helpful to describe the internal and external anatomy, as well as representing the position of drains and stomas. Clear postoperative instructions must be written, especially with regard to the frequency of observations, when the next blood tests should be done, management of drains or stomas, when or how to start feeding, plans for mobilisation and any tasks or issues specific to the case (see case scenario 10.1).

In addition, a description of anticipated complications or the warning signs indicate the need for prompt surgical review at an appropriate level, will prevent delay in the identification of deterioration, especially if the patient is admitted to the ICU or HDU.

When you are asked to assess the postoperative patient outwith your usual schedule of reviews, it is likely that they are deviating from their predicted course. From your knowledge of the preoperative presentation, such as the examples in Table 10.1, you should have suspicions of potential complications. However, you must use the CCrISP system of assessment to guide your management and prevent omissions; do not jump to conclusions and do not try to fit the findings to one of the known complications. If you are unsure of the cause, the three-stage assessment system will enable you to recognise if the patient is unstable or deteriorating, and help you to plan if senior surgical or ICU review is necessary. This way you can be confident in your findings and call for help as appropriate, and be clear about why you are asking for help.

### Anticipating a need for critical care

You should have observed that some patients are planned for critical care preoperatively because of factors that predict a need for more intensive support, such as:

- their age;

- critical nature of their diagnosis;

- preoperative comorbidity;

- acute physiological stress.

Current guidance from the National Emergency Laparotomy Audit recommends the completion of a postoperative assessment bundle to determine where the patient should be cared for in the initial postoperative period.

Pre-emptive transfers allow for early recognition of any complication and so minimise the delay in any additional treatment needed.

## Recognising deterioration on critical care

The benefit of more intensive patient monitoring is the early recognition of systemic changes, since these will raise a suspicion of new pathology developing, eg a rise in serum lactate in a blood gas sample may raise suspicions of intra-abdominal pathology and prompt intervention far earlier than waiting for the patient to develop signs when the abdomen is examined.

While the abdomen alone may seem a likely source when deterioration occurs after laparotomy, consider alternative causes such as sepsis from lines, urine or chest, or limb ischaemia in a prothrombotic state. Information from critical care monitoring can help you to work through these differentials. A missed intra- abdominal sepsis or ischaemia is often fatal and if other causes for the deterioration are being considered they have to be of sufficient magnitude to explain the deterioration – minimal findings on clinical and radiological examination of the chest should not be ascribed as the cause of major patient deterioration.

### Practice task

Consider previous ICU patients you have seen with abdominal pathology. Were there obvious abdominal signs or did you rely on the charts to identify clinical deterioration?

## Assessing the abdomen on critical care

Often clinical abdominal signs are unreliable in the ventilated or sedated patient and in the presence of a large laparotomy wound. It is easy to be lured into a false sense of security because the abdomen feels soft and non-distended; conversely, in non-ventilated patients, it is easy to overinterpret tenderness and guarding.

Careful analysis of the patient's observation charts, taking into account the degree of support the patient is receiving, will help you recognise whether the patient is making progress or deteriorating. For example, the charts may show a gradual increase in oxygen or ventilatory requirements, or an increasing dependence on inotropes to maintain perfusion. The urine output may be gradually diminishing despite adequate fluid filling.

### Practice point

Think of patients you have seen that have demonstrated features of deterioration. Was there a concern about reoperating, or a delay in return to theatre?

Patients' transport to theatre is often delayed by subtle and gradual clinical deterioration. Close liaison and good communication with the critical care team is vital in these circumstances if patients are to have good outcomes.

While it may be the systemic signs that show the patient's deterioration, the diagnostic question is whether this is due to bleeding, perforation, mesenteric ischaemia, pancreatitis or sepsis, and where the source might be. Within the abdomen there may be the temptation to confirm the diagnosis with imaging, but one should carefully appraise the benefits of this as opposed to direct intervention with a laparotomy. If a colonic anastomotic leak is suspected, abdominal and pelvic CT may be useful. It may reveal pathology that can be treated without further surgery; for example, it may reveal a collection that can be treated by radiological drainage. A negative scan does not exclude a leak completely, and the delay caused by transfer to and from the CT scanner should be weighed against the benefit of rapid drainage from an immediate return to theatre. The possibility of false-positive findings also need to be considered and imaging should be performed only if it will alter management, not to justify a decision that has already been made. Ultrasound scanning may show free fluid but will rarely result in a change in management; ultrasound is of little value in excluding diagnoses. Simple blood tests, particularly the white cell count and blood gases, may guide you towards a specific cause of deterioration, as shown in Table 10.2. Take all possible cultures (blood, pus, urine or sputum, etc) in order to direct therapy in the longer term. If you are not sure, seek senior help and advice, do not just organise more tests. A major focus of specialty training is to learn when decisions need to be made and who needs to make them.

Table 10.2 Warning signs of significant pathology

| Warning sign | Possible underlying surgically related causes |
| --- | --- |
| Neutropenia (neutrophil count $< 1 \times 10^9$/L) | Overwhelming sepsis/profoundly impaired host response |
| Grossly elevated WCC ($> 20–25 \times 10^9$/L) | Sign of infarction, presence of a collection<br>Also occurs post splenectomy<br>Consider *Clostridium* spp. infection if associated diarrhoea |
| Metabolic acidosis, elevated lactate | Tissue hypoperfusion from ischaemia or sepsis |

In patients with more subtle postoperative changes, contrast CT arterial imaging may exclude an ischaemic cause. Isolating a focus of infection may require a white cell labelled scan. However, in the case of acute deterioration there is no time to delay and a laparotomy may be indicated.

Occasionally, a laparotomy performed as part of a diagnostic process in a deteriorating surgical patient will be negative. This does not necessarily mean that laparatomy was the wrong course of action, but delaying the patient's return to theatre for a prolonged period will invariably lead to a worse outcome.

Case scenario 10.1

You are asked to assess a 45-year-old, 120-kg man on the ICU who underwent laparotomy for blunt abdominal trauma 10 hours previously. There is concern that, despite fluid resuscitation, he remains tachycardic and hypotensive. He is still ventilated. You arrive on the ICU and the nurse asks: 'Do you think he could be bleeding?'

## How would you manage this situation?

This is a difficult and complex assessment, especially since the patient remains ventilated. However, if you follow the CCrISP three-stage system, this patient can be assessed thoroughly and systematically in a similar manner to the non-ventilated patient (Figure 10.1). Your immediate management is as follows:

A: Intubated and ventilated.

B: ICU report increasing airway pressure required to ventilate. Inspired oxygen unchanged.

C: HR = 120 bpm, BP = 90/60 mmHg, CVP = 12 cmH$_2$O, though cardiac output is reducing.

No external signs of continued haemorrhage. Minimal reduction in Hb from 95 to 86 g/L in the last 5 hours though patient has had transfusion of 4 units of blood since theatre. Urine output in the last 7 hours was 200 ml.

D: Pupils respond appropriately. Patient is heavily sedated.

E: This patient is obese but you note that the abdomen appears distended.

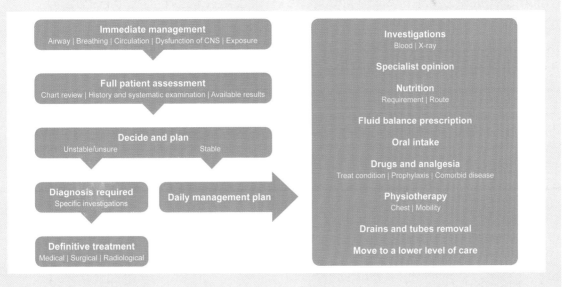

Figure 10.1 The CCrISP system of assessment.

**Is this patient stable or unstable and what would you do at this stage?**

The patient is clearly unstable. You need to consider whether more resuscitation is required or whether to call the surgical consultant for an immediate return to theatre. It is reasonable to gather more information and continue with the system of assessment while the ICU staff continue resuscitation. Using the CCrISP system, you would perform a full patient assessment. The available results are (all conventional units): Hb 86 g/L, WCC 18.9 × 10⁹/L, platelets 65 × 10⁹/L, amylase 240 units/L, $Na^+$ 128 mmol/L, $K^+$ 5.9 mmol/L, urea 12.5 mmol/L, pH 7.3, $PO_2$ 10.5 kPa, $PaCO_2$ 6 kPa, BE –7 mmol/L (increased from –3 mmol/L in last 3 hours). Chart review: the operation note reports the need for a splenectomy and extensive bleeding from the vena cava (Figure 10.2). An important part of this assessment is to clearly determine with the ICU staff whether the patient is having to have a lot of volume to maintain perfusion and what happens when boluses are given – repeated 'chasing' of volume may indicate on-going bleeding.

**Does this help you make a decision? Consider what your management plan would be and whether you need any other investigations**

A simple investigation is to check intra-abdominal pressure, which is now 28 mmHg (it was previously 18 mmHg). Therefore, this patient has abdominal compartment syndrome and should be immediately returned to theatre and his abdomen reopened. Further delay increases the risk of worsening organ dysfunction and further resuscitation or conservative measures will not be beneficial without immediate decompression. The decision to return the patient to theatre needs to be made by the surgical consultant in charge of the case; your role is to recognise that a decision needs to be made, by whom, and that this needs to be done without delay. In this case, the patient is returned to theatre and laparotomy reveals no on-going haemorrhage and a viable colon so the abdomen is left open as a laparostomy.

**Consider the problems that might be encountered when the patient is transferred back to ICU**

**Learning point**

- Abdominal compartment syndrome can lead rapidly to multiple organ failure which, without immediate decompression, is usually fatal.

2am   10/07/10
LAPAROTOMY FOR BLUNT TRAUMA
SPLENECTOMY. REPAIR OF GASTRIC AND CAVAL LACERATIONS
SURGEON- MR.Meanor/MR.R.S.Cue
ANAESTHETIST- DR.Gas
FINDINGS - Lacerated splen, Anterior Gastric Wall laceration
and midline retroperitoneal Haematoma.
PROCEDURE - Splenectomy with individual ligation of splenic vessels
2/0 PDS repair to gastric wall.
Exploration of Haematoma, massive blood loss.
Vascular surgery called.
At least 5 litre reported blood loss
Caval and iliac venous control by compression
3/0 prolene repair to large IVC defect with impingement of
proximal R iliac vein.
No arterial injury. R. Ureter intac

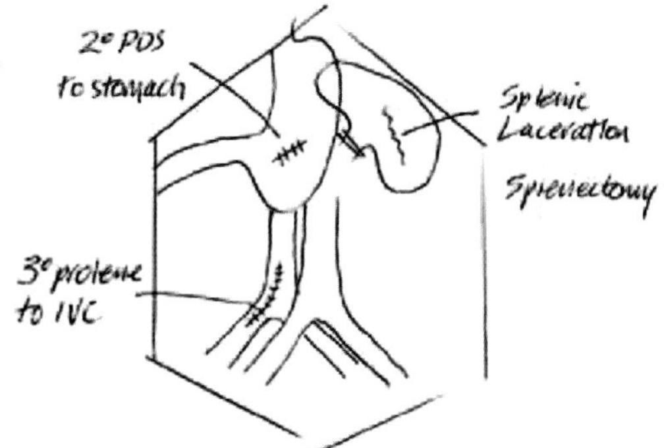

2° PDS
to stomach

3° prolene
to IVC

Splenic
Laceration

Splenectomy

Closure difficult. Intravesical pressure at the end 18mm Hg.
Post op.
     - Remain intubated.              - ICU support
     - NG Aspirate                    - Transfuse to Hb of 9g/dl
     - Massive blood loss so correct coagulopathy
     TED stockings

Figure 10.2 Operation note.

# Specific surgical site complications

## Abdominal compartment syndrome

Abdominal compartment syndrome or the presence of elevated intra-abdominal pressure is a significant cause of morbidity and mortality among critically ill surgical and medical patients. As shown in Table 10.3, major systemic effects occur with a rise in abdominal pressure.

Intra-abdominal hypertension (IAH) is a continuum of pathophysiological changes that begins with a disturbance of regional blood flow and culminates in frank end-organ failure, due to the development of abdominal compartment syndrome. The aetiology of IAH may be intra-abdominal, particularly in abdominal trauma patients (see scenario above), pancreatitis or following aortic surgery, but can also occur due to an extra-abdominal cause, such as burns or sepsis associated with aggressive fluid resuscitation.

Intra-abdominal pressure is expressed in mmHg, with the usual level being subatmospheric to 0 mmHg, though elevation to the range of 5–7 mmHg is common.

IAH is a sustained or repeated elevation of IAP > 12 mmHg and is graded as follows: I, 12–15 mmHg; II, 16–20 mmHg; III, 21–25 mmHg; IV > 25 mmHg. Grade IV requires surgical decompression.

The cardiac effect of IAH is due to elevation of the diaphragm and the subsequent rise in intrathoracic pressure, which in turn reduces the venous return and cardiac output.

Table 10.3 Systemic Effects Of Abdominal Compartment Syndrome

| System | Intra-abdominal pressure | | |
| --- | --- | --- | --- |
| | 10–15 mmHg | 16–25 mmHg | >25 mmHg |
| Cardiovascular | | Reduced preload and increased afterload<br>Reduced cardiac output | Reduced contractility<br>Gross reduction in cardiac output |
| Renal | | Oliguria | Anuria |
| Gastrointestinal | Slight intestinal and hepatic ischaemia | Marked intestinal and hepatic ischaemia | Bowel infarction<br>Hepatic failure |
| CNS | | Minimal effect | Increased intracranial pressure |

Such changes are far more likely in the hypotensive patient and so early signs of pressure elevation should be managed by fluid resuscitation.

Abdominal compartment syndrome is the progression of pressure induced end-organ changes and, if due to intra-abdominal causes such as trauma or acute pancreatitis, is characterised by rapid deterioration which if not recognised and treated is often fatal.

The treatment for ACS is to re-open or perform a laparotomy wound in order to decompress the abdomen. As in the scenario above, a thorough washout of all fluid/ blood should be performed, with a detailed inspection for sites of bleeding. The bowel should be carefully inspected for signs of ischaemia.

There are a number of options available at the end of the laparotomy though, usually, primary closure should not be considered. A large saline infusion bag can be opened up and sutured to the fascial edges in order to provide a temporary seal of the abdominal cavity (Bogota bag). Specific bowel bags can also be used in a similar way. Other temporary abdominal closure devices are available, including topical negative pressure systems and zippers. Leaving the abdomen open increases the risk of bowel damage and fistula formation, and care needs to be taken in this respect. Figure 10.3 shows a laparostomy in a patient who later underwent successful split skin graft closure.

Postoperatively, laparostomy patients can be challenging to manage, particularly from the nursing point of view. As the surgeon, you should liaise closely with the ICU staff and predict problems with fluid and temperature losses through the laparostomy wound and the potential for sepsis, especially with respect to any underlying vascular grafts, and make a plan to achieve wound closure.

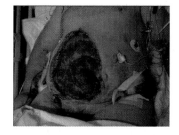 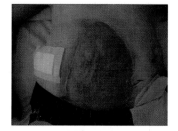

Figure 10.3 A laparostomy and outcome following mesh closure and skin graft.

## Case scenario 10.2

You are asked by the ICU staff to assess a 25-year-old man who, 14 hours following laparotomy for a penetrating abdominal stab wound, is becoming increasingly unstable with a base excess of −8 mmol/L. You follow the CCrISP system to assess and resuscitate the patient. Your findings from the initial management are:

A: Intubated.

B: Ventilated, parameters and oxygen requirement stable.

C: HR = 120 bpm; BP = 95/75; CVP = 6 cmH$_2$O, cold peripheries, pedal pulses not palpable, increasing dose of noradrenaline required, urine output 250 ml since return from theatre.

D: Pupils respond appropriately. Patient is paralysed.

E: Abdominal wound is laparostomy, with appearance of right-sided stoma.

Full patient assessment of available results: Hb 90, WCC 24, platelets 75, amylase 200, sodium 130, potassium 6.5, urea 16, pH 7.2, $PO_2$ 12.5 kPa, $PaCO_2$ 5 kPa, BE −8, lactate 5, creatine kinase 4000 u/L. Chart review showed the patient was stabbed in the abdomen and suffered significant blood loss at the scene. He had a systolic pressure of only 70 mmHg on arrival in the emergency department. He was immediately taken to theatre, where laparotomy findings were a distal aortic laceration and a small sigmoid laceration with minimal contamination. The sigmoid laceration was closed primarily but defunctioning ileostomy performed. Significant blood loss occurred before and during the aortic repair with repeated episodes of clamping. It was a long procedure; therefore, abdominal packing was inserted with a relook planned at 24 hours.

*What do you think might account for the deterioration and how would you manage the situation?*

It is unlikely to be abdominal compartment syndrome because of the laparostomy. You need to perform a thorough systematic examination, in particular looking at the patient's lower limb vasculature because of the history of aortic injury. Only femoral pulses are palpable; both feet are cold and poorly perfused. From toes to knees, the calves are very swollen and tense. The patient is clearly unstable and no further investigations are required to confirm the diagnosis of bilateral lower limb compartment syndrome. Arrangements are made for urgent fasciotomies to be performed. Upon performing the fasciotomies, all muscle groups are very oedematous and immediately bulge from the wounds. Some areas of muscle do not contract to electrical (diathermy) or physical stimuli, though other areas contract normally.

## Lower limb compartment syndrome

Limb compartment syndrome should always be considered when there has been a period of ischaemia and perfusion. Case scenario 10.2 highlights the need for thorough systematic assessment and prompt therapeutic action. A delay in recognising limb compartment syndrome can rapidly lead to irreversible muscle damage, resulting in permanent neuromuscular defects within 12 hours. This may necessitate amputations. Also, aggressive fluid resuscitation is required to minimise the effects of myoglobin from muscle breakdown that can cause acute kidney injury.

Lower limb trauma and associated hypotension may lead to reperfusion with a significant rise in interstitial pressure and subsequent compartment syndrome. Prolonged operation in the lithotomy position can also produce compartment syndrome and any delay in treatment minimises the chances of limb salvage. If there is any doubt in the diagnosis, compartment pressures can be performed with a needle inserted into each compartment, with the knowledge that tissue necrosis can occur with an interstitial pressure as low as 30 mmHg.

### Practice point

An old surgical adage is that if you are thinking of the need for fasciotomies, then you should perform them without further discussion. If you think about it, you should discuss it with an appropriate senior.

## Compartments to decompress

The lateral compartment/superficial posterior/deep posterior and anterior compartments of the leg all require decompression and this should be performed in a sterile environment in theatre.

After the procedure, as a result of the muscle oedema, there will be a lot of fluid discharge from the wounds. It is important that instructions for dressing are clear and that no compression should be applied to reduce blood or fluid loss from the wounds. Occasionally, brisk venous bleeding can occur from the wounds that may require further surgical exploration to control the source. Compartment syndrome can also occur in the thigh and upper limb and the management principles are identical.

## Burst abdomen

This complication is at the other end of the spectrum from compartment syndrome though the immediate management is similar to a laparostomy, with the aim being to keep the exposed viscera warm and moist and to minimise the loss of fluid and temperature. When it occurs, it is usually heralded by the so-called 'pink fluid sign', serosanguinous discharge, some 8–10 days after the initial surgery. If there were little systemic upset, and the wound can be brought together without undue tension, the abdomen may be resutured within 3–4 hours; however, if there is systemic instability, it would be better to manage the wound temporarily as a laparostomy.

## Postoperative bleeding

Despite anticipating bleeding problems, postoperative haemorrhage can be covert, with the only sign being progressive haemodynamic deterioration. An example would be after angiography with a high puncture of the common femoral artery, when a retroperitoneal bleed is common. Consider this as a potential complication, so it can be addressed with surgical correction if necessary.

Primary haemorrhage occurs at the time of surgery. If difficult to control – particularly if from the liver, pelvis or other inaccessible sites – consideration should be given to packing the affected area with a view to returning the patient to theatre at 48 hours for removal of packs and reinspection of the operative site.

Reactive haemorrhage occurs in the immediate postoperative phase and may present while the patient is in recovery or following return to the ward from theatre. Again, this requires a thorough systematic assessment of the patient to ensure prompt detection and return to theatre. As stated above, determining whether or not there is on-going bleeding can be difficult. The way to do this is to give the patient serial fluid challenges and make decisions based on the response. For example, if the patient responds, give them maintenance fluids and observe closely. Further deterioration may indicate on-going bleeding. This is a situation when more senior help should be sought early. Examples include a short gastric ligature coming loose after splenectomy. Even though the vessels are small, this bleed can still cause a rapid deterioration and cardiovascular compromise. Reactive haemorrhage may also occur after fluid resuscitation in trauma patients as the increased perfusion pressure may initiate bleeding.

## Case scenario 10.2 continued

You are asked to reassess the patient from case scenario 10.2, 4 hours after he was returned to the ICU because of blood-stained fluid appearing in the laparostomy bag and a 25 g/L fall in Hb (now 65 g/L compared with 90 g/L at the time of leaving theatre).

### How would you manage this situation?

This decision is often a difficult balance between returning the patient to theatre and controlling coagulopathy. This decision should be made in collaboration with the ICU staff. There are a number of factors that will predispose to coagulopathy, including the massive blood transfusion, hypothermia and reperfusion injury.

## Learning point

A coagulopathy is common in critically ill patients and should be considered as a cause of any overt or concealed haemorrhage. Any clotting problem should ideally be corrected prior to reoperation, and this may require close collaboration between surgeon, anaesthetist and haematology staff. Be careful not to ascribe surgical bleeding to a general bleed associated with a minor coagulopathy, as trying to correct the clotting will not improve the situation. Further delay may worsen the coagulopathy and cause a cycle of deterioration. It is better to control the source and correct the coagulopathy in theatre.

Other factors to consider with generalised bleeding problems are:

- effect of anticoagulant therapy;
- a recent large transfusion;
- the presence of sepsis or disseminated intravascular coagulation;
- previously unrecognised concomitant bleeding disorders, either congenital (eg Waldenström's macroglobulinaemia) or acquired (eg drugs).

Secondary haemorrhage occurs much later, often 7–8 days following a procedure. It is often related to infective complications but still may be unexpected and unheralded; control may be difficult to achieve. More proximal vascular control is often required and should be considered at the time of reoperation.

**Practice point**

Reversing a coagulopathy will not stop surgical bleeding. Correct the coagulopathy while addressing the source of the bleeding.

### Necrotising fasciitis

Necrotising infection can be difficult to diagnose; early diagnosis and targeted treatment is essential. Any diagnostic delay increases the mortality, which has a range of 25–73%. Immunocompromised patients on chemotherapy or steroids are vulnerable, but diabetes is the leading predisposing factor. The causative bacteria are synergistic and cause an infection involving the subcutaneous fascial layer, inducing extensive undermining of surrounding tissues. Presentation may be primary, in which no portal of entry or causative factor is found, or secondary, due to a precipitating event such as a perianal abscess.

The initial features may be subtle, including influenza-like symptoms and localised discomfort or pain. Subsequently, the limb or painful area begins to swell and may show a purplish rash. The skin marking will then blister with blackish fluid, and patients undergo severe systemic collapse due to sepsis. The surgical treatment required is prompt, aggressive debridement, with wide excision of all involved tissue back to bleeding edges. This may be quite extensive, and can take more than one operation. Patients usually require systemic support on critical care along with broad-spectrum antibiotics and consideration of immunoglobulin therapy.

## Anastomotic leakage

The signs of anastomotic leakage are of systemic instability with abdominal pain and/or rigid abdomen, tachycardia and fever. However, there may be a far more insidious presentation with low-grade fever, a prolonged ileus or failure to thrive. Therefore, anastomotic leakage should be considered as a cause for any unexplained postoperative deterioration following bowel surgery in which an anastomosis has been performed. It should be recognised that a defunctioning stoma does not exclude the possibility of an anastomotic leak; the presence of the stoma does not change the leak rate and the intention is to minimise the consequences of a leak.

In trying to anticipate anastomotic leakage, it is important to review the notes and the charts. For example, does the anaesthetic chart indicate preoperative dehydration or any episodes of perioperative hypotension? Does the operation note comment on the quality of perfusion in the mesenteric vessels? In an emergency case, does the chart show that inotropes/pressors were required, that may have caused mesenteric vasoconstriction? Factors that predispose to leak are shown in Box 10.1.

In trying to make the diagnosis of a leak, CT and contrast enema may have a complementary role, though CT with intravenous contrast is the radiological procedure of choice. If a collection is shown indicating a localised leak, CT- or ultrasound-guided drainage may be a therapeutic option. Major leakage has a significant mortality (10–15%) and so prompt reoperation is indicated with exteriorisation of suitable ends of small and large bowel. At this time, the need for nutritional support and the potential routes of access should be considered.

It is important to anticipate the difficulty of reoperative surgery on critically unwell patients and follow the principles shown in Box 10.2. A senior surgeon should be involved early in the decision-making, and in the surgery, together with a consultant anaesthetist.

## Box 10.1  Risk factors for intestinal anastomotic leakage

### Anastomotic technique

- Tension, poor anatomical blood supply (particularly after anterior resection), unrecognised mesenteric vessel damage, poor suture technique (eversion or mismatch)

### Local factors

- Obstruction, ischaemia or peritonitis

### Systemic factors

- Shock (excessive bowel preparation or excessive blood loss), age, malnutrition, immunosuppression

## Box 10.2  Principles of reoperative surgery for abdominal sepsis

- Prepare the patient as well as possible
- Involve a senior surgeon as early as possible in the patient's management
- Aim to deal with the source of the primary problem definitively
- Exteriorise leaking bowel
- Remove dead tissue
- Culture pus and drain sepsis
- Consider gastrostomy or jejunostomy for ease of future management

### The management of intestinal fistulae

The development of an intestinal fistula poses significant management challenges, which are likely to require high-dependency care even if there is no complicating infection or sepsis. The management involves the monitoring of significant fluid and electrolyte losses and their subsequent replacement along with nutritional therapy. Also involved is the physical management of the fistula; the surrounding skin requires protection by dressings or bags, and this will require the input of the stoma therapist.

When a fistula occurs postoperatively, assess by the CCrISP protocol and then utilise the 'SNAPS' (sepsis, nutrition, anatomy, procedure, skin care) protocol.

| S | Sepsis | Obtain adequate drainage |
| | | May involve CT-guided or surgical drainage |
| | | May involve defunctioning of the bowel |
| N | Nutrition | Provide nutritional support |
| | | Often this will be parenteral |
| A | Anatomy | Delineate by imaging the site of leak |
| | | CT with contrast is preferred choice |
| P | Procedure | Ultimately aim for reparative procedure |
| | | Delay until patient is well enough that success is likely (this may be months) |
| S | Skin care | Determine what is coming out of the fistula and protect the skin accordingly |
| | | Involve the stoma care and tissue viability teams |

---

## Case scenario 10.3

Consider the surgical patient in case scenario 10.1, who developed a compartment syndrome and required urgent laparotomy. The abdomen was washed out and closed primarily at 48 hours with a large-bore drain inserted via the left iliac fossa along the paracolic gutter into the splenic bed. The drain produces 50 ml of haemoserous fluid for 48 hours; however, before it can be removed it suddenly drains 300 ml of similar fluid.

How would you manage the patient? Could this be a fistula and if so what is the potential source?

Use the CCrISP system with simultaneous assessment and resuscitation. Following immediate management, you decide that the patient is stable and proceed to the full patient assessment. On review of the operation note, you should note the gastric repair and the splenectomy, and consider a missed injury to the pancreas or small bowel, or a leak from the gastric repair.

A pancreatic fistula (remember to send the draining fluid for an amylase level) may cause further problems due to the digestive actions of the pancreatic fluid, with concern for the various sites of surgical repair. A high small bowel fistula can cause high volume losses of fluids and electrolytes and rapid changes to acid–base balance. The initial fluid from a fistula can often be serosanginous and change to obvious faecal or small bowel content in the next 24 hours. These are complex problems and it is important to recognise them early. A diagnosis is essential and, while testing the fluid for amylase may suggest a pancreatic fistula, further radiological investigation is likely to be required, including contrast-enhanced CT. Having made a diagnosis, the SNAPS protocol should be used to manage the patient. Specialist senior help should be enlisted for the management of intestinal fistulae.

## Management of stomas and drains

There are various stomas that may form a part of the postoperative management of patients. Both on the ward and in critical care areas, this should be directed by the surgical team with the support of the stoma care nurse, or nutritional support team in the case of feeding stomas.

### Feeding gastrostomy or jejunostomy

The timing, content and volume of nutritional support should be planned depending on bowel function with the surgical team liaising with the dietitian or nutritional support team (see Chapter 13).

There must be clear advice given on timing of removal and obvious marking of the feeding stoma to prevent accidental removal if mistaken for a drain. Ten days is usually the minimum time required for an adequate seal to form.

## Faecal stomas

These may be temporary, loop or end type, as shown in Figure 10.4; their appearances are different, as are the difficulties in their management. Small bowel effluent from an ileostomy will irritate the skin and so the stoma is formed as a spout, whereas a colostomy will be flush to the skin since the effluent is more solid and less irritant. If a bridge is used for a loop stoma, the operation note should clearly state how long it should remain.

Irrespective of type, if there is concern with respect to the stoma's condition or function it should be inspected, which will require:

- removal of the stoma bag;

- assessment of the colour/perfusion of the stoma and the contents of the bag (Is the stoma functioning? is there any blood to indicate more proximal bleeding?);

- assessment of the skin around the stoma (Is there cellulitis or separation of the stoma from the skin? is the stoma in close proximity to the wound giving risk of contamination?);

- digital examination of the stoma (and the requirement for direct observation with a proctoscope to determine the extent of any discoloration).

A complication of the stoma may lead to systemic deterioration; conversely, systemic deterioration can lead to stoma deterioration.

(a)
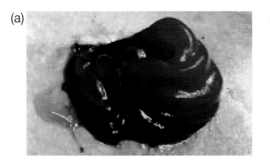

(b)
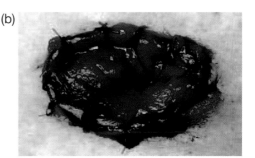

Figure 10.4 (a) End colostomy. (b) Loop ileostomy.

The small bowel effluent from an ileostomy is usually 500–700 ml/day but, initially, on starting to function, these volumes may be much higher, requiring careful electrolyte monitoring and replacement.

It is important to involve a stoma therapist as early as possible, especially for skin protection. The therapist also provides vital psychological support to the patients with a stoma and, if possible, this meeting should occur preoperatively with marking of potential stoma sites.

## Management of surgical drains

There is a continued debate as to the value and usage of drains; nevertheless, their presence in the critically ill surgical patient requires them to be assessed and managed effectively and appropriately.

In the assessment of the surgical patient, the amount and type of drainage, and whether that is expected, should be determined and documented. The drain site should be inspected and notes reviewed to determine the nature and positioning of drains, and the rationale for placement. Drains should be clearly marked if there is more than one, and it is the surgeon's responsibility to state when they should be removed.

## Post-surgical wound management

Surgical wound infections are a common hospital-acquired infection (~12%) and are subsequently an important cause of morbidity and mortality. Therefore, their prevention should be a primary management objective. The risk of infection should relate to whether the surgery was clean, clean with risk of contamination or contaminated. Prophylactic antibiotics should be used accordingly, guided by local policy. Ensure good hand-washing before and after the assessment of wounds to diminish the risk of direct contamination. The importance of environmental and hand hygiene is often underestimated and you can provide clinical leadership and set a good example.

A wound can be colonised by bacteria; there are bacteria present but there is no host response. This situation does not necessarily need any intervention other than considering the use of specific dressings, but be aware that the situation can progress to frank infection with or without surrounding cellulitis. In accordance with the CCrISP method of assessment, there should be a postoperative plan for all wounds, involving observation for the early signs of infection of redness, swelling, heat and pain. Depending on perioperative risk and/or the potential consequences of infection, the patient may have had prophylactic antibiotics. This and any postoperative regimen should be clear from a review of the charts. The majority of wounds are closed primarily; however, it may be prudent to leave a wound open if postoperative infection is likely. Collections of pus in the wound require adequate drainage rather than antibiotics and this may be achieved by suture removal alone or may require a return to theatre depending on the exact circumstances. Antibiotic usage should be reserved for the treatment of systemic disturbance or for the control of cellulitis. Empirical treatment while awaiting culture results should be based on the underlying procedure, not the site of the infection.

The timings of routine suture removal are a surgical decision and should be clearly documented within any surgical management plan.

## Summary

- It is sometimes difficult to assess the post-surgical patient, particularly on the ICU.

- The CCrISP process allows a structured assessment that will highlight the likely cause of any deterioration.

- By assessing the risk factors, many surgical site complications can be anticipated and prevented, or recognised early.

- Postoperative management plans should highlight which signs require early surgical review, such as the increasing abdominal pressure that would trigger the conversion to a laparostomy.

- There will always be surgical complications but the risk should be minimised and problems should be recognised and managed promptly and effectively.

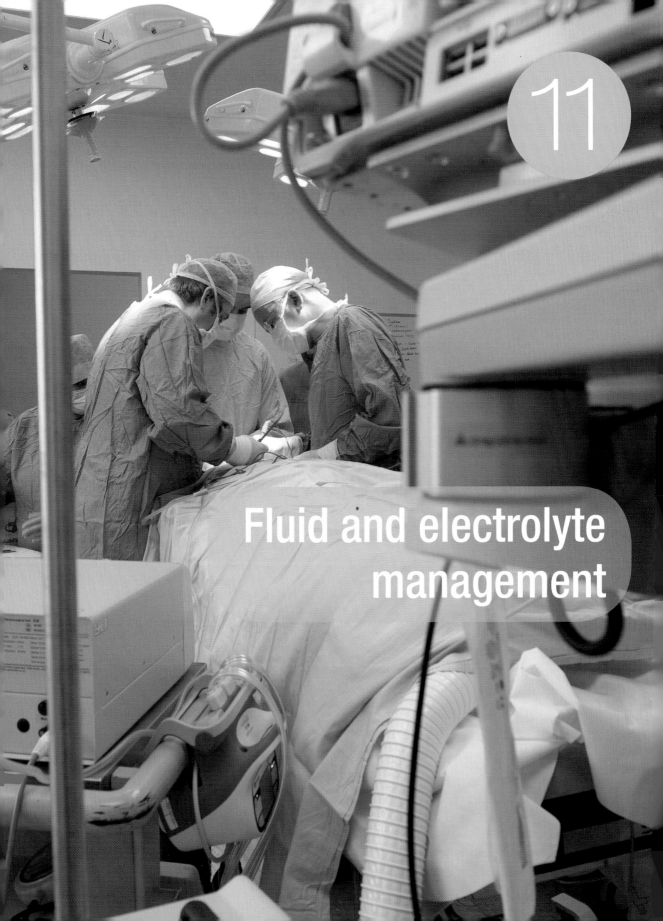

11

Fluid and electrolyte management

## Learning outcomes

This chapter will help you:

- describe the principles of management of complex fluid balance in surgical patients;

- avoid common pitfalls in fluid management in surgical patients;

- review water and electrolyte balance in the critically ill;

- manage common electrolyte abnormalities;

- list the properties of common intravenous fluids.

Assessing fluid balance and prescribing appropriate fluid is an important daily task for surgeons. As the registrar, it will be often be your responsibility to ensure that this is carried out safely and accurately. Do not delegate this task to junior members of the team without providing adequate oversight and ensure that the prescription of fluids in stable patients is performed by the owning team during the day and is not left to the out-of-hours teams – this often leads to inaccurate prescribing and complications. Conversely, do not attempt to write 24 hours' worth of fluid in unstable patients as predicting the circulatory status in such patients is not possible. In many surgical patients, the process becomes potentially complex because of multiple sources of fluid loss and several types of fluid input. However, with a logical approach and a clear understanding of a few basics, even complex cases can be dealt with. Conversely, poor prescribing remains a common cause of avoidable morbidity and mortality, from either inadequate resuscitation of the critically ill or excessive provision of fluids to elective patients.

## Patient groups

All patients are a different. Fluid needs are determined by baseline needs (dependent, in turn, on body weight), pre-existing fluid deficits and on-going abnormal losses. However, in the majority of surgical practice, there are two differing groups of patients who handle fluids differently. Patients may move between groups if complications develop.

## Critical illness and emergency surgery

In critical illness, and after complicated major surgery, the obligatory extracellular volume required to maintain adequate venous return to the heart rises as a result of the loss of salt, water and protein into sites of tissue damage, obstructed bowel, serous body cavities and the relaxation of the peripheral vascular bed. In some situations, such as sepsis, the amount of sequestered fluid may be large, owing to an enormous capillary leak, and sufficient to cause circulatory failure. This situation is often seen in critically ill surgical patients. Consequently, it is reasonable to suspect hypovolaemia in most patients and act accordingly.

Epidural anaesthesia causes vasodilatation, and this increased vascular space needs filling either by means of fluid boluses as the epidural is established or, once the patient is adequately filled, by controlling the degree of vasodilation by use of pressor agents. This is particularly the case if the patient has also been cold after surgery and experiences further vasodilation on warming up. In these patients, the commonest error is fluid resuscitation that is inadequate in terms of volume, fluid type or rate of delivery.

## Uncomplicated elective surgery

Major but uncomplicated surgery produces a different situation. Surgery causes activation of the antidiuretic hormone (ADH) and angiotensin–aldosterone, thereby retaining fluids and causing reduced urine output for 24–48 hours. In a well patient with otherwise normal parameters, isolated, modest oliguria can be acceptable. With fast-track recovery programmes advocating early and liberal oral intake and less in the way of bowel preparation (which dehydrates the patient significantly and causes electrolyte disturbances), the elective patient is less likely to be volume depleted. These patients often need less postoperative fluids. In these 'well' patients, excessive fluids cause more harm than good. Excessive provision of sodium and water is now recognised as the principal cause of avoidable problems, eg hyperchloraemic acidosis from excessive saline administration. This is a very different set of circumstances to the critically ill patient who frequently needs intravenous fluids rapidly for life-saving resuscitation. Fluid resuscitation from shock using an appropriate crystalloid was dealt with in the chapters on assessment and shock (Chapters 2 and 8).

## Clinical assessment

The patient should be fully assessed using the CCrISP system. Take particular note of indices of volume status and perfusion, including vital signs, skin perfusion as measured by capillary refill time and oedema (which appears on the sacrum if bed-bound). Note the patient's underlying age, BMI and lean body mass, general condition, operative treatment and timing, comorbid diseases and drugs.

Along with clinical examination, the fluid balance chart is the principal mechanism of assessment; however, their reliability is variable depending on the underlying pathology and should be used only as a general guide. Analysis of the fluid balance chart should be used in conjunction with the patient's response to fluid challenges to determine intravascular volume and cardiac filling. Insensible losses increase markedly with fever, respiratory rate and the breathing of dry $O_2$ – all of which can apply in the day or two after major surgery. As much as 500–1000 ml can be lost daily.

No single formula can be applied to all situations; regular frequent clinical assessment of the patient will be required to adjust the content and volumes of fluid replacement. This should be done at least daily, more often in the unstable. Occasionally with chronic overload, daily patient weighing, when feasible, can be of assistance and complements the fluid balance chart.

## Fluid compartments and control of volume

The total body water volume (~45 L) is distributed through the intracellular and extravascular compartments in a ratio of 2:1 (Figure 11.1).

The total volume of water is controlled by both central osmoreceptors and volume receptors that affect thirst and the release of ADH. Volume receptors will release ADH even in the face of hyponatraemia and a low plasma osmolality. Extracellular fluid (ECF) volume (of which blood volume is a special part) is maintained by the presence of sodium and its accompanying anions which are largely excluded from the intracellular compartment by the action of the Na/K pump. The body responds rapidly to a fall in central volume or renal perfusion by reducing renal sodium excretion to extremely low levels. There are two mechanisms for retaining water or sodium rapidly. Excretion is more passive and often slower, so the response to surgical stress favours fluid retention and overload. In critical illness this has some advantages, as

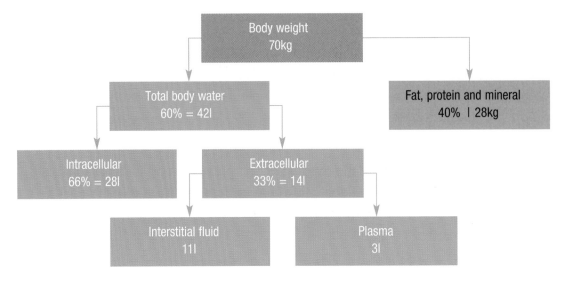

Figure 11.1 Fluid distribution in the body.

many of the effects of surgery cause fluid loss. When assessing patients, consider the following:

■ Assessment of fluid and electrolyte status requires both clinical and biochemical examination.

■ Intracellular volume is extremely difficult to assess clinically.

■ The extracellular compartment is easier to assess clinically as increased salt and water manifests itself as oedema and salt and water depletion by effects on the circulation.

■ The balance between blood volume and ECF is maintained by the oncotic pressure and the relative leakiness of the capillaries.

■ In haemorrhage, the plasma volume is partly replenished from the ECF.

■ In sepsis, gross capillary leak and a low oncotic pressure contribute to oedema and hypovolaemia.

## Biochemical assessment

Clinical assessment is assisted by biochemical measurement, primarily of blood, but also, on occasion, of urine and other fluid being lost from the body (eg fistula fluid).

## Water

Patients usually need 1500–2000 ml of water daily, depending on weight and fluid status. The basal water requirement is 30–40 ml/kg/day.

## Sodium

Normal basal requirements for sodium are 50–100 mmol/day but this can vary considerably with surgical illness. Drug solutions, eg intravenous antibiotics, can contain significant amounts of sodium. Care must also be taken to ensure that a false value for sodium is not obtained by venepuncture from a limb with a running fluid infusion or if there is frank lipaemia.

### Hyponatraemia

Often, the serum sodium gives a clearer idea of the relative water state of the body than of sodium status; hence clinical assessment is essential.

A patient with hyponatraemia, for example a serum level of 125 mmol/L, may be sodium depleted, sodium replete or sodium overloaded (oedematous due to cardiac, renal or hepatic disease) depending on the relative quantity of water in the extracellular space (Table 11.1). Dilutional hyponatraemia from excessive infusion of water (as 5% dextrose) is still seen on surgical wards.

The management of hyponatraemia may be sodium chloride infusion, water restriction or diuretic plus water restriction depending upon clinical assessment of volume status. Water cannot be excreted by the kidney in the presence of extracellular

Table 11.1  Hyponatraemia – types and causes

| | ECF volume low (NaCl – – –, $H_2O$ –) | ECF volume normal/slightly raised (NaCl normal, $H_2O$ +) | ECF volume high (NaCl +, $H_2O$ +++) |
|---|---|---|---|
| Urine Na high (>20mmol/L) | Diuretics (excessive) Salt-losing renal disease Mineralocorticoid deficiency | Glucocorticoid deficiency Hypothyroidism SIADH | Renal dysfunction |
| Urine Na low (<20 mmol/L) | Extrarenal loss: Outwith body Sequestration | | Dilutional (IV 5% dextrose, water ingestion) Cirrhosis Cardiac failure Nephrotic syndrome |

fluid depletion and the syndrome of 'inappropriate ADH secretion' (SIADH) can be diagnosed only once the patient has been shown to be in sodium balance.

Correction of hyponatraemia should be achieved at a similar rate to that at which it developed to avoid cerebral fluid shifts. Given normal renal function, water overload can be cleared by the administration of diuretic and 0.9% sodium chloride to replace the fluid excreted by the kidney. Hypertonic saline is seldom necessary unless the patient is fitting.

## Hypernatraemia

This can be caused by abnormal intake or administration of hypertonic fluid (eg 8.4% sodium bicarbonate), but is more commonly due to abnormal water loss (fever, diabetes insipidus or diabetes mellitus, osmotic diuretics) in a situation in which intake of water is impaired. Correction is with water (via the gut) or by intravenous 5% dextrose.

## Potassium

The usual requirement for potassium is 40–80 mmol/day.

## Hypokalaemia

Common causes of hypokalaemia in surgical practice include (i) renal losses; (ii) intestinal losses; and (iii) medical losses (eg high nasogastric outputs).

Plasma potassium is a poor reflection of the total body potassium content as plasma contains only 1% of the body total. The rate of change of the extracellular potassium concentration is more important than the absolute value. Hypokalaemia is usually the result of loss of potassium from the body via the kidney or bowel (diuretics, tubular disease, diarrhoea or laxatives). Acute changes in plasma potassium may occur as potassium moves into cells during the correction of an acidosis, secondary to the acute release of catecholamines (cerebral bleed or trauma), administration of salbutamol or upon refeeding with the start of anabolic activity. The level should be kept above 3.5 mmol/L by stopping any avoidable losses and the administration of potassium.

## Hyperkalaemia

A rapidly rising plasma potassium level is a medical emergency and will result in respiratory muscle weakness and cardiac arrest, resuscitation from which is extremely difficult.

The primary route of potassium excretion is via the kidney, in the distal nephron, under the influence of aldosterone. Renal failure, hypoadrenalism, distal nephron disease (eg chronic obstructive nephropathy) or drugs that affect the renin–aldosterone system (eg ACE inhibitors) will all impair the excretion of potassium. Where there is a sudden movement of potassium out of cells due to trauma, drugs (suxamethonium), ischaemic/hypoxic damage or a sudden rise in hydrogen ion concentration, patients with impaired renal excretion will be particularly vulnerable.

An example is the hypovolaemic patient with a metabolic acidosis plus respiratory compensation in whom anaesthesia is induced with suxamethonium and who is then underventilated, with consequent sudden fall in pH, and then suffers a cardiac arrest shortly after induction. There is no absolute level above which the signs and symptoms appear, and effects are related to the rate of rise as much as the plasma concentration. A chronic potassium level of 6.0 mmol/L will be well tolerated but may be fatal if the result of a rapid change from 4 mmol/L. Levels of this magnitude require rapid, specific treatment plus reversal of the primary condition and, if possible, the removal of any precipitant drugs.

## Calcium

The calcium level in the plasma is normally kept within a narrow range under the influence of parathyroid hormone, 1,25-dihyroxyvitamin $D_3$ and renal function. The active component is the ionised fraction, which is unbound to albumin. Total levels have to be interpreted in relation to the albumin level or the ionised fraction has to be measured directly.

## Hypocalcaemia

Apparent severe hypocalcaemia may be found in the critically ill if total plasma level is measured without reference to the albumin level. An absolute hypocalcaemia level is seen in acute pancreatitis, acute rhabdomyolysis and following thyroid or parathyroid surgery. Treatment is by the administration of calcium, treatment of the primary condition and, in post-parathyroidectomy syndrome or vitamin D deficiency, administration of activated vitamin D analogues. In situations of critical illness with intact parathyroid function, administration of calcium should be limited to where there is clinical evidence of hypocalcaemia or where the ionised calcium level is very low (usually <1 mmol/L). Symptoms include tetany, numbness and paraesthesia. Signs include Chvostek's sign, Trousseau's sign and seizures. Arrhythmias may also occur.

## Hypercalcaemia

Severe hypercalcaemia will affect neural tissue and damage renal tubular function. In the critically ill, this is most often due to paraneoplastic hypercalcaemia, but it can be caused by primary or secondary hyperparathyroidism. Hypercalcaemia diminishes the kidney's ability to retain salt, and the resultant hypovolaemia reduces the ability of the kidney to excrete calcium. Symptoms include malaise, abdominal pain and possible ureteric colic. Dysrhythmias may occur. Establishing a saline diuresis will normally help reduce the level. If this fails, the administration of a bisphosphonate intravenously will reduce the level of calcium. Effective treatment of the primary cause will also bring the level back to normal. The development of hypercalcaemia in association with recurrence of a solid tumour is usually an indication of a poor prognosis.

## Magnesium

Magnesium is the second most important intracellular cation after potassium. Magnesium is essential for the normal functioning of nerve and muscle. Depletion causes confusion and seizures and is associated with a range of dysrhythmias, while excess causes muscle paralysis and central nervous depression. In the critically ill, hypomagnesaemia is common in the early recovery period following severe insults such as peritonitis. Chronic losses from the bowel (diarrhoea) or kidney (loop diuretics) and alcohol abuse contribute. As with potassium, plasma levels reflect total body magnesium poorly, but a plasma level below 0.6 mmol/L associated with a condition likely to cause magnesium deficiency or the presence of symptoms should precipitate supplementation. This is best done intravenously in the acute stage to avoid the purgative effects of magnesium salts. The plasma level should not exceed 1.5 mmol/L. Critically ill patients with dysrhythmias should have magnesium levels checked as treatment with magnesium contributes to the control of several dysrhythmic states.

Significant hypermagnesaemia is almost always secondary to iatrogenic administration in the presence of impaired renal function.

## Phosphate

Phosphate is present in any protein-containing food and is absorbed from the gut. The kidney excretes phosphate under the influence of parathyroid hormone. High levels are seen in renal impairment or following massive muscle or bowel necrosis. In the short term, this is usually not a major problem unless large quantities of calcium are administered.

Hypophosphataemia is commonly seen during recovery from critical illness. As cell function is restored, phosphate is taken back into cells with potassium and magnesium. When the phosphate level falls below 0.6 mmol/L, there are measurable effects on skeletal muscle function and on the immune system. Replacement will come with feeding but, with levels below 0.6 mmol/L, intravenous supplementation will need to be given slowly over 24 hours.

## Trace metals

There are many trace metals that are essential to normal cellular function and the healing process (zinc, copper and selenium). In situations where there is prolonged dependence upon parenteral feeding or prolonged gut dysfunction, consideration must be given to their measurement and supplementation.

## Approach to the prescription of fluid and electrolytes

This should be read in conjunction with the section in Chapter 13 on nutrition. In the critically ill, fluid replacement will be guided by the clinical situation, which is constantly changing. Requirements will be dependent upon many factors, but with three main headings: (i) basal requirements; (ii) existing fluid and electrolyte excess or deficit; and (iii) continuing abnormal losses.

Basal requirements (1500–2500 ml of water, 100 mmol Na and 80 mmol K) are influenced by a number of factors, including body weight (Box 11.1). Age and cardiac or renal disease can jeopardise the patient's ability to correct imbalances so greater care is then needed. Intravenous fluids should be used for as short a period as possible, eg after uncomplicated elective surgery.

Pre-existing fluid and electrolyte excess or deficit needs to be taken into account in fluid calculations, eg potassium deficit takes some time to correct. Oedema also takes days to resolve, as a patient recovers from major surgery. The patient's recovery is often accompanied by a diuresis, which can be one of the clues that the patient is getting better.

Abnormal losses usually cause change gradually. These might include insensible loss of water dependent upon fever, continuing loss from the gastrointestinal or renal tract, or other effects of recent surgery, with fluid redistribution or loss from open wounds. As well as noting yesterday's outputs, your clinical assessment should help you predict, to some degree, how these losses might change today. For example, a patient recovering from laparotomy with a soft abdomen and passing flatus may be expected to successfully tolerate more oral intake. Previous nasogastric losses will probably resolve and the need for intravenous fluid will decrease as oral intake increases.

You should be realistic about tolerance of oral intake in unwell patients. Just because it is prescribed or permitted, does not mean it will be taken or tolerated by the patient. If, at this point, the fluid balance is no longer charted, then problems may develop.

## Box 11.1 Some considerations for fluid therapy

- Fluid isotonic for sodium will be required to maintain adequate extracellular volume
- Water (oral or 5% dextrose) is needed to maintain intracellular volume and provide sufficient volume to excrete the renal load of solute waste
- The volume of clear intravenous fluids will need to be reduced depending on the volume being given by other routes or forms (drugs, oral intake, nutrition, blood, etc)
- Electrolyte deficiencies will need to be corrected as well as basal needs being met

## Replacing abnormal losses

As a general rule, abnormal losses should be replaced with a fluid with the same composition as that which is being lost, and in a similar volume. However, matching the fluid exactly is not always necessary as the kidneys compensate efficiently under many circumstances.

Losses can be divided into those that consist more or less of ECF, or its equivalent, and those that are mainly or purely water (Box 11.2). Some conditions have elements of both.

When there is loss of an ECF-equivalent fluid, there is a decrease in the total ECF volume, and this includes the plasma volume.

### Box 11.2 Fluid losses

**Losses that approximate extracellular fluid**

- Blood loss
- Vomiting
- Diarrhoea
- Gut fistulae
- Unwell patients (eg sepsis, burns, pancreatitis)
- Diabetes mellitus (hyperglycaemia)

**Losses that are principally water**

- Fever
- Increased respiratory rate
- Prolonged water deprivation
- Diabetes insipidus

This deficit should be replaced promptly to restore perfusion to cells and vital organs. Abnormal losses of water with or without electrolytes (particularly sodium and potassium) will result in not only a reduction in plasma volume but also a marked change in intracellular fluid volume and the concentrations of important ions across cell membranes. Restoration of the plasma volume always takes precedence, and should be accomplished with a 'balanced salt solution' (see below).

Restoration of the water deficit and other electrolyte deficits can then be addressed. This should be accomplished gradually so that rapid shifts of water across membranes, especially the blood–brain barrier, are avoided. It takes much longer for electrolytes to equilibrate between some compartments, and the resulting osmotic gradient can lead to fatal cerebral oedema or other complications if therapy is too hasty. Aim to correct these over 48–72 hours.

## Replacing extracellular fluid loss

Central to the replacement of ECF deficits (blood volume, interstitial volume) is the use of a 'balanced salt solution'. This term refers to a crystalloid solution that is isotonic (and remains so) and has constituents that are similar to the ECF (normal saline or 0.9% sodium chloride, lactated Ringer's buffer – also known as Hartmann's solution). When a balanced salt solution is given, it will distribute itself throughout the extracellular compartment (~14 L) over several minutes.

Only about a third of the volume given will remain in the vascular space. Understanding this phenomenon will prevent undertreatment of blood volume deficits when using balanced salt solutions. As reduced intravascular volume is usually accompanied by an ECF deficit, redistribution of balanced salt solution into the interstitial space is usually desirable. Normal saline contains too much chloride for physiological needs and, with overprescription, hyperchloraemia and acidosis occur. Hartmann's solution does not cause this.

If the volumes required are large, maintenance water and electrolytes are often forgotten. This seldom matters in the first 24 hours or so because the volume shifts are so large and the kidney can usually sort out what it wants to keep or excrete. However, as time goes on, maintenance water needs to be thought about or the patient will become hypernatraemic and hyperosmolar.

## Vomiting, diarrhoea and intestinal fistula losses

These gastrointestinal conditions cause losses of fluid that resembles ECF but is typically of a lower osmolality (ie more water is lost relative to sodium). The result is blood volume depletion, dehydration and large electrolyte losses. If water only has been taken orally to try to compensate, hyponatraemia may be present. If serum sodium is normal or even high, the possibility of a significant sodium deficit must not be overlooked.

In some conditions (eg vomiting from complete upper small bowel obstruction, diarrhoea due to cholera) the volumes lost can be huge and rapidly life-threatening. Potassium depletion is universal, and may be severe with marked diarrhoea. Metabolic acidosis may mask the extent of total body potassium deficit by causing potassium to move from within cells to the extracellular compartment in exchange for extracellular hydrogen ions.

Additionally, vomiting or nasogastric drainage leads to loss of hydrogen ($H^+$) and chloride ($Cl^-$) ions from the stomach. This can produce a marked metabolic alkalosis but, despite this, it is rare that $H^+$ needs to be given intravenously. Adequate chloride replacement, in the form of normal saline, will usually correct the deficit, as endogenously produced acid ($H^+$) will be retained by the kidney.

By using fluid balance charts and clinical assessment logically to keep total volume and key ions, particularly sodium and potassium, in balance, you can achieve success in the great majority of cases. However, there is no single formula for success and patients change continually – so reassess.

### Case scenario 11.1

A 58-year-old, 70-kg man, otherwise fit except for long-standing AF controlled with digoxin, underwent a cystectomy for bladder cancer 3 days ago. An ileal urostomy was constructed, necessitating a small bowel anastomosis. Presently, he is on the HDU, is apyrexial and his chest is clear (respiratory rate 16/min), but his abdomen is rather distended. Although his urine output is rather low, he has a normal capillary refill time, pulse and blood pressure. The monitor shows AF at a rate of 118 bpm. It is Saturday and you are on call – the HDU nurse has asked you to sort out his fluid balance for the weekend. Review the fluid balance chart below and prescribe his intravenous fluid. His consultant wished him to stop antibiotics after 72 hours.

- What further information do you require?

- What would you prescribe and how?

- Are blood tests necessary today?

- When should you review further?

## Data

| Intake summary (last 24 h) | CVP line | Peripheral line (R) | Peripheral line (L) | | Oral |
|---|---|---|---|---|---|
| | Normal saline (975 ml) | Dextrose 5% (1800 ml) | Antibiotics (600 ml), PCA (125 ml) | | Sips (120 ml) |

| Losses summary (last 24 h) | Nasogastric tube | Pelvic drain | Urostomy | Bowels |
|---|---|---|---|---|
| | 1450 ml | 720 ml | 640 ml | Nil, no flatus |

## Case scenario 11.1: answers

This is a complex patient who is not clinically stable. In addition to making your own clinical assessment, you should review the fluid charts from the previous day or two to look for patterns and for accumulating losses or excesses. Look at the operation note for any specific postoperative orders. Urinary anastomoses may leak for a few days so urine appears through the drain as well as the catheter and/or urostomy. Ileus can be prolonged and nutritional support may be needed but, again, this is not pressing at 72 hours postoperatively. You need to review yesterday's biochemistry results (Na+ 138 mmol/L, K+ 3.1 mmol/L, urea 5.2 mmol/L) and repeat these today. Summate the data above and include insensible losses – about 750 ml is probably reasonable here, but revise the factors which influence this.

His needs are probably about 3500 ml – the water requirement (5% dextrose 2000 ml) will be unchanged – the excess volume should be normal saline (1500 ml) to replace the nasogastric losses. His antibiotics will be stopped, but his PCA will continue. He is hypokalaemic and you should aim to give 80 mmol $K^+$ over the next 24 hours – you may modify this when you review with the blood results later. This need is more pressing because of his AF and digoxin therapy. Remember that hypokalemia potentiates digoxin toxicity. The magnesium level should also be measured and corrected as necessary. If potassium replacement and digoxin fail to control the rate and any hypoxia or hypovolaemia has been corrected then alternative pharmacological interventions (eg a beta blocker and amiodarone) should be considered.

It is inappropriate to prescribe for the whole weekend just now. Some losses – the nasogastric loss for example – may increase or decrease and clinical and biochemical reassessment is needed. Plan to review with your team at the end of today and again at 8am tomorrow.

## Summary

- Fluid and electrolyte imbalance is common and detrimental to surgical patients if not addressed.
- Accurate fluid balance is achievable with a logical approach.
- Consider basal requirements based on patient size and age.
- Consider abnormal on-going losses, pre-existing deficits or excesses, fluid shifts.
- Normal renal and cardiovascular function protect against fluid intolerance.
- Look at the fluid balance chart for last 24 hours.
- Are all fluids given or lost included? Do the volumes seem right from other available information? Check previous charts for insidious changes.
- Aim to correct abnormal electrolyte values.
- Consider measuring urine electrolytes and plasma osmolality if blood results and patient clinical examination do not add up.

## Further reading

National Institute for Health and Care Excellence (NICE). *Intravenous Fluid Therapy in Adults in Hospital*. NCE Guideline 174. NICE, London; 2013.

Powell-Tuck J, Gosling P, Lobo DN et al. *British Consensus Guidelines on Intravenous Fluid Therapy for Adult Surgical Patients (GIFTASUP)*. NHS National Library of Health, London. Available at http://www.ics.ac.uk/downloads/ 2008112340_ GIFTASUP%20 FINAL_31-10-08.pdf.

# 12

# Sepsis and multiple organ failure

## Learning outcomes

This chapter will help you to:

- describe the clinical pathophysiology of the septic process;

- recognise that prevention, early diagnosis and prompt treatment of sepsis is more beneficial for patient survival than treatment of established septic shock;

- outline the essential features of the Surviving Sepsis Campaign;

- describe the linkage between organ dysfunction, sepsis and patient outcomes;

- describe a system for managing the septic patient.

Sepsis and hospital-acquired infections remain major healthcare issues in the developed world. Patients with indwelling devices, those in ICU or HDU, and those being treated with chemotherapy or steroids, are at particular risk. In addition, an ageing population and the ability to treat patients with major chronic illness increases the complexity of management of patients with sepsis. In the US in 2011, 5.2% of total hospital costs were attributable to sepsis, and it remains a leading cause of mortality of surgical patients worldwide.

The signs and symptoms associated with sepsis are caused by the release of endogenous mediators. This mediator release may be caused by a variety of insults, including infection and trauma. The mediators involved include nitric oxide, bradykinin, histamine, prostaglandins and cytokines, all of which have vasoactive properties. They produce a state of vasodilatation, enhanced capillary leak and, eventually, myocardial depression.

Cytokines involved include interleukin 1 (IL-1, an endogenous pyrogen), tumour necrosis factor and IL-6. These are released from the patient's own white blood cells, and contribute to the pyrexia and hypermetabolic state found in sepsis. While production of mediators is needed to combat infection, an excessive, prolonged and unregulated activation of such cellular and humoral mediator pathways is thought to contribute to the development of multiple organ dysfunction (MODs) sometimes seen in patients with sepsis.

A balance exists between inadequate and excessive responses to infection. Inter-individual variation in the pattern of mediator release and of end-organ responsiveness (probably related to genotype) plays a significant role in determining the initial physiological response to sepsis and this may be a determinant of outcome. Other important prognostic features include the severity of the initial 'trigger event', the timeliness and adequacy of treatment of the underlying condition and the patient's general state of health.

## Definitions

Understanding of sepsis is constantly developing. In February 2016, the European Society of Intensive Care Medicine and the Society of Critical Care Medicine's Third International Consensus Definitions for Sepsis and Septic Shock (Sepsis-3) were published (see Further reading). This work has attempted to simplify the understanding of sepsis and to focus attention on the groups most at risk of death from sepsis. The prognostic value of these definitions has been retrospectively tested in large cohorts of patients in whom outcomes were known and, in this way, the definitions have a greater evidence base than the earlier approach. As part of this approach, the previous focus on the recognition of systemic inflammatory response syndrome (SIRS) is no longer useful as it does not identify those at high risk of mortality. SIRS is now recognised as an appropriate, regulated non-specific response to infection and, along with the term 'severe sepsis', is no longer recommended for use. Sepsis is defined as a 'life-threatening organ dysfunction caused by a dysregulated host response to infection'. Septic shock is a condition characterised by profound circulatory, cellular and metabolic abnormalities and is associated with a greater risk of mortality than is sepsis alone.

Clinically, sepsis is recognised by looking for signs of organ dysfunction in patients who are suspected of having an infection. Signs of organ dysfunction can be determined using the Sequential Organ Failure Assessment (SOFA) methodology but, as this is really only suited to patients already in a critical care environment, a modification of this for use early in a patient's illness has been developed. The quick SOFA (qSOFA) assesses respiratory rate, blood pressure and mentation. A respiratory rate over 22, a systolic BP of less than 100mmHg and altered mentation all score 1 point each; organ dysfunction is defined as a score of 2 or more and puts the patient into a group with a predicted 10% risk of death.

Recognising septic shock clinically is more difficult, as it can be assessed only by response to treatment. Patients who have infection and persistent hypotension after fluid resuscitation, or a persistent lactate of more than 2 mmol/L after resuscitation, or a vasopressor requirement to maintain a mean arterial pressure (MAP) of ≥65 mmHg in the absence of hypovolaemia are all considered to have septic shock. Septic shock is associated with a 40% mortality rate. In a ward setting, a definitive diagnosis of septic shock is difficult as it not possible to be sure that someone is not hypovolaemic without invasive monitoring, but the message is to understand these definitions and treat the patient appropriately.

## Implications for screening and management of infection (adapted from SSC)

The Surviving Sepsis Campaign (SSC) has offered the following clarification on the implications of current definitions.

### Step 1: screening and management of infection

The appropriate first step in screening should be identification of infection. In those patients identified as having infection, management should begin by obtaining blood and other cultures as indicated, administering tailored antibiotics as appropriate, and simultaneously obtaining laboratory results to evaluate the patient for infection-related organ dysfunction.

### Step 2: screening for organ dysfunction and management of sepsis

Patients with sepsis should be identified by the organ dysfunction criteria (including lactate level greater than 2 mmol/L). Organ dysfunction may be identified using the sepsis-related qSOFA, as outlined above.

Importantly, evidence of two out of three qSOFA elements in patients who have screened positive for infection may be used as a secondary screen to identify patients at risk for clinical deterioration. Consider closer monitoring of these at-risk patients.

If organ dysfunction is identified, ensuring that the step 1 elements have been initiated continues to be a priority. For instance, patients with organ dysfunction require blood cultures if only non-blood cultures had previously been obtained and administration of broad-spectrum antibiotics if only narrow-spectrum antibiotics had previously been administered in step 1.

### Step 3: identification and management of initial hypotension

In those patients who have infection and hypotension or a lactate level greater than or equal to 4 mmol/L providing 30 ml/kg crystalloid with reassessment of volume responsiveness or tissue perfusion should be implemented.

## Quick SOFA clarification for the practitioner

Sepsis-3 introduces qSOFA as a tool for identifying patients at risk of sepsis with a higher risk of hospital death or prolonged intensive care unit (ICU) stay both inside and outside critical care units.

Note that qSOFA does not define sepsis (but the presence of two qSOFA criteria is a predictor of both increased mortality and ICU stays of more than 3 days in non-ICU patients). NICE guidance has also been released, which stratifies the risk criteria when assessing sepsis (Table 12.1).

## How to proceed once sepsis is suspected

The keys to sepsis management are early recognition and prompt and accurate treatment. To aid management of what can be a complex situation the Surviving Sepsis Campaign has recommended the concept of care bundles.

The SSC includes two recommended management packages or 'care bundles' – the 3-hour care bundle and the 6-hour care bundle.

## The SSC care bundles

### The 3-hour care bundle

The 3-hour care bundle aims to optimise the care of patients with sepsis during the first 3 hours after presentation. It starts with the 'Sepsis Six' – six tasks easily performed by non-specialist staff that form the crucial first steps in delivering the care bundle. These should be completed within 1 hour of presentation/suspicion of sepsis

Table 12.1 Risk stratification tool for adults, children and young people aged 12 years and over with suspected sepsis

| Category | High risk criteria | Moderate to high risk criteria | Low risk criteria |
| --- | --- | --- | --- |
| History | Objective evidence of new altered mental state | History from patient, friend or relative of new onset of altered behaviour or mental state | Normal behaviour |
| | | History of acute deterioration of functional ability | |
| | | Impaired immune system (illness or drugs including oral steroids) | |
| | | Trauma, surgery or invasive procedures in the last 6 weeks | |
| Respiratory | Raises respiratory rate: 25 breaths per minute or more | Raised respiratory rate: 21–24 breaths per minute | No high risk or moderate to high risk criteria met |
| | New need for oxygen (more than 40% $FiO_2$) to maintain saturation of more than 92% (or more than 88% in known chronic obstructive pulmonary disease) | | |
| Blood pressure | Systolic blood pressure 90 mmHg or less or systolic blood pressure more than 40 mmHg below normal | Systolic blood pressure 91–100 mmHg | No high risk or moderate to high risk criteria met |
| Circulation and hydration | Raised heart rate: more than 130 beats per minute | Raised heart rate: 91–130 beats per minute (for pregnant women 100–130 beats per minute) or new-onset arrhythmia | No high risk or moderate to high risk criteria met |
| | Not passed urine in the previous 18 hours | Not passed urine in the previous 12–18 hours | |
| | For catheterised patients, passed less than 0.5 ml/kg of urine per hour | For catheterised patients, passed 0.5 ml/kg of urine per hour | |
| Temperature | | Tympanic temperature less than 36°C | |
| Skin | Mottled or ashen appearance | Signs of potential infection, including redness, swelling or discharge at surgical site or breakdown of wound | No non-blanching rash |
| | Cyanosis of skin, lips or tongue | | |
| | Non-blanching rash | | |

and contribute to the 3-hour bundle. Note also that the Sepsis Six and associated care bundles fit well into the CCrISP three-stage assessment process, and that completing a CCrISP assessment will ensure that you do not miss elements of the care bundles.

## The Sepsis Six

- Give high-flow oxygen
- Take blood cultures
- Give intravenous antibiotics
- Start intravenous fluid resuscitation
- Check haemoglobin and lactate levels
- Measure accurate hourly urine output

Additional elements of the 3-hour care bundle include:

- Ensure broad-spectrum antibiotics have been given.

- Administer 30 ml/kg crystalloid for hypotension or lactate ≥4 mmol/L.

Following the 'Sepsis Six', the SSC recommends that patients with persistent hypotension or increased lactate should be managed with early goal-directed therapy (EGDT). EGDT will require input from your critical care colleagues or other senior doctors, but the principles used are important to recognise and are outlined below.

These recommendations are encompassed in the 6-hour care bundle.

### The 6-hour care bundle

- Apply vasopressors (for hypotension that does not respond to initial fluid resuscitation) to maintain a MAP ≥65 mmHg.

- In the event of persistent hypotension after initial fluid administration (MAP <65 mmHg) or if initial lactate was ≥4 mmol/L, reassess volume status and tissue perfusion and document findings.

- Remeasure lactate if initial lactate is elevated.

## Further management of patients with sepsis

The above measures are all supportive and, although important, are only part of the management of sepsis. Source identification and control are vital if patients are to have good outcomes. These two things need to be achieved as quickly as possible, and this is the remit of the surgical team. The CCrISP three-stage assessment process will help to achieve this, as will be illustrated in the cases described below.

## Management of multiple organ dysfunction

Owing to the severity of the initial insult or when there is a persistence of an activated systemic inflammatory response, a patient may develop dysfunction or failure of one or more organ systems (cardiovascular, pulmonary, renal, gut, liver, haematological, CNS). If three or more systems have failed, the ensuing mortality risk approaches 80–100%. Once one organ system has failed, others typically follow (see case scenarios). It is important to appreciate the phenomenon of multiorgan dysfunction and to support each organ system to avoid further adverse events (eg ventilation, haemofiltration/haemodialysis, inotropic support, nutritional support, use of blood products).

Respiratory failure may be the result of infection (often added to pre-existing chronic airway disease) or adult respiratory distress syndrome (ARDS). ARDS is a diffuse, inflammatory process, usually involving both lungs, and is often seen associated with sepsis. The lungs become 'waterlogged' as a result of extravasation of inflammatory fluid and cells. Patients may develop ARDS quickly, deteriorating rapidly over a few hours. Pulmonary signs are often minimal or non-specific: patients are breathless, becoming progressively tachypnoeic and hypoxic. A chest X-ray will show bilateral infiltrates but this may lag behind the clinical picture. Respiratory support is almost always needed (usually mechanical ventilation) and expert critical care help should be obtained at an early stage. Suspicion is the key to diagnosing ARDS.

Cardiovascular failure in sepsis results from three main factors: (i) loss of peripheral vascular tone (vasodilatation); (ii) loss of circulating volume due to leaky capillaries (hypovolaemia); and (iii) myocardial depression (pump failure from circulating cytokines). Arrhythmias can exert a further effect. Close monitoring of cardiovascular status is essential to guide treatment adequately. Fluid resuscitation may prove successful, although inotropic and vasopressor support is often required. Many intensivists use noradrenaline to increase peripheral vascular tone, often in conjunction with other agents to increase cardiac contractility. Renal dysfunction in the form of acute kidney injury is common in sepsis and is often established during the early stages of the condition before hypovolaemia is corrected. Circulating nephrotoxins may compound this. Although renal function usually improves when the patient recovers, renal replacement therapy may be required during the period of septic shock and for some time afterwards. Failure of other systems (gut, brain, clotting system) may be due to direct effects of the pathology or to systemic inflammation and hypoxia. For there to be any prospect of recovery, the underlying cause or source of sepsis must be treated.

## Other causes of patients being unwell

Many patients showing signs of tachycardia, tachypnoea, raised WBC and hyper- or hypothermia will recover uneventfully with good surgical care. However, the presence of such signs, particularly when persistent, serves as a warning of the potential for deterioration in the absence of prompt treatment, and if you see a patient with these signs you should actively exclude sepsis as a cause. These signs may result from an infective process and, with organ dysfunction, may represent sepsis although other conditions can also cause this inflammatory response. These include pancreatitis, ischaemia, multiple trauma and haemorrhagic shock.

You should also be actively looking for clinical evidence of organ derangement to prevent potential future problems (eg dyspnoea, hypoxia, oliguria, jaundice, thromobocytopenia) in all susceptible patients.

The essential points of management of these patients also include:

- early recognition;
- immediate resuscitation;
- localisation of pathology;
- appropriate management of the primary problem including the use of surgical or radiological drainage;
- on-going reassessment to ensure that the patient continues to improve.

Failure to accomplish any of these promptly will markedly worsen the prognosis.

Table 12.2 shows some causes that you will encounter. The classification might help you remember them but a number of the causes could appear in different boxes depending on the stage (eg ischaemic gut). Surgical causes often require a surgical solution but all causes occur in surgical patients.

Table 12.2 Potential causes of abnormal patient physiology

|  | Infective (actively exclude sepsis) | Non-infective |
|---|---|---|
| Non-surgical | Pulmonary<br>Urinary and catheter-related<br>Intravenous lines, especially CVP<br>Soft tissue infection | Acute pancreatitis<br>Reperfusion injury |
| Surgical | Anastomotic leak<br>Biliary, especially if obstructed<br>Urinary with obstruction<br>Collection/abscess<br>Infected prosthesis (hip, aortic graft,<br>heart valve, neurosurgical shunt)<br>Necrotic tissue | Ischaemic gut<br>Ruptured aorta<br>Major haemorrhage<br>Trauma |

# Patient assessment and management

## Immediate care

The CCrISP immediate assessment may reveal that the patient has tachypnoea and cardiovascular changes consistent with the presence of two organ dysfunctions. Treatment with high-flow oxygen via a facemask and establishment of IV access with volume expansion is appropriate. Rapid volume expansion with crystalloid (30 ml/ kg lean body mass) is appropriate. An arterial blood sample to assess lactate level should be taken at this point.

## Full patient assessment

### Chart review

Vital signs should be reviewed carefully: tachypnoea, tachycardia, altered mentation and hypo- or hyperthermia are all consistent with sepsis. A normal capillary refill time and a urine output greater than 30 ml/h are reasonable guides to the adequacy of initial fluid resuscitation, but changes in urine output are slower to occur than changes in capillary refill time. If hypotension or inadequate perfusion persists despite adequate fluid replacement in the presence of a lactate concentration >4 mmol/L, then escalation of organ support should be considered, which will require input from colleagues experienced in critical care and involve additional monitoring. Your role is to recognise these patients, to try to identify the source of sepsis and to escalate their care.

### History and systematic examination

An assessment of the patient's presenting complaint may help to establish the likely source of sepsis:

- Breathlessness and a productive cough may indicate a pulmonary source.

- Abdominal pain or bowel symptoms may point to an abdominal source. An abdominal or pelvic abscess may cause diarrhoea or an ileus: anastomotic leaks after bowel surgery can be subtle.

- Frequency, dysuria or haematuria are common in urinary sepsis. Beware the combination of obstruction with infection (usually due to a stone), as sepsis may be severe and permanent renal damage can occur rapidly.

- Headache and neck stiffness may point to a source in the central nervous system.

Altered mentation is common in the unwell septic patient and does not necessarily indicate a source in the CNS.

The systemic review should also evaluate chronic health problems and current medication that may suggest a susceptibility to sepsis (eg use of steroids) or may indicate the need for more intensive monitoring (eg recent myocardial infarction).

The history and examination may be very useful in helping to indicate the source of the problem. Common things occur frequently: chest infection, anastomotic leak and central venous line infection are often implicated in the recovering surgical patient. The timing of events can also help: the chest is a common early cause of postoperative fever or sepsis from day 1 onwards while anastomotic leak, as mentioned previously, usually occurs from day 4 and central line infection becomes more frequent in lines more than 48 hours old or those that are being used for TPN.

### Case scenario 12.1

As the surgical trainee on the HDU 8am ward round, you review a 73-year-old woman with mild COPD who had a left hemicolectomy with primary anastomosis for colonic carcinoma 5 days ago. You are told that her WCC yesterday was $16.3 \times 10^9$/L, increased from $8.5 \times 10^9$/L the day before.

## What would you do?

Systematic assessment shows that her immediate observations are stable and she is alert. Her systolic BP is over 100 mmHg and her respiratory rate is 18/min. The charts show an increased heart rate (was 70 bpm, now 95 bpm), a temporary pyrexia of 38°C overnight and decreased urine output (only 25 ml/h for the last 3 hours). The patient has no specific complaints but has been generally slow to recover, which is why she is still on the HDU. The CVP line from theatre is still in situ, as is the urinary catheter. Examination of her chest reveals that it is unchanged from previously; a few basal crackles are present, but gas exchange is stable, lactate is not elevated and she is able to expectorate adequately without pain. Her abdomen is slightly distended, and she has been passing flatus but no faeces. There is no evidence of a DVT. Macroscopically and on 'dipstick', her urine is clear.

## What would you do now?

Now is the time to decide and plan. The patient is not quite right but has no definite signs of pathology and you suspect sepsis.

There are a number of potential sources of infection (chest, CVP line, urine, urinary catheter, abdomen, anastomosis). Peripheral blood cultures and cultures through the central venous line should be sent, as should urine and sputum cultures. A chest X-ray should be ordered if there is not a recent one, a fluid challenge started and the physiotherapist called.

When reviewing such a case, the operation performed (which includes a primary colonic anastomosis), the stage of recovery and the fact that her gut has still not started working again should make you consider an anastomotic leak. You discuss the case with your consultant and arrange contrast- enhanced CT after adequate fluid resuscitation. A small, localised leak is suspected. Your consultant thinks that the patient may settle and takes a conservative approach to further management. Antibiotics are prescribed to cover a possible leak and the patient is fasted.

### On review

Overall, the patient's condition appears to be unchanged throughout the next 24 hours. There is one further flicker of pyrexia (37.8°C). The heart rate remains at 95–100 bpm. The next morning, her abdomen is still distended and her ileus persists. The urea has climbed to 10.4 mmol/L from normal and the patient had a run of fast AF at 5am despite a CVP of +9 mmHg and normal oxygen saturations and lactate of 2.3 mmo/L. Twelve-lead ECG and cardiac enzymes were normal but the Mg level was low. This has been corrected.

Your consultant joins you and together you decide that the failure to respond (abdomen, heart rate) and the recent cardiac and renal effects warrant further surgery to deal with the leak. After appropriate resuscitation, she is taken to theatre, where the anastomosis is taken down and the ends exteriorised. The patient returns to HDU and makes an uncomplicated recovery.

### Learning points

- Where sepsis is suspected, management along Surviving Sepsis principles using the CCrISP three-stage assessment helps to prevent further deterioration and to plan care.

- Decisions to return a patient to theatre after surgery are complex and the presence of overt sepsis is not a prerequisite.

### Available results

Review available results and arrange new investigations.

Do not forget that the white blood cell count may be abnormally high ($> 10 \times 10^9$/L) or low ($< 2 \times 10^9$/L) in sepsis and a coagulation screen should be checked, particularly if surgery is contemplated. Thrombocytopenia and coagulopathies are common in sepsis and should be corrected before surgery.

The urea and electrolytes should be reviewed with particular attention to evidence of acute kidney injury. Liver enzymes may be abnormal, particularly when the biliary tree is the primary source of sepsis or as part of the multiorgan dysfunction of sepsis. An ECG should be checked for evidence of ischaemia or arrhythmia. ABG analysis should be taken if not already done so and may show hypoxaemia, with or without a metabolic acidosis, and evidence of raised lactate levels.

Aerobic and anaerobic blood cultures are obligatory but will be positive in only about 20% of cases. A higher positive culture rate can be achieved if the primary source of sepsis can be cultured (eg pus from an abscess, urine from an infected system). Sputum, urine, drain fluid and pus from wounds should be sent for culture and sensitivity to antibiotics. Cultures should also be taken through indwelling central venous catheters. Fungal infection should be considered, particularly when the diagnosis is proving elusive, there is an upper GI source of pathology, eg pancreatic necrosis, or there have been multiple previous courses of antibiotics. Empirical treatment with antibiotics can be started on an 'educated guess' basis (with advice from the microbiologists locally, remembering that broad-spectrum cover is recommended if organ dysfunction has been identified). These can be changed (de-escalated) when results of culture and antibiotic sensitivity become available.

Further evaluation of possible sites of sepsis include the use of ultrasound (remember that this investigation does not exclude collections), CT and laparotomy. Remember the adage, 'pus somewhere, pus nowhere, pus under the diaphragm'. Patients who are immunocompromised (eg transplant patients) may develop opportunistic infections which may require very specific investigation, eg bronchoalveolar lavage, or induced sputum sampling for those with unusual pneumonias such *Pneumocystis jirovecii* (formerly called *Pneumocystis carinii* (PCP)).

## Daily management plan: the stable patient

A daily management plan is needed for all patients and this is particularly important in patients who have or have had sepsis, no matter how stable they appear. This ensures that the patient and all members of the multidisciplinary team know what is going to happen. A list of clear, positive decisions in the patient record provides a plan for genuine progress as well as advice in the event of deterioration, eg latest microbiology results and recommendations for antimicrobials if required. The aim is to ensure progress through attention to detail and gives the patient the best chance of avoiding further deterioration. Features to consider include the following.

## Fluids

Consider the need for IV fluids on a daily basis. It is important to facilitate good tissue perfusion, and this needs to be balanced against the principles of enhanced recovery after elective surgery. Patients who were on an enhanced recovery programme may have been encouraged to regulate fluid balance themselves, relying on oral intake, but, when sepsis develops or is suspected, IV fluids will be required. Crystalloids are usually appropriate fluid replacement in cases of sepsis as there is concern that use of artificial colloids may worsen the outcome.

Large volume fluid resuscitation is likely to require guidance by using additional monitoring (CVP or cardiac output monitoring) and the patient is likely to need a higher level of care.

### Case scenario 12.2

A 61-year-old, previously fit, woman was admitted to the ward 4 days ago with acute sigmoid diverticulitis. Initial signs included minimal tenderness in the left iliac fossa. Treatment was started with co-amoxiclav and metronidazole and her fever and leucocytosis settled within 48 hours. She has suddenly become acutely unwell, with recurrent tenderness in the left iliac fossa, pyrexia of 39.2°C, tachypnoea, tachycardia and hypotension.

**What would you do at this stage? What is your differential diagnosis?**

It is clear that the patient has deteriorated markedly despite initial treatment for her presumed diagnosis: a change of treatment is needed, including review of the diagnosis. Following resuscitation (including performing the Sepsis Six, blood cultures and biochemical tests) and after discussion with her consultant, the patient is taken to theatre for an emergency sigmoid colectomy. There is a 7-cm pelvic abscess beside the inflamed sigmoid colon, which is drained and a sample of pus sent for urgent microbiological examination and culture. A Hartmann's procedure (sigmoid colectomy with colostomy and closure of the rectal stump) is carried out and the patient returned to HDU in a stable condition. Perioperative antibiotics were given and continued for a further 5 days.

**Learning points**

Recognise the patient who deviates from their anticipated recovery plan, use care bundles appropriately and involve your seniors when making decisions about source control.

## Oxygen

It is essential that the patient does not become hypoxaemic: oxygen should be administered as required to correct hypoxaemia. If facemask oxygen is inadequate, consideration should be given to additional respiratory support, which will usually require help from critical care colleagues.

## Nutrition

It is essential to ensure adequate metabolic and nutritional support of the patient in order to optimise the patient's endogenous immune function. This can be by the enteral or parenteral route.

## Antibiotics

Antibiotics must be given as early as possible when sepsis is suspected. Empirical treatment on a 'best-guess' basis should be started with microbiological advice. It is important to review the microbiology after 48 hours when cultures are available and sensitivities obtained: discussing cases with the microbiologist can be very helpful and is to be recommended.

Prolonged 'prophylaxis' is not recommended, as 'superinfection' by fungi and antibiotic-resistant organisms is encouraged. Finally, remember that enteric streptococci account for 10–20% of severe infections related to the abdomen and that they are not sensitive to all common prophylactic antibiotics.

## Additional considerations

Instructions for physiotherapy, DVT prophylaxis and, in a patient with ongoing abdominal sepsis, drain management should also be included in the daily management plan.

## Diagnosing the cause of deterioration: the unstable surgical patient

In a patient with new or on-going sepsis, deterioration may be elicited by an increase in the patient's NEWS supplemented by other information such as clotting disturbances, a metabolic acidosis, a raised lactate and/or organ dysfunction. Alternatively, the patient may simply fail to progress (see case scenario 12.1). The presence of such a pattern demands careful clinical review of symptoms and signs, repeat microbiology and review of antibiotic sensitivities and may require further radiological evaluation with either percutaneous or operative drainage of localised sepsis. Failure to diagnose significant sepsis will prove fatal.

## Definitive treatment

Definitive treatment is the single most important factor in securing survival. Localised collections of pus generally need either operative or percutaneous drainage and dead tissue should be excised. Specific soft tissue conditions such as necrotising fasciitis need to be borne in mind. Sometimes the diagnosis is obvious, but the presentation can be more subtle: suspect the diagnosis in a patient with sepsis, pain out of proportion to the physical signs and skin blistering.

In spreading soft tissue infection, it is important to establish adequate drainage and vital to excise necrotic or devitalised tissue as well as giving antibiotics. Repeated examination under anaesthesia with further debridement is usually needed.

Abdominal sepsis, if localised, may be treated initially with antibiotics or percutaneous drainage, but generally the primary source of sepsis must be removed. You should be alert to the development of recurrent sepsis during subsequent assessments of the patient.

The use of a laparostomy and/or a planned, second-look laparotomy may be useful, particularly in patients with equivocal bowel perfusion during previous procedures or if there is a significant risk of intra-abdominal hypertension.

Obstruction of the biliary or urinary system must be relieved. An infected prosthesis will usually need to be removed (eg peripheral or central venous cannulae, urinary catheters, prosthetic metalwork).

Sometimes, such decisions are difficult and will require discussion between different medical teams. Vigilance around the possibility of catheter-associated sepsis, particularly in patients in the HDU or ICU, is essential and can be avoided by adherence to vascular device care bundles.

MRSA infection is becoming more common in all patients. It is important to distinguish between patients who are colonised carriers and those with MRSA sepsis. Whereas MRSA colonisation does not present major problems in most patients, it may do so in those patients with prostheses (aortic valves, aortic grafts, hip replacements), among whom it is associated with a very high mortality. Often, the only treatment is removal of the prosthesis and long-term antibiotics. Microbiological help is essential.

## Case scenario 12.3

You are asked to review the patient discussed above (case scenario 12.2) 72 hours following surgery. She had improved for 48 hours and was returned to the ward, but is now breathless and pyrexial again (38.3°C). Her blood pressure is normal but she is tachycardic (115 bpm), tachypnoeic (28/min) and poorly perfused. Urine output has fallen off over the last 4 hours to 12 ml in the last hour. Her chest seems clear but her abdomen is distended and quiet. The stoma has not worked properly yet. The pelvic drain has produced 40 ml serous fluid today only. You suspect sepsis and give high-flow oxygen (15 L/min) and start a fluid challenge of 500 ml of Hartmann's stat and recognise the need to complete the full CCrISP three-stage assessment.

The foundation year doctor had checked bloods and a chest X-ray. Apart from a leucocytosis ($17 \times 10^9$/L), the blood results are unremarkable. There are no diagnostic features on the chest X-ray. There are no signs of DVT and prescribed DVT prophylaxis (SC heparin and anti-thrombosis stockings) are in place. You perform a cautious rectal examination but find no obvious abnormality. Blood gases are now reviewed and show $PaO_2$ (on $FiO_2$ of 0.6) 11.4 kPa, pH 7.29, BE −7.2 mmol/L and lactate 4.5 mmol/L. After 1000 ml of saline, there is a little improvement in perfusion, but no change in heart rate and urine output is only 15 ml in the hour since you were called.

## What would you do now?

The patient remains breathless and you have neither a diagnosis nor any further intervention of obvious help at your disposal. You request an urgent review by the critical care team and, as the patient still seems underperfused, give a further fluid challenge, while the foundation year doctor checks an ECG (normal).

The critical care team arrive and assess the patient. They share your concern and think ventilation will be needed – transfer is arranged. You inform your consultant, who asks to be kept informed. During transfer, the patient becomes more breathless and is intubated shortly after arriving in ICU. The positive-pressure ventilation reduces cardiac filling and, despite further fluid loading, inotropes are required to support the cardiovascular system. Urine output tails off. A chest X-ray shows some diffuse bilateral shadowing suggestive of ARDS. You update your consultant, who comes to examine the patient. No cause for deterioration has yet been found.

Given the previous operation and the leucocytosis, recurrent abdominal sepsis is suspected. The patient is too unstable for CT, so repeat laparotomy is arranged and carried out by the consultant. The bowel is intact but two abscesses are found between loops of small intestine and a left subphrenic abscess is identified: these are drained and lavaged. More pus is sent for culture.

The patient returns to ICU for full cardiac, respiratory and renal support. The culture result from the pus taken at the first operation has grown a coliform resistant to prescribed antibiotics but sensitive to netilmicin. Treatment is changed accordingly and the patient slowly begins to improve over the succeeding 72 hours.

## Learning points

- Patients can deteriorate despite receiving appropriate initial adequate treatment.
- A diagnosis that accounts adequately for any septic deterioration is essential – this allows definitive treatment ('source control').
- Early cultures can help target later treatment – the right antibiotic is important.

Nosocomial (hospital-acquired) infection is common in patients treated in ICU and may compound multiorgan failure. The decision to give antibiotics for a positive culture (eg of *Pseudomonas* spp.) should be carefully balanced by the presence of a host response to such bacteria, the site of the potential infection and the need to avoid superinfection or antibiotic resistance. Such issues should be discussed with the microbiologist.

The recognition of the role of endogenous mediators in sepsis syndrome and the advent of biotechnology resulted in several, large, multicentre, randomised trials using monoclonal antibodies or antagonists to various sepsis mediators including activated protein C, endotoxin, tumour necrosis factor and IL-1. However, it remains clear that these treatments are unlikely ever to replace the established basic principles of management, although time will tell whether a substantial adjuvant role can be identified.

## Case scenario 12.4 (continuation of case 12.3)

Four days after her admission to ICU, the patient again deteriorates overnight, needing increased vasopressors, inotropic support and oxygen, and the critical care team suspect sepsis. A full infection screen has been taken by the time you arrive and the central lines have been changed by your ICU colleagues. There are no clinical features to suggest recurrent intra-abdominal sepsis: abdominal CT confirms that there is no new intra-abdominal collection. The patient has had several recent courses of antibiotics and there is no clear 'best-guess' antibiotic to use.

Six hours later, the patient is no better and a joint discussion is held between surgeons, ICU staff and the microbiologist. No cultures are available but Candida was seen on samples from the urinary catheter and one of the removed central lines. It is decided to start treatment for presumed candidaemia.

After a 4-week course of antifungal therapy and several other complications, the patient is discharged to the ward.

## Learning points

- Surgical patients on ICU with sepsis and organ dysfunction run a roller-coaster course, often with a range of complications – some surgical and some medical.
- Active surgical input to care helps manage these effectively.

- Multiple courses of antibiotics, gastrointestinal perforation, critical illness and multiple monitoring lines are all risk factors for fungal sepsis – many of these factors exist in surgical patients.

- Fungal sepsis may present with non-specific signs such as a failure to progress. Identification of fungi within the blood, abdomen or urine (or at any two other sites) would prompt many intensivists to discuss antifungal therapy with their microbiologist and surgeon.

Established septic shock or multiorgan dysfunction is thus really treatable only by prevention through attention to detail.

Preoperatively, the general health of the patient should be optimised (coexisting diseases, nutrition) and any focus of sepsis should be treated.

Perioperatively, prophylactic antibiotics should be given and surgery executed in a rapid, clean and haemostatic manner in order to prevent complications. Operations should be performed electively whenever possible.

Postoperatively, assess clinically and monitor closely to detect problems at an early stage, and deal with any problems found quickly and comprehensively. Be alert to 'occult' hypoxia and hypovolaemia. Use prophylactic measures such as chest physiotherapy and reinstate oral intake/enteral feeding at the earliest opportunity. Remove lines and tubes as soon as possible, and employ short courses of targeted antibiotics. In the event of a septic complication, adequate resuscitation and early definitive treatment should reduce the chance of full-blown sepsis developing.

## Summary

- Sepsis is a mediator disease.

- Prevention is better than cure.

- Clinical signs may be obvious but are often covert.

- Survival is improved by suspecting the diagnosis and treating the patient at an early stage.

■ The principles of management are:

- rapid resuscitation to restore oxygenation and perfusion;
- continued optimal organ support;
- diagnosis and eradication of the source of sepsis;
- judicious and appropriate antibiotic treatment after cultures;
- reassessment to ensure continued progress.

■ The SSC guidelines, particularly the 'Sepsis Six', are a useful starting point in the management of the patient with severe sepsis.

## Further reading

National Institute for Health and Care Excellence (NICE). *Sepsis: Recognition, Diagnosis and Early Management*. NICE Guideline 51. NICE, London; 2016.

Seymour CW, Liu VX, Iwashyna TJ et al. Assessment of clinical criteria for sepsis: for the Third International Consensus Definitions for Sepsis and Septic Shock (Sepsis-3). *JAMA* 2016; **315**: 762–774.

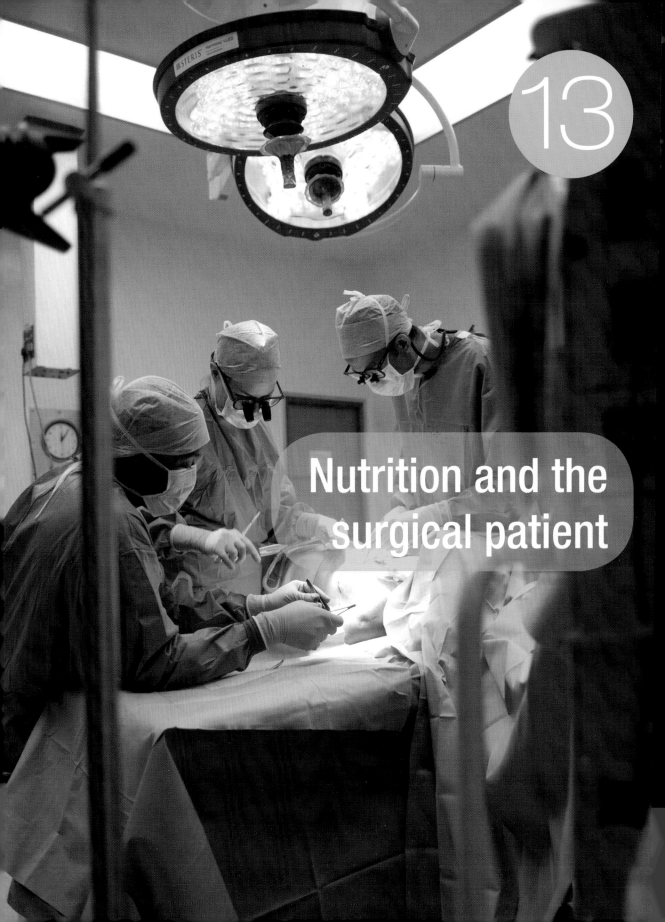

13

Nutrition and the surgical patient

## Learning outcomes

This chapter will help you to:

- identify the underlying mechanisms and consequences of malnutrition in critically ill surgical patients;

- use screening and assessment procedures to identify both patients with established malnutrition and those who are at risk;

- describe basic nutritional requirements and how critical illness affects these needs;

- understand the various methods of delivering nutritional support and choosing the most appropriate option;

- recognise the potential complications of the different methods of nutritional support, and how these can be minimised.

## Malnutrition

Malnutrition represents a deficiency, excess or imbalance in nutrient supplies to the body, typically of multiple components such as energy, protein, vitamins and minerals. This results in adverse effects on body composition and function. Most surgical patients will have a nutrient deficiency.

The National Institute for Health and Care Excellence (NICE) defines malnutrition using the following criteria:

- body mass index (BMI) $< 18.$ kg/m$^2$;

- unintentional weight loss $> 10\%$ within the last 3–6 months;

- BMI $< 20$ kg/m$^2$ and unintentional weight loss $> 5\%$ within last 3–6 months.

Malnutrition is present in up to 60% of surgical patients upon admission to hospital, and may either contribute to, or be a result of, the underlying disease process. Furthermore, people who are admitted in a good nutritional state may go on to develop malnutrition as an inpatient. This may be directly related to their surgical pathology, the metabolic response to illness, or simply inadequate oral intake whilst in hospital. Patients should be considered 'at risk' of this if they have:

■ poor oral intake for more than 5 days and/or likely to have on-going poor intake for 5 days or longer;

■ poor absorptive capacity and/or high nutrient losses and/or increased nutritional needs from causes such as catabolism.

It is crucial to consider nutritional support for those with established malnourishment and to identify and treat those at risk. If left untreated, malnutrition is associated with increased postoperative complications, infection, increased length of hospital stay and greater mortality.

## Pathophysiology

In order to address the problems of malnutrition in the acutely unwell surgical patient, you should have a knowledge of the metabolic changes that occur with starvation (see Box 13.1), as well as the effect of the stress response to surgery.

### Starvation and malnutrition

Under normal circumstances, the body utilises carbohydrate as its primary energy substrate, creating adenosine triphosphate (ATP) via the citric acid cycle and oxidative phosphorylation. Insulin is the major anabolic hormone, whose key roles include stimulating glycogenesis, promotion of intracellular glucose uptake/storage, protein synthesis and lipid synthesis.

Box 13.1 Overview of the main metabolic responses to starvation

- Insulin ⬇
- Glucagon ⬆
- Hepatic glycogenolysis ⬆
- Protein catabolism ⬆
- Lipolysis and ketogenesis ⬆
- Basal metabolic rate ⬇

During fasting, insulin levels fall and glucagon levels rise; subsequently, hepatic glycogen stores (approximately 200 g) deplete rapidly over 24–48 hours. Muscle contains an additional 500 g of stored glycogen, but this cannot be directly utilised by other tissues. Instead, it is converted in the muscle to lactate, which is then transported to the liver and converted to glucose via the Cori cycle.

As carbohydrate supply diminishes, the body adapts to use fatty acids as its main fuel source. Protein is preserved where possible; however, some breakdown remains necessary to supply amino acids for gluconeogenesis, as fatty acids cannot be used for this purpose. Certain cells, including erythrocytes and renal medullary cells, can only use glucose as an energy substrate. The brain is also largely reliant on glucose metabolism, but can adapt over time to use ketone bodies for approximately 30% of its energy requirements.

Fatty acids undergo a process called beta-oxidation to form acetyl-coA. In normal health, acetyl-coA can enter the citric acid cycle, by combining with oxaloacetate. However, in starvation, oxaloacetate stores become depleted, as it is also required for essential gluconeogenesis. As a result, the acetyl-coA formed from beta-oxidation is converted to ketone bodies. With continued starvation, the liver increases its capacity for ketone body production, and the brain adapts, partly using ketone bodies for energy. This allows some protein sparing, with the result that losses eventually fall to around 20 g/day.

Metabolic rate also falls over time, with reduced conversion of thyroxine to its active compound, triiodothyronine. This reduces resting energy requirements from around 1800 to 1500 calories per day (in an average 70-kg man).

*Stress response to surgery/trauma*

The 'stress response' describes a myriad of metabolic and hormonal changes that occur in response to trauma, the magnitude of which reflect the extent of the injury. These adjustments create a 'catabolic state', designed to increase the availability of energy substrates and preserve body fluids during the period of increased metabolic demand.

Sympathetic nervous system stimulation causes adrenal catecholamine release, resulting in tachycardia and vasoconstriction. The renin–angiotensin–aldosterone system is activated, promoting sodium and water retention.

Levels of adrenocorticotrophic hormone (ACTH) rise, resulting in glucocorticoid release. Cortisol promotes breakdown of fat and protein, and increases gluconeogenesis. Growth hormone (GH) secretion is stimulated, promoting protein synthesis, increasing lipolysis and antagonising the effects of insulin. Cortisol and GH both impair peripheral glucose uptake, whilst catecholamines inhibit insulin release, limiting the usefulness of glucose as an energy source by creating a state of 'insulin resistance'. These changes mean that hyperglycaemia is common. Many critically ill patients require a variable-rate insulin infusion to maintain normoglycaemia, typically 8–10 mmol/L, as this has been shown to improve outcome after major surgery, particularly cardiac surgery. Hypo- and hyperglycaemia have been associated with increased morbidity and mortality, so titrating insulin to very restrictive blood glucose limits is more likely to result in significant swings in plasma levels and you should aim to ensure that the patient has a moderate target for blood glucose.

Whilst the body cannot use glucose effectively, fatty acids released via lipolysis once again act as the primary energy substrate.

As the stress response subsides and insulin resistance falls, there is a move towards net anabolism, making up the lost reserves of protein and energy. This usually coincides with the resumption of eating/adequate nutritional intake and increased mobility, both of which are required to restore muscle mass. Although some forms of anaesthetic technique, eg epidural anaesthesia, have been shown to moderate the stress response to surgery for a short time, there is little else that can be done to reduce this response.

## Metabolic changes in sepsis

The metabolic changes that develop with the onset of sepsis are complex and are an exaggeration of the stress response. The key changes are development of a hypermetabolic state and increased protein breakdown. There may be marked glucose intolerance with the development of a diabetes-like state. As with the stress response, insulin resistance develops, and the septic patient has a greater reliance on fat as fuel.

The rate of protein breakdown may reach a substantial 250 g/day. Muscle and visceral protein is consumed for gluconeogenesis, despite the frequently elevated plasma glucose concentration. Although some of this exaggerated muscle protein breakdown might be due to the hormonal environment, the release of cytokines such as IL-1, IL-6 and tumour necrosis factor (TNF) may also be implicated.

## Screening and assessment

### Screening tools

Potential or established malnutrition can easily be missed, particularly among critically ill patients. As a result, numerous screening tools have been developed to help with early identification of 'at-risk' individuals. All hospitalised patients should undergo nutritional screening by an appropriately trained professional on admission, and at least weekly thereafter during their inpatient stay.

The most commonly used, and validated, nutritional screening tool in the UK is MUST (Malnutrition Universal Screening Tool), which uses similar indicators to those described by NICE in its criteria (Figure 13.1).

As with many screening tools, the outcome is operator dependent and subject to variability. BMI measurements alone will not be able to identify all malnourished patients. Excessive oedema or ascites can influence results, as a 'dry weight' is needed for accurate calculation (see Table 13.1), and the practicalities of obtaining measurements can be an issue with obtunded or immobile patients. It is also important to remember that a high BMI does not exclude nutrient deficiency, as the effects of acute illness and poor diet may still result in significant depletion of various nutritional components.

Therefore, it is helpful to use additional methods of assessment in conjunction with screening.

Table 13.1 Estimated contributions to body weight from ascites or oedema, based on severity of clinical findings

| | Ascites (kg) | Oedema (kg) |
| --- | --- | --- |
| Mild | 2.2 | 1.0 |
| Moderate | 6.0 | 5.0 |
| Severe | 14.0 | 10.4 |

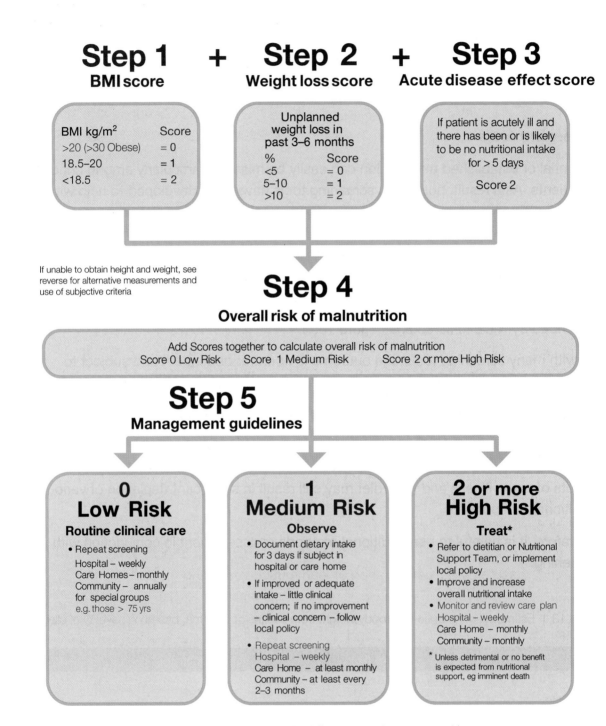

Figure 13.1 Malnutrition Universal Screening Tool (from www.bapen.org.uk).

## History and examination

A detailed history may be difficult to get from a critically unwell patient, but information regarding weight loss, altered/poor nutritional intake or increased gastrointestinal losses may be found from the patient's relatives or medical records.

Non-specific examination findings such as cachexia, oedema, skin changes and muscle wasting may be seen in extreme malnutrition, but there may be little to find in milder cases.

## Anthropometric and functional measures

Anthropometry studies the quantitative measurement of the human body, and numerous measurement techniques to assess nutritional status have been developed. The procedures are inexpensive and non-invasive, but must be performed by a trained practitioner in order to achieve consistent results.

BMI is an example of an anthropometric measure, but, as discussed, it has limitations and does not provide a comprehensive picture of body composition. Calliper measurements of skinfold thickness (eg triceps, subscapular, biceps) give an indication of subcutaneous fat stores that correlates closely with overall body fat percentage. Mid-arm circumference (MAC) and mid-arm muscle circumference (MAMC) can be useful adjuncts to estimate fat/muscle ratios. Typical values are shown in Table 13.2. Again, changes seen in fluid distribution in critical illness can render these measures inaccurate and must be taken into consideration. MAC can also be used to estimate BMI in patients in whom height or weight cannot be measured – if less than 23.5cm, the BMI is likely to be less than 20mg/m$^2$.

Functional measures of nutritional status include hand grip and respiratory muscle strength. These provide an indication of lean muscle mass and may be useful in

Table 13.2 Typical adult values for commonly used anthropometric measures in nutritional assessment

| Anthropometric measures | Typical adult values |
| --- | --- |
| Triceps skinfold thickness (TSF) (mm) | Male: 12.5<br>Female: 16.5 |
| Mid-arm circumference (MAC) (cm) | Male: 29.3<br>Female: 28.5 |
| Mid-arm muscle circumference (MAMC) (cm)<br>MAC – 3.14 × (TSF/10)] | Male 25.3<br>Female: 23.2 |

monitoring of clinically stable patients. However, in critical illness, a number of factors, such as impaired consciousness, critical illness polyneuropathy/myopathy and oedema, will contribute significantly to reduced muscle strength.

## Investigations

Laboratory investigations are rarely helpful during initial assessment. Albumin is used in the wider population as a marker of protein deficiency in chronic malnutrition. However, hypoalbuminaemia is commonly seen as a consequence of the stress response, making it unhelpful for assessing nutritional status in the critically ill, in whom it is more of a reflection of illness severity.

Identification of any major blood glucose or electrolyte abnormalities is important, and a renal profile will help in assessment of hydration status, which is often also compromised in the acutely unwell patient. More detailed studies of other vitamins/minerals and trace elements may be recommended following dietetic involvement.

## Basic nutritional requirements

The typical daily nutritional requirements of an average, healthy adult are shown in Table 13.3.

These requirements are markedly altered in critical illness, where the response to stress and injury results in a significant rise in basal metabolic rate (BMR), and hence

Table 13.3 Typical daily nutritional requirements in a healthy adult

| Component | Typical daily requirement in a healthy adult |
| --- | --- |
| Energy | 30–40 kcal/kg |
| Carbohydrate | 10 g/kg |
| Protein | 0.5–1 g/kg |
| Fat | 1 g/kg |
| Water | 30–40 ml/kg |
| Nitrogen | 0.2 g/kg |
| Sodium | 1 mmol/kg |
| Potassium | 1 mmol/kg |
| Calcium | 0.1–0.2 mmol/kg |
| Magnesium | 0.1–0.2 mmol/kg |

Table 13.4 Increases in BMR observed in various clinical conditions

| Condition | Stress factor (% increase in BMR) |
|---|---|
| Infection | 25–45 |
| ICU admission | |
|   Ventilated | 0–10 |
|   Sepsis | 20–60 |
| Surgery | |
|   Uncomplicated | 5–20 |
|   Complicated | 25–40 |

nutrient demand. Table 13.4 provides estimates of increases in BMR associated with various conditions: even in uncomplicated surgical procedures, the metabolic rate may rise by an additional 20%. Stress hyperglycaemia, loss of muscle mass, concurrent infections and organ failure can also have a significant effect on energy expenditure (EE), and the body's ability to use different substrates. Various equations have been formulated to calculate EE and guide replacement, but these are often inaccurate, resulting in under- or over-feeding when used in the critically ill population.

Management of nutrition in surgical and critically ill patients must be tailored to the individual, and involve early specialist dietetic input. Other vitamins, minerals and trace elements in addition to those listed above are also required for maintenance of health, and should be accounted for when devising a plan of nutritional support.

## Treatment

### Methods of nutritional support

The options available for providing nutritional support in patients with malnutrition, or at risk of malnutrition, are:

- enteral nutrition:

  - supplementation of oral intake
  - nasogastric feeding
  - nasojejunal or nasoduodenal feeding
  - tube enterostomy

- parenteral nutrition.

## Enteral nutrition

### Supplementation of oral intake

Where possible, feeding by the enteral route should be maintained. In compliant patients who have no swallowing problems and are still maintaining some oral intake, a dietetic review and adjustment of the meal plan to accommodate the patient's clinical condition may be sufficient.

The use of oral nutritional supplements may also be of benefit. These are available in a variety of forms, such as juices, soups and mousses, providing from around 1 to 2.4 kcal/ml depending upon the preparation (typically with carbohydrate as the predominant energy source). They also contain vitamins, minerals and trace elements. These supplements should be used in conjunction with an oral diet, not as a meal replacement therapy, in order to maximise their benefit. Despite the variety of preparations available, some patients do not find these palatable, and, in the critically ill, regular adequate oral intake is often not possible or is insufficient to meet increased requirements.

### Nasogastric feeding

Nasogastric feeding is commonly used when oral intake is deemed insufficient or unsafe, such as in patients with swallowing difficulties or impaired consciousness. Successful feeding by this route requires access to a functioning gastrointestinal tract.

Absolute contraindications to nasogastric feeding are mechanical bowel obstruction, suspicion of ischaemic bowel, massive gastrointestinal haemorrhage or patient refusal (if the patient has capacity). Relative contraindications include severe diarrhoea/ vomiting, circulatory shock states (where there may be a risk of intestinal ischaemia), proximal small bowel fistula and conditions in which nasogastric tube placement may be unsafe (eg following major maxillofacial surgery, skull base fracture or oesophageal varices). Paralytic ileus is a common relative contraindication that is often identified following failure to absorb nasogastric feed, and may be managed without discontinuing feed altogether (see below).

Nasogastric feed can be delivered as a bolus over mealtimes, or continuously over 16–24 hours. The latter is used in critically ill patients, as they will often be sedated and receiving intravenous insulin infusions, with the result that continuous

Table 13.5 Advantages and disadvantages of nasogastric feeding

| Advantages | Disadvantages |
| --- | --- |
| Physiological | May be difficulty with placement |
| Effective, cheap and safe | Misplacement may occur |
| Reduced incidence of hyperglycaemia, cholestasis and hypertriglyceridaemia compared with the parenteral route | Potential complications |
| | Pulmonary aspiration |
| | Discomfort |
| | Pressure necrosis |
| | Diarrhoea |

administration is safer and more practical. Maintenance of 30–45° head-up positioning during feeding is important in these patients. Even ventilated patients with cuffed endotracheal tubes are susceptible to aspiration. Tracheal intubation prevents aspiration of most oropharyngeal secretions, but small creases in the cuff/balloon will permit some leakage, which can result in the development of ventilator-associated pneumonia. Head-up positioning and above-cuff suctioning can help to reduce this risk.

Each hospital will each have its own feeding protocols, with different feed rates and definitions of 'high' aspirates. An example of a typical regime involves commencement of a 'standard' feed at 30 ml/h. The nasogastric tube is aspirated after 4 hours, and if less than 250 ml gastric fluid is aspirated, the feed rate can be increased to 65 ml/h and 4-hourly aspirates continued. If repeatedly high aspirates (eg >250 ml) are obtained, management options include reducing the feed rate and, if this fails, introducing prokinetic medications.

Gastroparesis is common in critically ill surgical patients and is caused by a multitude of factors such as the underlying illness, altered gut perfusion and the use of medications that delay gastric emptying (eg opioids, sedatives).

The use of prokinetics is common, to increase luminal transport and strengthen smooth muscle contraction in the gut. Treatment regimens may use of one or more of the following drugs:

- metoclopramide 10 mg IV tds
- erythromycin 250 mg IV bd
- domperidone 10 mg IV tds.

Typically, a response to treatment will be seen within 24 hours. Ongoing high aspirates warrants consideration of alternative feeding methods, such as post-pyloric or parenteral nutrition.

## Nasogastric tube insertion

Patients may struggle to comply with the discomfort of feeding tube insertion, particularly if they are confused or agitated. If a surgical patient is likely to need postoperative nutritional support, consideration should be given to intraoperative insertion of a nasogastric tube (NGT), whilst the patient still has the benefit of general anaesthesia. Preoperative feeding may also be indicated in patients undergoing major elective procedures who have established malnutrition.

In 2005, the National Patient Safety Agency (NPSA) issued an alert regarding injury/death occurring in patients who were fed via misplaced NGTs. Despite this, between 2005 and 2010, a further 21 deaths and 79 cases of harm occurred (see Table 13.6). As a consequence, since 2009, **feeding via a misplaced NGT is a Never Event**.

Any NGT used for feeding should be radio-opaque along its entire length, and have clear markings for measurement of external length. Measurement of nose to ear to xiphisternum distance should be performed prior to insertion, to estimate the appropriate tube length.

Table 13.6 Incidents related to misplaced NGTs reported to NPSA September 2005 to March 2010

| Checking method where error occurred | Total number of incidents | Number of reported deaths |
|---|---|---|
| X-ray misinterpretation | 45 | 12 |
| Fed despite pH aspirate 6–8 | 7 | 2 |
| Fed after obtaining pH 1–5.5 (Note – almost none of these pH levels were contemporaneously recorded) | 9 | 1 |
| Water instilled down NGT before pH testing | 2 | 0 |
| Not checked at all | 9 | 1 |
| Apparent migration after initially correct placement | 8 | 1 |
| No information obtained re. checking method | 17 | 4 |
| Other | | |
|    Placed under endoscopic guidance | 1 | 0 |
|    Visual appearance of aspirate | 1 | - |
| Bubble test | 1 | 0 |
| **Total** | **100** | **21** |

Once in place, correct positioning must be confirmed and clearly documented prior to use, with one of the following methods:

- pH testing (first line): pH should be between 1 and 5.5, as determined using pH paper manufactured to test human gastric aspirate;

- X-ray (second line): must be adequate to confirm the tube position, and this confirmation should be made only by someone assessed as competent to do so.

Figures 13.2 to 13.4 show X-rays of correctly placed (Figure 13.2) and incorrectly placed (Figures 13.3 and 13.4) NGTs.

Feeding should be discontinued and repeated testing performed following any episodes of vomiting and retching, if there is suspicion of tube displacement, or the patient develops unexplained respiratory symptoms. Regular pH testing is also recommended: at least once daily and prior to feeding or administering medication. The latter may not be practicable in critically ill patients receiving continuous nasogastric feed (which will raise the pH of any aspirate) and being treated with anti-reflux medications. Most units will have protocols based around external inspection and regular documentation of external tube length and condition of the fixation tapes.

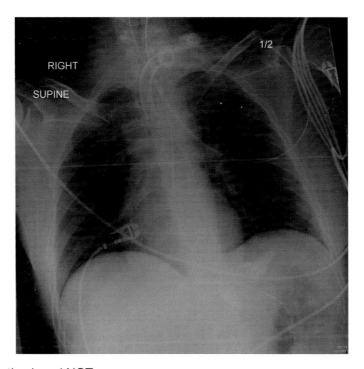

Figure 13.2 Correctly placed NGT.

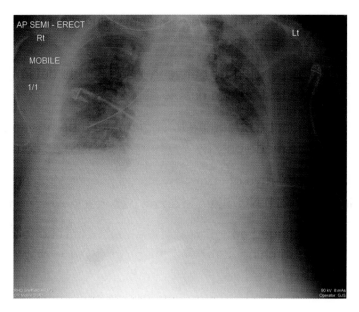

Figure 13.3  Right main bronchus placement.

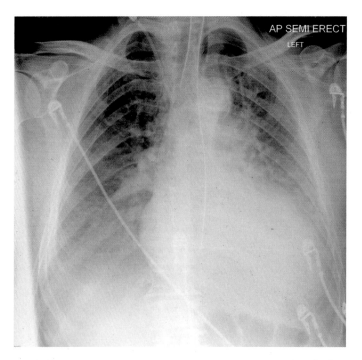

Figure 13.4  Oesophageal placement.

A large proportion of critically ill patients develop delirium and agitation, pulling out their NGTs, resulting in the need for repeated tube reinsertions and X-rays, which is neither pleasant nor optimal for their care. In such patients, a bridle device may be of use. These devices use catheter-mounted magnets to allow passage of a length of tape behind the patient's vomer nasal bone, which can then be secured to the tube where it exits each nostril, making the NGT more difficult to remove.

## Nasojejunal and nasoduodenal feeding

Post-pyloric feeding may be appropriate in some patients in whom the nasogastric route is relatively contraindicated, such as those with gastroparesis that fails to respond to prokinetics or postoperative patients with upper gastrointestinal tract anastomoses. Otherwise, the contraindications for nasojejenual/nasoduodenal nutrition are the same as for nasogastric feeding.

Post-pyloric feeding tubes are largely similar to nasogastric tubes, although may have adaptations such as weighted tips and artificial 'cilia' to promote transit into the small bowel. Double-lumen varieties are available, with an additional gastric opening for decompression and/or aspiration if indicated.

They can be inserted at the bedside, but will always require radiological confirmation of placement. More common methods of tube insertion involve siting under direct vision during surgery, endoscopic placement and fluoroscopically guided insertion. Correct positioning can be tricky, and requires the input of an experienced clinician. Therefore, although there is some evidence that feeding critically ill patients via this route may result in lower pneumonia rates than with nasogastric feeding, it is not practicable to use this as a first-line method for enteral nutrition.

Feed regimens are similar to that used for the nasogastric route. Regular aspiration is not routinely performed with post-pyloric tubes, so patients must be observed carefully for signs of abdominal distension or vomiting, which may suggest outward tube migration. In patients with a multi-lumen tube, the presence of feed in the gastric aspirate may also suggest misplacement. If concerned, feed should be discontinued pending radiological confirmation of tube position.

## Tube enterostomy

Tube enterostomy (gastrostomy, jejunostomy or duodenostomy) should be considered in patients expected to require prolonged nutritional support (>4 weeks), or if access via the oral/nasal route is not feasible in the short term. This may be following complex elective abdominal surgery (eg oesophagectomy, gastrectomy or pancreatoduodenectomy), major intra-abdominal trauma, following resection of oropharyngeal tumours, or in those at chronic risk of aspiration (eg neuromuscular disorders).

There are a few absolute contraindications to tube enterostomy, which include uncorrected coagulopathy, distal mechanical bowel obstruction, and peritonitis/ infection over the insertion site. Relative contraindications include the presence of intra-abdominal malignancy (due to the potential for seeding), massive ascites, hepatosplenomegaly, gastric varices, and peritoneal dialysis – many of these prohibit percutaneous tube placement, but the associated risk can be attenuated by choosing different insertion methods.

Enterostomy tubes can be placed using surgical (open or laparoscopic), endoscopic or radiological techniques; numerous varieties are available, as demonstrated in Figure 13.5. Surgical placement can be performed, where appropriate, as an adjunctive procedure in patients undergoing major elective surgery. Fluoroscopically-guided insertion may be indicated in cases where oral access is not possible.

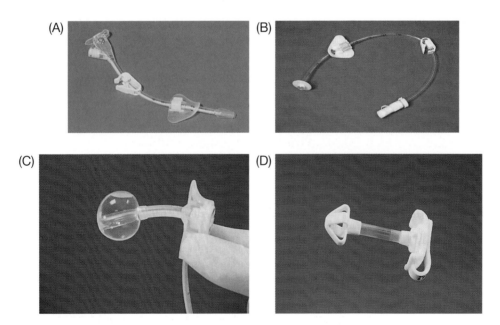

Figure 13.5 Examples of enterostomy tubes. (A) Standard percutaneous endoscopic gastrostomy (PEG) tube. (B) Radiologically inserted gastrostomy (RIG). (C) Button PEG – low profile, held in position by water-filled balloon. More convenient for longer term use than a standard tube. (D) Alternative low profile PEG, held in position with a distal flange.

In postoperative/non-surgical patients, percutaneous endoscopic gastrostomy (PEG) using local anaesthetic infiltration and endoscopic guidance is the most commonly used method, as it has a lower complication and mortality rate (2%) compared to surgical insertion. PEG tubes which have been inserted without complication can be used for feeding 4 h after insertion. Feeding regimens are similar to those used for other enteral routes, with bolus or continuous feeds being possible.

## Parenteral feeding

Parenteral nutrition should be considered in patients with, or at risk of, malnutrition and in whom:

- oral and/or enteral intake is unsafe or inadequate to meet nutritional requirements;

- there is a non-functional, inaccessible or perforated gastrointestinal tract.

Common surgical indications include: proximal small bowel obstruction or intestinal fistulae, short bowel syndrome (<300 cm functional small bowel), or refractory inflammatory bowel disease.

Feed is usually supplied as total parenteral nutrition (TPN), an all-in-one preparation that can be administered via continuous infusion, and its components adjusted to meet a patient's specific and complete nutritional requirements.

TPN must be administered into a central vein because of to its high osmolality, which can otherwise precipitate thrombophlebitis. 'Peripheral' parenteral nutrition (PPN) is available as a temporary alternative until central access is obtained; PPN has a lower osmolality than TPN, but remains hyperosmolar to plasma, so can still cause vascular injury in a similar way. Furthermore, PPN does not provide equivalent nutrient replacement to TPN.

Many critically ill patients will have central venous catheters (CVCs) in jugular or subclavian veins which can be used to commence parenteral feeding (femoral CVCs should be avoided as there is greater risk of introducing bacteraemia). These lines are routinely changed every 7 days to minimise the risk of catheter-related bloodstream infection (CRBSI); in cases where prolonged TPN may be required, insertion of a PICC (peripherally inserted central catheter) or tunnelled central line should be considered.

Regardless of catheter type, TPN should be administered via a dedicated lumen to reduce contamination risk. Feed should be introduced gradually, under dietetic guidance, with the rate of infusion increased over a 24- to 72-hour period.

Careful monitoring of metabolic status and specialist dietetic input is crucial and regular blood glucose measurement is required; the carbohydrate component of TPN is supplied as glucose, and hyperglycaemia is common. Daily urea, creatinine and electrolyte measurements (ie sodium, potassium, chloride, magnesium, phosphate and bicarbonate) are also required, particularly when there is a risk of refeeding syndrome (see later). TPN is presented as a lipid emulsion; therefore, regular monitoring of triglyceride levels is also needed. Abnormal liver function tests (LFTs) are also common. In the short term, these do not reflect permanent damage, although this may occur in patients receiving long-term treatment (ie >4 weeks). A 2010 National Confidential Enquiry into Patient Outcome and Death (NCEPOD) investigating inpatients receiving parenteral nutrition found that 43% of all patients studied were not adequately monitored clinically and biochemically. As a result, 39% experienced some form of electrolyte disturbance, in half of whom it was deemed to have been avoidable.

## Complications of different nutritional support methods

### Complications of enteral feeding

#### Related to intubation of the gastrointestinal tract

##### Tube displacement

This is a common complication that can have serious consequences. Hospital protocols for enteral feeding should incorporate regular checks for correct tube positioning, and instructions as to how to manage suspected displacement.

In patients with a displaced tube enterostomy, continuing feeding may result in peritonitis. If suspected, feeding should be stopped and appropriate contrast imaging arranged to confirm tube position. In the event that an enterostomy tube is completely removed, a Foley catheter can be temporarily inserted via the stoma site to prevent tract closure whilst specialist input is sought for definitive management.

## Pressure necrosis/fistulation

Pressure necrosis of the nasal mucosa is common when nasoenteric tubes remain in place for long periods, hence the importance of considering whether tube enterostomy is appropriate.

In extreme circumstances, more distal necrosis can lead to fistula formation. In patients with both endotracheal and nasoenteric tubes, tracheo-oesophageal fistula can develop, which may become apparent by the presence of feed on tracheal suctioning. Gastrocolocutaneous fistulae can also occur in patients with tube enterostomies, usually following injury to the large bowel at the time of insertion.

## Wound infection/dehiscence/bleeding

This occurs more commonly in patients with tube enterostomy, and can usually be managed conservatively with appropriate antimicrobial treatment of correction of any underlying coagulopathies.

## Related to nutrient delivery

### Tube blockage

Tubes can easily become blocked, particularly after the delivery of crushed medications. Post-pyloric feeding tubes are typically of a finer bore than NGTs and are more susceptible to blockage. Most blockages can be resolved by flushing with sterile water, or specific commercial solutions are available if this fails.

### Pulmonary aspiration

This may be a result of tube misplacement, but can also occur with correctly positioned tubes. Nasoenteric tubes may impede gastro-oesophageal sphincter function; delayed gastric emptying also increases patient vulnerability. Maintaining a head-up positioning during feeding can reduce the risk of aspiration, and the use of proton pump inhibitors or H2-receptor antagonists increases the pH of any aspirated gastric contents, which may reduce the resulting harm. Prokinetics may be indicated if delayed emptying is suspected; and more distally positioned tubes can be considered if there is likely to be long-term aspiration risk.

## Diarrhoea

This has been reported in up to 68% of critically ill patients receiving enteral feed, and is usually multifactorial in aetiology. Concomitant antibiotic administration is the commonest identifiable cause. Villous atrophy occurs when there are prolonged periods without enteral nutrition and may also contribute; this can sometimes be attenuated by the early introduction of even small volumes of enteral nutrition ('trophic feeding', eg 10 ml/h nasogastric feed), if full feeding is not possible.

Infections of the gastrointestinal tract (eg *Clostridium difficile*) should be considered, and appropriate samples for culture obtained. Where no infective source is found, reducing feed rates or using pharmacological agents to slow gut transit (eg loperamide, codeine) may help.

## Complications of parenteral nutrition

### Catheter related

#### Infection

Catheter-related bloodstream infection. is a major source of hospital-acquired bacteraemia and mortality, with many cases (approximately 42%) arising from central venous catheters. TPN further increases the risk of CRBSI, so a high index of suspicion should be maintained.

The risk can be reduced by adopting strict aseptic techniques during the insertion and handling of central lines, the use of antimicrobial-impregnated catheters, and by allocating a dedicated lumen for the administration of TPN.

In cases of suspected CRBSI, ideally the catheter should be removed and the line tip sent for culture and sensitivities. However, if the risk of line removal outweighs the benefits (ie if there are difficulties in obtaining alternative venous access), then paired blood cultures should be taken, from the central line and a peripheral site. Microbiology input should be sought early, particularly in the latter scenario, to ensure early and appropriate antimicrobial management.

#### Line blockage

Line occlusion may be due to a blockage within the lumen of the catheter (eg clotted blood, precipitate from drugs or TPN), external venous thrombus, or secondary to line positioning (eg the exit port pressing against the vein wall, external kinking of the line). Intraluminal occlusion can often be remedied by flushing with sterile 0.9% sodium chloride; occasionally thrombolytic agents (such as urokinase and alteplase) are used, under specialist guidance.

## Central venous thrombosis

This is a particular risk in patients with long-term CVCs, those with recurrent CRBSIs and those in whom multiple line changes are required. Many thrombi only cause partial vessel occlusion and are asymptomatic. Occlusive thrombi may cause facial or ipsilateral limb swelling, localised tenderness and pain. The diagnosis can be confirmed with Doppler ultrasonography, and managed with anticoagulation under haematology advice. The duration of treatment will depend upon the extent of the thrombus and whether or not the central catheter is still required.

## Metabolic

### Fluid overload

Critically ill patients are particularly vulnerable to fluid overload. Careful monitoring of fluid input and output is crucial to their care, as is ensuring that intravenous fluids are discontinued when appropriate (maintenance fluids are not usually required once a patient is fully established on TPN). The consequences of fluid overload (such as pulmonary oedema, hyponatraemia) can significantly delay patients' recovery and increase their morbidity.

### Hyperglycaemia

This is secondary to the high glucose load. In most critically ill patients, hyperglycaemia is controlled with a variable rate intravenous insulin infusion although dextrose intake can also be adjusted. Conversely, when discontinuing TPN, hypoglycaemia is a potential complication.

### Hypertriglyceridaemia

Critically ill patients often have reduced lipid clearance, and may be receiving medications other than TPN with a high lipid content (eg the sedative agent propofol, which is used on the ICU). In sedated patients, using alternative sedative agents to reduce the propofol infusion rate may be sufficient to restore triglyceride levels to within normal limits. Alternatively, fat content can be adjusted in TPN, and some lipid-free emulsions are available. Note that pancreatitis, although associated with hypertriglyceridaemia, is not a contraindication to TPN.

## Refeeding syndrome

Refeeding syndrome occurs following the rapid reintroduction of carbohydrates (either enterally or parenterally) in malnourished patients. It is characterised by marked hypophosphataemia, and may be fatal if unrecognised.

As previously discussed, during starvation/malnutrition, fat and protein metabolism provides the predominant energy supply. Intracellular mineral stores become severely depleted over time, although serum levels are relatively well preserved.

Resumption of carbohydrate intake prompts insulin release, resulting in stimulation of glycogen, fat and protein synthesis. These processes require a supply of minerals (including phosphate, magnesium, calcium and potassium) and vitamins such as thiamine (an essential cofactor in carbohydrate metabolism). As they are taken up by cells, the serum levels of these minerals/vitamins fall significantly, and marked fluid shifts can occur as a result of changing osmolalities. Serum phosphate is transported to the intracellular space to utilise in carbohydrate phosphorylation, resulting in profound hypophosphataemia. This leads to depletion of ATP and 2,3-DPG levels in red blood cells, inhibiting cellular oxygen utilisation.

The clinical effects of refeeding syndrome are broad in type and severity (see Table 13.7), and can easily be misdiagnosed unless a high index of suspicion is maintained. There is no diagnostic test for refeeding syndrome; treatment should be started based upon a suggestive history or clinical picture.

The key treatment goals are:

- Correction of mineral and vitamin deficits: central venous electrolyte replacement may be required in cases of severe depletion or in those with worrying clinical signs.

- Safe initiation of feeding under dietetic guidance: this involves a slower reintroduction of feed, to reduce the magnitude of the carbohydrate load, and possibly vitamin supplementation.

- Close observation for the development of clinical features, and appropriate management of these.

Table 13.7 Clinical manifestations of refeeding syndrome

| Organ System | Clinical features |
|---|---|
| Cardiovascular | Arrhythmias<br>Cardiac failure<br>Sudden death |
| Respiratory | Dyspnoea<br>Respiratory muscle weakness<br>Ventilator dependency |
| Neurological | Weakness<br>Paraesthesia<br>Altered conscious level<br>Seizures<br>Tetany<br>Wernicke's encephalopathy |
| Gastrointestinal | Abdominal pain<br>Nausea and vomiting<br>Ileus |
| Renal | Acute tubular necrosis |
| Musculoskeletal | Myalgia<br>Osteomalacia<br>Rhabdomyolysis |
| Haematological | Leucocyte and platelet dysfunction<br>2,3-DPG depletion<br>Haemolysis |

## Nutrition as a component of enhanced recovery after surgery programmes

Enhanced recovery after surgery describes a package of care for patients undergoing major elective surgery that aims to obtund the normal stress response to surgery, which in turn reduces complications and speeds recovery. The approach was initially applied in colorectal surgery by Henrik Kehlet, a Danish intestinal surgeon, and the basic principles have now been extended to several other specialties with specific modifications. Evidence gathered to support this practice comes from the multimodal approach, and individual elements of the pathway have not been shown to be effective in isolation.

This section considers the basic principles of enhanced recovery rather than procedure specific regimens, which differ between hospitals.

The aim of an enhanced recovery programme is to reduce complication rates, improve patient experience and, as a result, reduce hospital length of stay. Patients undergoing major surgery experience a major stress response resulting in salt and water retention, stress hormone release, catabolism and insulin resistance, which lead to a loss of function in the short and medium term. Details of the metabolic response have been described above. Traditional approaches to surgery with prolonged periods of preoperative fasting, fluid restriction and bowel preparation followed by a further period of nil intake by mouth, restricted mobility and the excessive use of opiate analgesia do not address these issues. The basic principles of enhanced recovery programmes aim to maximise the patient's physiological status preoperatively, to interfere with normal physiology as little as possible intra- and postoperatively, and to restore normal function as quickly as possible.

## Nutritional elements of enhanced recovery

### Preoperative phase

#### Bowel preparation

Purgation with powerful laxatives leads to dehydration, electrolyte imbalance and prolongation of the period of preoperative starvation and is now considered to be unnecessary. A single enema given on the day of surgery for left-sided colonic and rectal resections can still be used.

#### Preoperative fasting

Traditional wisdom was that patients needed to be nil by mouth for a considerable time prior to surgery. It is now accepted that the last intake of food can be 6 hours before surgery and that clear fluids can be taken up to 2 hours prior to surgery. Preoperative oral carbohydrate loading with a glucose solution means that patients go into surgery in the 'fed state', which reduces the stress response to surgery by decreasing insulin resistance and catabolism.

### Postoperative care

Recovery is promoted by attention to the following in the postoperative period:

- avoidance of opiates and using paracetamol and non-steroidal anti-inflammatory drugs (NSAIDs) aimed at restoration of gut function;

- early commencement of postoperative diet;

▪ early and structured postoperative mobilisation;

▪ early catheter removal;

▪ administration of restricted amounts of intravenous fluid.

The success of enhanced recovery programmes depends on a coordinated multidisciplinary approach, and best outcomes are observed if the programme is led by a designated individual who ensures compliance with all aspects of the programme with regular audit of outcomes.

## Summary

▪ The importance of nutritional support in critically ill patients is often underrecognised, and this can have a significant impact on their morbidity and mortality.

▪ Elective surgical and critically unwell surgical patients are undergoing major metabolic changes, which means that maintaining an adequate nutrient supply is vital.

▪ It is essential that nutritional assessment and screening forms a routine part of patient care. Many patients will have a degree of malnutrition upon admission, and many more are at risk of developing nutrient deficiencies as an inpatient, whilst they spend several days 'nil by mouth' or managing only a minimal oral intake.

▪ Assessment must not be a 'one-off' process. The nutritional status of these patients is dynamic and must be reviewed daily.

▪ Numerous methods of support are available and, whilst these may be associated with complications, many can be avoided with careful assessment and monitoring.

▪ Remember there is a wealth of support available to you to help guide management (including dietitians, pharmacists and specialist surgical nurses).

▪ Calculating nutritional requirements and assessing nutritional status is a complex process, so expert input should be sought early to optimise patient care.

▪ Enhanced recovery programmes can improve patient outcomes and patient experience and reduce length of stay, and managing nutrition is an important part of this.

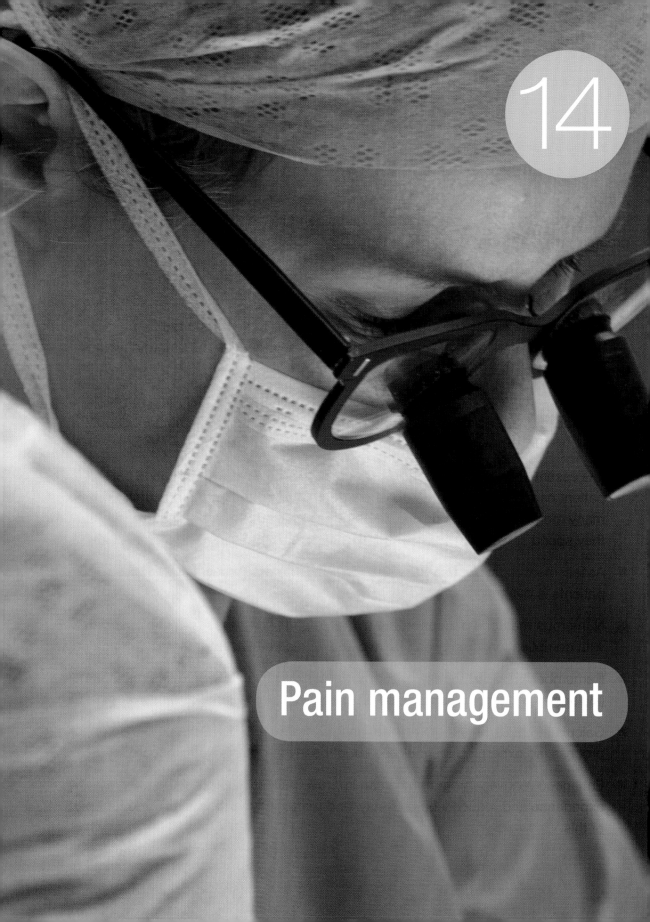

14

Pain management

## Learning outcomes

This chapter will help you to:

- understand the pathophysiology of pain and the need for effective treatment;

- appreciate the risks of inadequate pain treatment and its effects on the recovery of surgical patients;

- understand your role as a part of a multidisciplinary team to relieve pain in the surgical patient;

- evaluate the benefits and limitations of commonly used analgesics and techniques;

- recognise that poorly treated acute pain can result in long-term persistent pain.

## Introduction

Pain is defined as 'an unpleasant sensory and emotional experience associated with actual or potential tissue damage, or described in terms of such damage'. Acute pain is of recent onset and could be due to illness, injury or surgical procedures. If it persists beyond the time of healing, then it is described as chronic pain.

Physiological pain includes nociceptive or inflammatory pain (eg musculoskeletal, visceral pain) whereas pathological or maladaptive pain includes neuropathic pain (eg entrapment neuropathy, neuroma pain): both pains usually exist together in some patients. *Nociception* is the perception of the stimuli by the somatosensory system, whereas *pain* is the experience of the patient. Pain is a product of the interaction between biological, psychological, social and environmental factors.

In critically ill surgical patients, pain can be complex and patients may need an integrated multidisciplinary approach to help with management. As a member of the surgical team, you will be managing patients with significant painful conditions caused either by illness or by interventions carried out in hospital. Safe and effective management of acute pain is an integral part of a good surgical practice.

## Physiology of pain

Peripheral nociceptors (sensory nerve endings) detect noxious stimuli and turn them into electrical activity. These signals are conducted by C and A-delta nerve fibres of the peripheral nerves to the dorsal root ganglion in the spinal cord. Various neuropeptides modulate the transmission of these signals in the spinal cord. Ascending spinal tracts project to the thalamus and then to the sensory cortex. Some of these pathways also track to the medulla and midbrain linked with homeostatic and autonomic responses as well as the emotional component of the pain. Descending tracts from the brain to the spinal cord inhibit the noxious stimulus and modulate the pain pathway (Figure 14.1).

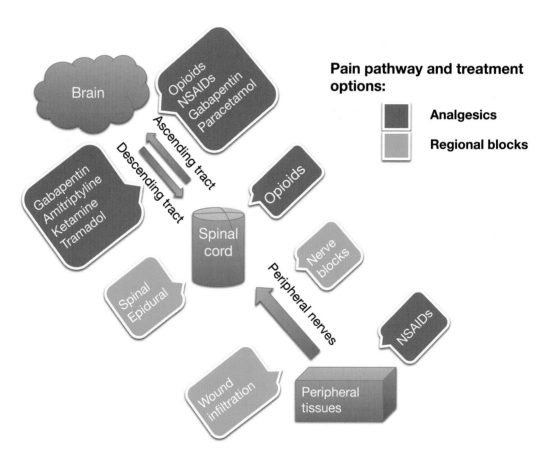

Figure 14.1  Pain pathway and treatment options.

## Why should acute pain be treated?

Control of pain is important not only for humanitarian reasons but because uncontrolled pain has poor effects on body physiology, which in turn will affect the outcome of surgery.

Pain causes sympathetic stimulation resulting in increased heart rate, peripheral vascular resistance and visceral vasoconstriction. These changes increase the cardiac workload and oxygen demand with consequences such as myocardial ischaemia and reduced blood flow to other vital organs. Pain restricts mobility and increases the chances of developing DVT. Conversely, some forms of analgesia can reduce hypercoagulability.

Major surgery such as laparotomies and thoracic procedures already carry a risk of adversely affecting pulmonary function. Anaesthesia and surgery can reduce the functional residual capacity of the lung and predispose to atelectasis. Poorly managed pain can further compound the effects by restricting respiratory excursion, impairing the ability to cough and clear secretions, and predisposing to chest infections.

Poorly managed pain also negatively affects hormonal, metabolic and immune systems, which can be attenuated by some combinations of systemic analgesics and regional analgesic techniques. Intense pain can modify the nervous system, described as 'neuroplastic changes', and this phenomenon can lead inadequately treated acute pain to become chronic persistent pain. Persistent post-surgical chronic pain is relatively more common following certain procedures including thoracic, breast, inguinal hernia, knee and amputation surgery.

Acute pain can affect the patient psychologically causing anxiety, helplessness, sleep problems, mood problems and loss of autonomy. Elderly critically ill patients can also develop postoperative cognitive dysfunction due to various causes, pain being one of the most important among these.

## Principles of acute pain management

An element of pain is inevitable following trauma or surgery. Complete elimination of pain in the immediate postoperative period is unrealistic, but the aim should be to reduce symptoms to an acceptable level such that the patient can function, eg move in bed, cough and comply with physiotherapy to enable recovery and rehabilitation.

## Preoperative education

It is important to inform and involve the patient regarding pain relief before an operation to get optimal results. Higher levels of preoperative anxiety regarding the extent of pain can lead to higher postoperative pain levels. Setting realistic expectations and engaging a patient in the pain management plan can give the patient the confidence needed to mobilise early and participate in rehabilitation.

## Prevention

The most important principle in surgical pain control is prevention. The magnitude of noxious stimuli is proportional to the severity of the tissue disruption, so avoiding tension in the surgical wound and preventing drains or other tubes causing drag on tissues or sutures is important. The choice of site of the surgical incision and the type of incision is important in the critically unwell surgical patient with limited respiratory reserve not just in terms of surgical access, but in relation to the degree of analgesia and also the risk of postoperative morbidity.

'Pre-emptive' analgesia is a method by which analgesic medications are administered and/or local anaesthetic procedures are performed prior to the surgical trauma. Although there is little evidence for how successful the pre-emptive measures are, the consensus is that proactive management of pain before it gets too severe has potential advantages in both the short and long term.

## Use multimodal analgesia wherever possible

Systemic analgesic medications in isolation are unlikely to achieve satisfactory pain relief. A combination of medication and regional analgesic techniques is desirable for many patients in the immediate postoperative period. Studies have shown significant improvement in pain control with local anaesthetic infiltrations along the wound, use of devices to infuse local anaesthetic along the wound edges (local anaesthetic 'bombs') as well as by using specific regional anaesthetic block techniques.

## The pain management team

Whenever you are called to the ward for postoperative analgesia problems, the three-stage assessment process is helpful: you need to know the patient's physiological status and further details, including the surgery and interventions they have undergone. Usually the anaesthetic chart and the drug prescription chart give adequate detail in addition to the clinical notes. Discussion with the ward nursing staff will help in understanding the present problem. It is essential to examine the patient, record the vital signs and discuss with the patient before a proper plan is made. It might be necessary to give some immediate pain relief before the patient can settle to give further details.

Multidisciplinary pain teams include surgeons, anaesthetists, nursing staff and pharmacists. The use of more sophisticated methods of analgesia require you to discuss with the pain team to make a proper plan. Acute pain team nurses have huge experience in dealing with postoperative patients and are available for advice in most hospitals. Out-of-hours, this role might be done by the on-call anaesthetist, who can provide some immediate advice and assistance. Most hospitals have local protocols and guidelines for pain management and you need to be aware of these. It is better to adhere to local protocols given that the nursing staff and other ward staff will be more familiar with these.

## Assessment of a patient with acute pain

### Is this pain due to a new problem?

Whenever you are called to assess a patient with a recent change in the type and intensity of pain, it is vital to rule out new surgical problems. Using the CCrISP three-stage assessment system can help you to do that quickly and reliably. Surgical conditions that can lead to new or increased levels of pain include ischaemia, bleeding, anastomotic leak or compartment syndromes. 'Breakthrough pain' in a patient whose pain was stable before should always be treated as a surgical complication unless proven otherwise at the end of your three-stage assessment.

### Airway

Sedative drugs such as opioids can cause sedation and airway obstruction, especially in the older person, the obese and patients with obstructive sleep apnoea. The risk is higher when sedative drugs are coadministered. It is important to check that unintubated patients are able to maintain a patent airway and have intact protective reflexes.

## Breathing

Check the respiratory rate, pattern, depth of breathing, and the ability to cough effectively. Remember that oxygen saturation may not fall until the patient develops profound respiratory depression.

## Circulation

Tachycardia in a patient with pain could have many causes including sepsis, myocardial ischaemia, hypoxaemia, hypovolaemia, cardiac arrhythmias or anxiety. Hypotension in a patient receiving continuous epidural analgesia could be attributed to sympathetic blockade causing vasodilation but there may also be other causes. For example, low blood pressure due to hypovolaemia can be exacerbated by epidural block. Meticulous attention to fluid balance charts, measurement of surgical and other drain losses and a high index of suspicion for concealed bleeding or fluid losses helps in this situation.

## Disability

Analgesic medications and techniques can also contribute to clinical deterioration. Level of consciousness and sedation scores are useful guides in patients who have had intrathecal opioids or are presently receiving epidural or intravenous infusions of analgesic medications. In less communicative patients, behavioural observation such as facial expressions, verbal expressions, and restriction of mobility is invaluable.

After ensuring that the general status of the patient is stable in the ABCDE assessment, focused assessment of pain can be made when you do the full clinical examination. A popular acronym to use is SOCRATES:

S: Site of pain. Is this pain described in the surgical site or in a remote location (eg calf pain due to deep venous thrombosis or chest pain due to PE)?

O: Onset. Was the onset acute or gradual (chest pain following central line insertion may be due to pneumothorax)?

C: Character. Is the pain aching, burning or shooting (chest wall pain following rib fractures can be musculoskeletal or neuropathic; the choice of drugs is different for these two presentations)?

R: Radiation. Sound anatomical knowledge and pattern of spread of symptoms can help to identify the source of pain (for example, shooting pain to the legs can be due to nerve root irritation at the level of spinal cord). Pain is described as 'referred' if discomfort is perceived in a location remote from the source of pain (for example, shoulder pain following diaphragmatic irritation).

A: Associations. These include nausea, vomiting and fever (abdominal pain with distension and vomiting may be due to obstruction).

T: Time course. Duration of pain – intermittent or continuous.

E: Exacerbating/relieving factors. This includes association with any movement, bowel or bladder functions

S: Severity. Documenting the pain score is crucial to describe the severity, assess the response to the interventions and monitor any progress.

Patient-reported pain assessment is also completed in the chart review.

## Measuring pain-scoring systems

Pain is the 'fifth' vital sign; local protocols will guide the surgical trainee in the appropriate use of the pain and sedation scoring systems used. Most of these systems measure pain at rest and during movement to predict effectiveness of pain relief to facilitate functional restoration. Functional assessment such as the ability to walk, move, breath deeply and cough is an important integral component of measuring pain.

### Numerical rating scale (NRS)

The NRS is a commonly used 11-point scale for self-reporting of pain with reference to the patient's individual experience; zero represents no pain, 1–3 mild pain, 4–6 moderate pain and 7–10 disabling severe pain.

### Verbal rating scale (VRS)

Patients verbally rate the pain with descriptions such as no pain, mild, moderate or severe pain. This is an easy method to assess the efficacy of an intervention compared with previous scores in the same patient.

### Visual analogue score (VAS)

The VAS is a measurement instrument on a 100-mm horizontal line, often used by researchers. Patients indicate a position in the scale to describe the intensity of their pain; zero represents 'no pain' and the maximum 100 represents 'the worst pain imaginable'.

## Communication and documentation

Effective communication and good record-keeping are important in the provision of a high-quality pain service. If, having properly assessed the patient, you feel that the issue is solely attributable to pain then consider why the method of analgesia failed:

- Is it due to inadequate medication or dosage?

- Is it due to the technique used or its incorrect implementation?

- Is it because there is a surgical complication you have not yet recognised?

- Is it because other supplemental analgesic techniques are not used appropriately?

It is essential you confirm any plan for changes in analgesia to the patient and the ward staff. Once satisfactory analgesia is achieved, methods should be put in place to continue this and review it in a timely manner.

## Management of acute pain – the clinical aspects

The choice of pain management strategy depends on different factors including the site and nature of the surgery, type and intensity of pain, comorbidities and the on-going clinical condition of the patient.

Whilst satisfactory pain relief is essential for patient recovery, care should be exercised to ensure that the analgesic techniques do not make the patient worse (eg hypotension with an epidural, respiratory depression with opioids, renal impairment with NSAIDs).

The management options (Figure 14.2) can be categorised into:

- analgesic medications (eg paracetamol, NSAIDs, opioids);

- regional analgesic techniques (local anaesthetics with or without opioids).

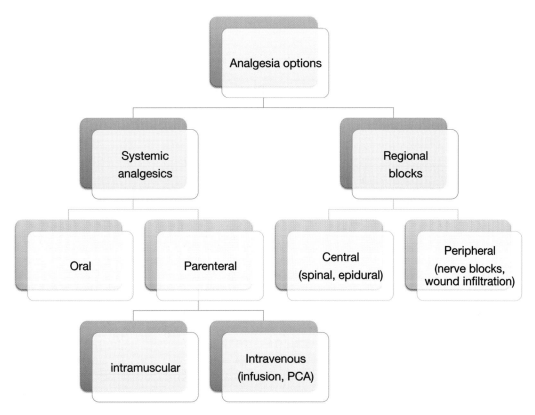

Figure 14.2 Analgesia options.

Often, a combination of medications/local anaesthetic techniques is employed for safe and effect pain relief. The World Health Organization analgesic ladder was introduced to improve cancer pain control. The concept has been extrapolated to other pain conditions as well – as the intensity of the pain increases, the complexity of the interventions also increases. As described below, this may not be applicable in the acute setting as rapid and effective pain relief is the goal of treatment.

- step 1: simple analgesics (paracetamol with or without NSAIDs);

- step 2: weak opioids (such as codeine) with or without simple analgesics;

- step 3: stronger opioids (such as morphine) with or without simple analgesics.

One of the fundamental principles of the pain ladder is to deliver the analgesic medications on a regular basis – 'by the clock' rather than as required: PRN for pain relief as required may also mean 'pain relief nil'.

If the initial presentation of acute pain is severe and difficult to control, an alternative analgesia ladder recommended by the World Federation of Societies of Anaesthesiologists (www.wfsahq.org) is useful. In this approach, initially effective pain control is facilitated with stronger opioids and local anaesthetic techniques. Once controlled, the simpler options such as regular oral opioid analgesics and then simple analgesics are introduced.

## Analgesic medications and techniques

Medications used for pain management can be grouped as:

- paracetamol;

- NSAIDs, eg ibuprofen, diclofenac, naproxen, ketorolac;

- opioids, eg codeine, morphine, fentanyl, alfentanil, oxycodone and miscellaneous opioids such as tramadol;

- co-analgesics such as gabapentin, ketamine.

### Paracetamol

Paracetamol is an analgesic and antipyretic, but its exact mechanism of action is not fully understood. The drug is well absorbed orally and is metabolised by the liver. When limited to the recommended dosage, paracetamol has few side-effects. Regular administration, as a part of multimodal analgesic technique, can contribute to effective pain management. The dose needs to be adjusted in patients with hepatic dysfunction and in malnourished/underweight people. Paracetamol is available in oral, suppository and intravenous infusion (over 15 minutes) formulations and is administered at the dose of 1 g, 4- to 6-hourly up to a maximum dose of 4 g in 24 hours. In patients weighing less than 50 kg, intravenous paracetamol is limited to 15 mg/kg per dose and a maximum of 60 mg/kg in 24 hours. There is no significant benefit to intravenous paracetamol over the oral form, which is considerably cheaper and should be used in preference to the intravenous form whenever possible.

### NSAIDs

This group of medications have analgesic and anti-inflammatory properties. Examples include ibuprofen, diclofenac, ketorolac and naproxen. Extreme care should be taken when considering these drugs in critically ill patients and the elderly because of unfavourable side-effects, particularly in the presence of other comorbidities. Their mechanism of action is mainly inhibition of prostaglandin synthesis by inhibiting the enzyme cyclooxygenase. Prostaglandins are the chief mediators of inflammation. Prostaglandins also have a crucial role in physiology including renal regulation, gastric protection and platelet function. A subgroup of NSAIDs, COX-2 inhibitors, was developed to selectively block the cyclooxygenase 2 enzyme to enable pain relief with minimal systemic side-effects. However, in critically ill patients, they still have significant adverse effects (see below), thereby limiting their routine use in pain management. Examples of COX-2 inhibitors include celecoxib, etoricoxib and parecoxib.

NSAIDs are available in different formulations, such as oral tablets, suppositories and injections for intramuscular and intravenous use. Whilst they may have a useful role in stable patients, their therapeutic index is narrow in patients who are volume depleted or dehydrated, have pre-existing renal dysfunction or are prone to bleeding. The incidence of adverse effects can be similar regardless of the route of delivery. In patients with deranged physiological parameters, NSAIDs can also predispose to acute kidney injury and bleeding. It would be prudent to seek senior advice and thoroughly assess the risks and benefits if contemplating use of NSAIDs for managing pain in critically unwell patients.

## Opioids

Opioids are derived from opium alkaloids and exert their analgesic effects by acting on mu-opioid receptors. Despite their long list of side-effects including nausea and vomiting, constipation, itching, bladder retention, drowsiness and respiratory depression, opioids are still the mainstay approach for treating moderate to severe pain. Based on their potency, opioids are arbitrarily classified as weak (eg codeine) or strong (eg morphine). Tramadol has some mu-receptor actions along with other mechanisms of action including serotonin and noradrenaline reuptake inhibition.

Opioids are available in different formulations including oral preparations, injections for intramuscular and intravenous administration, lozenges and buccal preparations. In monitored care areas, infusions (eg morphine, fentanyl, alfentanil) are also used and doses can be titrated depending on the severity of the patient' s pain, respiratory and hepatorenal parameters.

## Patient-controlled analgesia

Patient-controlled analgesia (PCA) is a well-established method that enables patients to control their pain and is likely to be the most common way to administer intravenous opioids you will encounter on the ward. If the patient is capable of using a simple hand-held device, opioid medication can be self-administered through an intravenous cannula in small boluses. This concept is appealing as individual requirements of opioids vary considerably, and with a PCA technique patients can titrate the dose to their own end-point of pain relief. In theory, unlike clinician-administered intramuscular or intravenous boluses, which lead to fluctuations in plasma opioid levels, in PCA, the plasma level of analgesic will be fairly constant within a therapeutic range providing the patient continues to make requests through the hand-held device. A typical PCA regimen consists of 1- to 2-mg boluses of morphine with a lockout interval of 5 minutes. The purpose of the lockout interval is to ensure that unintentional overdose is avoided. The potency of all other opioid medications is compared with that of morphine. Oxycodone, a synthetic opioid, is twice as potent as morphine and may sometimes be used in a PCA device if morphine is not working well.

Codeine is commonly given for mild to moderate pain when a patient can tolerate oral medications. It is prescribed at a dose of 30–60 mg by mouth 4- to 6-hourly, often as a co-drug with paracetamol. Constipation is an important side-effect and may be undesirable, particularly if the patient is recovering from abdominal surgery. In older patients, eg elderly patients with a fractured neck of femur, it may be sensible to prescribe regular laxatives along with the codeine prescription.

## Monitoring of patients on opioids for pain relief

Opioids have many side-effects and vigilance is essential for timely recognition of these potentially deleterious effects. In the case of continuous infusions and PCA, initial monitoring includes hourly recording of pain score, infusion pump checks, assessing sedation score, respiratory rate and vital parameters (heart rate, oxygen saturation, blood pressure) (Table 14.1). The frequency of monitoring can eventually be reduced (to 2- to 4-hourly or so) once the general condition of the patient improves and stabilises. In patients with PCA devices or who are receiving other opioid intravenous infusions, additional oxygen should always be administered as a safety in case the patient develops respiratory depression from the opioids.

Table 14.1  Tool for monitoring pain and side effects

| Pain score | Sedation score | Nausea score |
|---|---|---|
| 0 = None | 0 = Awake | 0 = None |
| 1 = Mild | 1 = Drowsy | 1 = Mild |
| 2 = Moderate | 2 = Asleep but rousable | 2 = Moderate |
| 3 = Severe | 3 = Unrousable | 3 = Severe |

If the patient is nauseated or vomits, after ruling out causes such as hypovolaemia, hypoxia or surgical reasons (intestinal obstruction etc), antiemetics such as ondansetron 4 mg or cyclizine 50 mg can be administered intravenously to manage opioid-induced nausea and vomiting.

## Co-analgesics

When patients have uncontrollable nociceptive (musculoskeletal or visceral pain) or neuropathic pain (post-thoracotomy, post-amputation, etc, where nerves are injured), conventional analgesics may not provide satisfactory relief. The issue is further compounded if the patient has a past history of chronic pain. Regional analgesic techniques (discussed below) can help. When traditional interventions fail, co-analgesics such as anticonvulsants (eg gabapentin), antidepressants (eg amitriptyline) or ketamine (5–10 mg per hour as an intravenous infusion) may be used. It is prudent to seek help from the hospital acute pain team prior to embarking on less conventional approaches to manage pain.

## Regional analgesic techniques

Local anaesthetics (eg bupivacaine, laevo-bupivacaine, ropivacaine) can be deposited along the pain pathway to provide effective analgesia by selectively blocking the neural structures and interrupting the pain impulses generated. Depending on the level of neural blockade, the techniques can be categorised as:

- neuraxial (intrathecal, epidural);

- paraxial (eg thoracic paravertebral block);

- peripheral (eg brachial plexus nerve block, transversus abdominis plane block);

- local (eg wound infiltration, periarticular infiltration after joint surgeries).

Regional analgesic techniques have the benefit of providing pain relief without the side-effects of systemic pain medications. Opioid receptors are located in the spinal cord and hence neuraxial blocks commonly involve administration of a combination of local anaesthetic and opioids. Other peripheral blocks are performed with either a one-off injection or continuous infusion of local anaesthetics. Local anaesthetics block the nerves by inhibiting the sodium channels in the neuron, preventing transmission along it. Epidural analgesia, apart from blocking sensory nerve fibres, also blocks sympathetic nerve fibres, resulting in hypotension (which can be undesirable in critically ill patients). With careful calculation of local anaesthetic doses, peripheral techniques have a favourable safety profile. When used judiciously, techniques such as thoracic paravertebral block for rib fractures and transversus abdominis plane block for abdomino-pelvic surgeries have an important role in managing pain in unstable surgical patients and can provide analgesia that is as effective as an epidural in some cases. Continuous catheter techniques are mostly initiated by anaesthetists in the operating room and the infusions are continued in the postoperative period.

## Care of patients receiving epidural infusions

Patients undergoing major thoracic procedures or upper abdominal surgery and those with bilateral multiple rib fractures can benefit from epidural analgesia. Effective epidural analgesia helps minimise postoperative respiratory complications. A combination of local anaesthetic and opioids (eg bupivacaine 0.1% + fentanyl 2 µg/ml) is infused through a catheter placed in the epidural space. Although this method gives better analgesia, complications can arise from either the technique itself or the effect of the medications.

Complications associated with the technique include damage to the nerve roots or spinal cord, accidental dural puncture (resulting in headache), haematoma formation and infection risks. Local anaesthetics can cause sensory/motor blockade and hypotension. Epidurally administered opioids can cause nausea, vomiting, pruritus, bladder retention and respiratory depression. Some epidurals fail because of technical issues, and insertion can be difficult in patients with degenerative spinal conditions. Epidural insertion and removal need to be coordinated with the administration of prophylactic anticoagulants; insertion should not be performed within 12 hours of administration and removal within 4 hours. Epidural anaesthesia is contraindicated in patients who are fully anticoagulated.

When caring for patients with an epidural infusion running, observe for any above-mentioned complications secondary to the neuraxial block and inspect the catheter insertion site for redness, tenderness or leakage. Check for the sensory block height to ensure that it is a functioning epidural infusion and the appropriate dermatomal levels are covered. Suitable evidence that the epidural is working properly include the patient being able to cough and clear their respiratory secretions and engage with physiotherapy.

The Bromage score is used to evaluate motor weakness.

0 = full flexion of knees and feet;

1 = just able to move knees;

2 = able to move feet only;

3 = unable to move feet or knees.

Contact the acute pain team/anaesthetist if there are any major changes in motor function or if the Bromage score is 2 or 3.

A 'functioning epidural' can produce an element of hypotension (as sympathetic nerve fibres are blocked before sensory nerve fibres). This hypotension is managed with a combination of intravenous fluids and vasopressors such as metaraminol infusions, which might require the patient to be cared for on an HDU-type environment. In some patients, extreme care should be taken, as both fluid overload and too much vasoconstriction can be deleterious, and other causes of hypotension (such as bleeding, sepsis) can be masked. Meticulous examination and comprehensive evaluation of the clinical situation is a matter of paramount importance. Chasing the numbers (such as blood pressure, central venous pressure, respiratory rate, urine output) without consideration to the clinical context can be misleading. When in doubt, complete the CCrISP three-stage assessment and, if still unsure, call for help.

## Care of patients receiving local anaesthetic infusions

Ultrasound guidance is frequently used to place catheters close to peripheral nerves and in fascial planes to provide safe and effective analgesia. For example, high-risk patients with a fractured neck of femur may receive a fascia iliaca block as part of their anaesthetic management. Peripheral regional blocks have the dual benefit of avoiding the systemic side-effects of opioids as well as the adverse effects of central neuraxial blocks such as respiratory depression and sympathetic block-related hypotension.

These patients may be at risk of local anaesthetic toxicity. Manifestations of toxicity include metallic taste, tingling fingers and tongue, agitation, decreased conscious level, hypotension, convulsions, apnoea, cardiac arrhythmias or cardiac arrest. If toxicity is suspected, stop the local anaesthetic infusion immediately and use the 'ABCDE' approach to assessment. Call for assistance, including the on-call anaesthetist who will help with haemodynamic support and may give intravenous lipid emulsions to combat the toxicity.

## Conclusion

- Pain assessment is considered to be the fifth vital sign in the management of surgical patients.

- Effective pain management is essential to facilitate recovery from critical illness.

- Pain may be a symptom of other more significant problems in unwell surgical patients, and you should aim to use the CCrISP three-stage assessment to ensure you have identified all the relevant issues.

- Documentation is important for supporting this evaluation and planning should encompass the overall pain management plan, any consultations from the pain team received, and periodic review of the pain score of the patient.

# 15

# Communication, organisation and leadership in surgical care

## Learning outcomes

This chapter should enable you to:

- describe the facets of professional behaviour which are important in good surgical practice, including NOTSS (non-technical skills for surgeons) and the role of medical ethics in decision making;

- recognise the importance of clear and effective communication in surgical critical care;

- identify the key components you may wish to develop in your transition to specialty training.


## Introduction

Medicine evolves as a result of the development of effective treatments for new diseases. Against this backdrop of change there is one constant: the need for you to act professionally at all times.

Professionalism, in any setting, encompasses integrity, expertise and an excellent standard of work, but when applied to medicine it also embodies a raft of other qualities including compassion, confidentiality, teamworking and continuous professional development. The Royal College of Physicians defines medical professionalism as, 'a set of values, behaviours, and relationships that underpins the trust the public has in doctors'.

Twenty-first century medicine is practised with a patient-centred approach, in contrast to previous ideas of medical paternalism, a move that has seen the erosion of the idea that doctors are infallible. Professionalism is not inherited with a medical degree; it needs to be developed as your career progresses. The apprenticeship system that has dominated surgical education for so long is still important in helping trainees to develop professional behaviours but it is naive and outdated to think that role modelling alone is sufficient. Passive learning through observation of your seniors occurs less frequently with reduced working hours, and so training opportunities must be maximised. There is a growing emphasis on teaching non-operative skills through simulated scenarios and subsequent debriefing. This method is integral to the

CCrISP course and throughout the face-to-face sessions participants will have the opportunity to discuss and practise a variety of non-technical skills.

## NOTSS (non-technical skills for surgeons)

Non-technical skills describe the interpersonal and cognitive domains that complement technical ability in allowing safe and efficient task performance.

Medicine owes a debt of gratitude to the aviation industry, which first introduced training in non-technical skills for pilots on the back of research suggesting that most accidents were a result of human factors rather than equipment failure. These 'Crew Resource Management' programmes led to improved performance and fewer adverse events. Extrapolating from this, human factors training was embraced by anaesthetists as part of 'Anaesthesia Crisis Resource Management' courses, and there is an increasing body of evidence showing the link between improved non-technical skills and better clinical outcomes.

Non-technical skills can be broadly divided into the following four domains.

### Situational awareness

This describes the ability to perceive and respond to changes in one's environment and can be summarised as detection, diagnosis, prediction. It is a dynamic process that relies upon concentration and a good working memory. Situational awareness can occur at an individual and a team level, with both relying upon excellent communication. Consider the example of a patient undergoing a carotid endarterectomy with awake testing who shows signs of neurological deterioration upon clamping. This change in the patient's neurological state must be recognised by the team and communicated to the surgeon, who may then decide that a shunt is required. This relies upon a coordinated effort from all members of the team resulting from a shared appreciation of the problem. From an individual perspective the surgeon will be aware that the use of a shunt makes the procedure more difficult. They must ensure that the scrub nurse and assistant understand the sequence of events involved in inserting a shunt, and the need to perform this part of the operation as quickly as possible to minimise any period of cerebral hypoperfusion. This highlights how good situational awareness allows the prediction of future difficulties.

## Decision-making

This refers to the process by which an individual chooses a course of action from the options available using a combination of new information and past experiences to balance risks. It is dynamic because continual re-evaluation is necessary to assess the outcomes of previous decisions. Good decision-making is linked to good situational awareness but the latter does not guarantee the former. Returning to the example above, imagine if the surgeon, having correctly identified the need for a shunt, allowed a junior trainee with minimal experience of carotid surgery to perform the procedure.

Decision-making in medicine frequently involves consideration of an ethical dimension to a decision. The 'four principles' approach of Beauchamp and Childress can be useful in identifying and considering the issues around the decision.

- **Autonomy.** Individuals have the right to self-determination. Doctors must respect this by explaining all available treatment options so that patients can make informed decisions about their care. In situations where patients lack capacity, and there are no advance directives to suggest which treatment they would want, then they should be treated in accordance with their best interests.

- **Beneficence.** This describes actions carried out for the benefit of others. In the context of medical ethics it means serving the best interests of patients at all times.

- **Non-maleficence.** This is encapsulated in the Latin phrase *primum non nocere*, which translates as 'first do no harm'. Patients should not be exposed to risks of harm where there is no clear benefit to them.

- **Justice.** This refers to fairness and equality of treatment and access. This simple definition belies its complexity, particularly when one considers the concept of 'distributive justice', which is concerned with the allocation of scarce resources and who gets what treatment.

Treating patients who are nearing the end of their lives can be incredibly challenging; clinical decisions are often emotionally distressing and far from straightforward, and may have moral uncertainties. The law surrounding end of life care varies from country to country, and it is not the aim of the CCrISP course to discuss legal frameworks; however, the ethical considerations do warrant some discussion. Doctors have an obligation to administer effective palliative care to patients who are terminally ill.

The provision of adequate opioid analgesia to dying patients is a clear example of beneficence but the respiratory depression associated with these medications may shorten the life of the patient and could be viewed as contravening the principle of non-maleficence. This introduces the notion of 'double effect', which describes how an intervention can have both intended and unintended consequences. It can be argued that an action with two opposite outcomes is morally justifiable if the intention is to achieve the good effect, even if the possible negative effect is foreseen.

Another example of a clash of ethical principles concerns the patient who is bleeding but does not want a blood transfusion owing to religious beliefs. In this case there is a conflict between autonomy and beneficence. However, if the patient is mentally competent, then his or her wishes should be respected, particularly since a breach of autonomy may deter similar patients from seeking medical attention in the future, reducing the ability to carry out beneficent acts.

## Task management

This describes the combination of planning and prioritisation which allows work to be carried out to the highest standards using the resources at one's disposal.

## Teamworking

Unlike the other cognitive skills, teamworking is rooted in the interpersonal domain. It refers to the way in which an individual can function as part of a group to achieve a goal, and requires the reciprocal qualities of followership and leadership depending upon one's role within the team. Effective teamwork relies upon accurate exchange of information and supporting others, with excellent communication skills. The importance of the multi-disciplinary team in patient management is not in question but a team of experts does not automatically translate into an expert team. This realisation has led to a greater emphasis on interprofessional team training using simulated patients, wards and operating theatres to improve communication skills and enhance patient safety.

Within this classification the ability to deal with stress and fatigue is not included as a discrete non-technical skill but its influence in each of the four domains should not be underestimated.

Being an effective communicator is a vital skill for surgeons. Large numbers of people, coming from different branches of the healthcare professions, are now involved in the care of a single patient and this process needs to be actively managed by the surgical consultant and his/her team, who have ultimate and continuing responsibility for each individual patient. Patients and relatives expect good outcomes from surgical interventions and expect to be kept informed about details of their care at each stage. It is vitally important to understand patients' expectations from the outset so that all concerned can understand what a realistic outcome for that patient may be. It is easy to make assumptions of what other people think and believe, which may reflect the surgeon's own beliefs rather than the reality for that individual. Many problems arising in surgical care are the result of poor communication, and often serial episodes, rather than a lack of knowledge or an incorrect decision.

Evidence suggests that adverse outcomes, iatrogenic injuries, failure to provide adequate care, mistakes or system errors are more likely to lead to litigation or complaints if there have been preceding communication problems. Other international data on litigation have shown adverse outcomes occurring in 3.7% of admissions, with one in four (1% of the total admissions) due to negligence. However, two out of three claims come from patients with no adverse outcome or an adverse outcome not due to negligence. Another study found that only 3% of patients who suffered negligence filed a lawsuit. Reasons given for instigating litigation include a desire to correct apparently deficient standards of care, to find out what happened and why, to enforce accountability and to gain compensation for accrued and future costs of care. A further study has shown that 70% of medical litigation is related to poor communication, citing patient feelings such as desertion, devaluation, lack of information and lack of understanding. In one study, over half of patients who commenced litigation claimed that they were so unimpressed by the doctor that they wanted to sue him or her before the alleged event occurred.

Communication matters, therefore, not just with the patient and relatives, but also with colleagues, so that clinical information can be provided quickly and accurately. Furthermore, good communication skills allow you to be able to respond to psychological and emotional issues in colleagues and detect the possibility of tension or distress building up within the team as well as how to respond to this.

A comprehensive account of basic communication skills is outside the remit of this chapter, although certain relevant communication skills are discussed and practised on the CCrISP course. You should develop an awareness of basic communication skills including the appropriate use of open, focused and closed questions, knowledge and avoidance of leading and multiple questions, knowledge of and methods to overcome responses such as denial and blocking, and the use of empathic statements (see Glossary).

## What are the specific communication problems in critically ill surgical patients?

Often, surgical critical care takes place in an environment where background obstacles to communication are more likely. The patients are ill and frightened, and the staff are often incredibly busy. The patient may be unable to concentrate, especially if there is pain, severe illness or complications of medication. Equally, operational fatigue on the part of staff is also important. It is often easier for others to recognise the signs than for individuals to identify themselves. Signs of operational fatigue include loss of clinical sharpness and reduction in the quality of decision-making. Other obstacles to communication may include irritability and anger, high tension, confusion (most obvious in organic brain syndromes but may also occur in functional disorders), distress and tearfulness, and high expectations from patients, relatives, colleagues and oneself.

## Specific communications strategies

### The critical care setting

Critical care settings can be bewildering for patients and their relatives, with a lot of unfamiliar equipment, background noise and sometimes with limited access to natural light. It is easy to assume that patients, relatives and doctors have a greater knowledge and experience of these environments than they actually have. It is especially important that, at each stage of care, explanations are provided. These can be very simple tasks, such as explaining the role of a particular piece of equipment, an account of the next intervention or an explanation of where a specific issue fits into the overall management plan. It can be helpful to try to predict what may happen and have a plan for the different possibilities. An environment with limited natural light may increase disorientation, especially in elderly patients. Readable clocks or other ways of helping to overcome this are important. Where there is a degree of organic confusion, aids to orientation can be important, such as photographs of loved ones and easy-to-read name badges. Acute confusional states (delirium) are common, and the three-stage assessment process can be used to address the causes rather than immediately resorting to sedative-type medications.

It may be necessary to repeat both questions and explanations at different times. Being prepared to go back over the history after the immediate crisis is good clinical practice and may reveal issues that were previously unconsidered. You have probably realised that many communication situations are not single episodes of communication but rather a continuous process involving multiple episodes over time. Similarly, it is helpful to reduce fear by offering repeated explanations and using check-backs to assess that a patient and relatives have understood. Patients can often recall only small amounts of the information provided from a single communication episode.

## Breaking bad news

There is no perfect way to communicate – what works well in some situations can fail in others. However, some general principles are helpful. It can be useful to think about this in terms of what educators call the 'set'. This includes the environment in which the communication episode will take place and who will be present. It also includes an introduction as to the purpose of the episode, the details of the episode itself and then a summary of the salient points of the discussion. When speaking to relatives, it is important to confirm that the patient has given permission for relatives to be informed of their condition. Understanding intra-family dynamics can also help manage communications with relatives. For example, in some circumstances it may be necessary for the medical staff to talk to several family members together, while in others a family 'spokesperson' may be the best person to talk to.

When breaking bad news, it is important to talk, and to listen. The barriers to doing this may come from patients (or relatives if they are receiving the communication) or from us. Some things are hard for us to talk about but, in this setting, it is important to be able to tackle these. One way of starting such a conversation is to ask an open question such as 'what is your understanding of the present situation?' or 'what have you been told so far?'. In this way, you are giving the patient or relative the first opportunity to have a say and it may help you understand their expectations and how much they wish to be told. Some patients want a lot of detail, others only a broad outline. If you are unaware of the patient's expectations at the outset, you will not be able to meet them and you should not make assumptions. Starting in this way also gives you the opportunity to show that you are listening and to pick up on any verbal or physical clues as to the patient's or relative's underlying emotions. These can be subtle and you need to consciously look for them. You need to be prepared to use direct and understandable language. It is a great temptation to 'beat around the bush' in an attempt to soften the blow, but it is important to say difficult, emotive words such as 'cancer' or 'death', should they be appropriate. People find uncertainty difficult to handle; once they know what they are facing, they can start to deal with it and patients will often thank you for being frank and honest. Clearly, however, this can still be a delicate situation. A good tip is to avoid the urge to fill silences with your words and to avoid pushing your own agenda. It is often a good idea to say the minimum, allow silences for information to be absorbed and then for more information to be exchanged in a question and answer manner, with the patient and/or relatives asking the questions.

Attitudes have changed substantially in the last two decades, but the work of John Hinton in the 1970s with people who had terminal illnesses is useful. He found that, in an inpatient unit, although staff believed that only a small minority of patients knew of their diagnosis and prognosis, a substantial majority had a very good understanding. This knowledge was acquired in various ways, including overhearing bedside conversations or reading case files. Patients were able and willing to share this with Hinton in a way that they had not done with the other staff. When asked why they did not discuss their knowledge with staff, patients often indicated that they did not want to cause the staff distress. In other words, patients chose silence partly to protect the staff working with them. From this, the concept arose of being prepared and able to give the patient permission to talk about bad news. To be able to give permission effectively requires good listening skills. Listening is an active process, interspersed with signs of encouragement. We all do this differently but should use attitude, facial expression, body language or verbal acknowledgements to show interest and encourage further disclosure.

The use of **empathic statements** can be a straightforward way of identifying feelings and showing support. These are statements in which the interviewer tries to identify a current feeling such as sadness, anger or fear and then ties it to what has been happening, such as 'It sounds as if this news has made you feel more fearful than anything else'. This can allow the person to talk about feelings and it also gives the interviewer a chance to check if what he or she perceives is correct. In contrast,

**sympathetic statements**, such as 'I know just how you feel', should be avoided. It is very unlikely that you could really feel the same and such statements can lead to aggressive reactions from patients or relatives.

The most important aspects of helping people talk about feelings is to allow time and space. The setting should be quiet and private. The interviewer should give a sense of having time to talk. Often it will not take much time (in general, more skilled communicators take less time than less skilled communicators) but it does require planning to ensure, for example, that discussions like this are not started a few seconds before a ward round or some other fixed event. There is evidence to show that if a person is left to talk freely that they will speak for between 40 and 80 seconds. Allowing them to do so will start things off on the right footing and help the patient appreciate that you are focused on their problem. Sitting down to talk to the patient is good body language and gives the impression of more time being available. In a study where a doctor, who was either sitting or standing, spoke to patients for a set length of time, the patients' estimation of how long the doctor had spent with them was doubled if the doctor was sitting down.

An important part of communication is the use of 'mirroring'. The doctor mirrors what the patient is doing in terms of tone and speed of speech, and body language. For example, if a patient sounds timid and scared, using a similar tone may reassure the patient that he or she is being listened to and dealt with appropriately. If the patient leans forward, you should lean forward. It is not suggested that everything a patient does should be mirrored but doing the opposite to what the patient is doing can send a message that you are not listening or concerned about them.

A further issue, for more junior doctors in particular, is the way they handle their own uncertainties. In general, patients want definite statements and guarantees of outcomes. Clearly, there is much uncertainty surrounding surgical outcomes and you need to be able to appear confident in your knowledge, yet not lead patients to have unrealistic expectations.

At the end of the discussion, make it clear that further meetings can be arranged and give details of how this can be done. Giving the family a 'liaison' person can often provide reassurance that it should be easy to talk again. It is also important to document in the patient's notes that a discussion has taken place, to provide a brief outline of what was said and to record any issues that may be relevant in the future.

## Medical mistakes

Occasionally, people come to harm following a medical complication or a medical error. This raises quite different communication issues. In addition to breaking bad news, there is the additional matter of handling guilt and fear of litigation. It is not possible to make absolute statements but, in general, you should provide a frank and full explanation and, if an error has been made, offer an apology. Not only is this in keeping with current thinking in the NHS but, since a sense of injustice often drives litigation, it is probably also a part of good risk management. It is important to be clear that one cannot apologise for the actions of others; you can state that you are sorry to hear of any concerns/worries and that a full reply to questions/complaints will be provided in time. Recent developments in the UK have led to the introduction of the concept of the Duty of Candour, which places a duty on a hospital to ensure that patients are informed if mistakes in their care have led to significant harm. Your role as the trainee may be to recognise where a patient has suffered a harm that would require a disclosure under the rules of Duty of Candour.

It is also important to realise that you should not criticise the actions of others without very careful consideration. General Medical Council guidance stresses the importance of collegiality, and it is very easy to comment on something without knowing the full details. Criticism of others is easy to imply by the most innocent off-hand remarks or ill-guarded body language. In certain cases, such actions can lead the patient to feel justified in making a complaint or seeking legal advice.

## Working with colleagues

Staff relationships are of particular importance in critical care settings. Not only does the work involve vulnerable and dependent patients, it also carries with it a lot of work-related emotional issues. It is easy for these pressures to translate into aggression and lack of respect. They may be made worse when interprofessional rivalries intervene or when people normally outside the unit are involved with particular patients.

Ideally, there needs to be some way for these issues to be dealt with on a team basis – identifying problem areas and finding supportive and effective ways of achieving change. Methods of achieving this cannot be prescribed but must vary with the situation. Deficient communication must be addressed, whether within or between professional groups, either by individual or group meetings, and formally or informally. These techniques often remain alien to the medical profession but can help greatly in the development of efficient and good-humoured units. Individuals should also show respect in their own behaviour and learn how to use assertive rather than aggressive or passive interaction (see Glossary). It is important to remember that the communication issues when talking to patients outlined above also apply to communication with colleagues. It is easy to make assumptions about colleagues' knowledge of a situation or their attitudes and motivations towards work. Try not to make assumptions but approach situations with the view of exploring and confirming facts and be clear about what has been agreed and who will action any agreements by confirming actions at the end of conversations.

## Coping with adverse events

Emotionally charged events are common in everyday life, and particularly so in the critical care setting. This holds true for relatives and staff as well as for patients. Coming to terms with these everyday events is a largely automatic process. In simple terms, it seems to include having an awareness of the emotional reaction and somehow returning towards a normal balance. Traumatic stressors are events that produce intense pressure or tension and are associated with the negative emotions of fear and sadness. In normal circumstances, these emotional reactions gradually decline and each subsequent recall of these feelings is rather less intense until eventually, as a new equilibrium is reached, the emotional reaction fades completely and the individual adapts.

Faced with events that are perceived to be especially traumatic, this adaptive mechanism may be overwhelmed. The initial emotional reaction may be so intense that the only viable reaction is to attempt to prevent or avoid (blot out) these painful feelings. This may be achieved by avoiding places or objects that remind the person about the trauma, or through suppression of emotions in general – 'emotional numbing'.

These defensive reactions will rarely be completely successful and the individual is left with painful intrusive recollections, which alternate with defensive avoidance. This cyclical reaction of intrusion and avoidance is the central element of post-traumatic stress disorder (PTSD). It is possible that, as the emotions are suppressed because they are too extreme, they are not held in awareness and do not decline. The condition becomes chronic and may be disabling. Stress disorders are not rare:

some symptoms of PTSD are seen in the majority of patients who are involved in significant accidents and features occur in relatives of the victims and staff. Patients may report recurrent and intrusive distressing recollections of the event including flashback episodes. These can be precipitated by cues, which symbolise or resemble an aspect of the traumatic event (eg hearing a car's brakes on TV or even driving past the hospital). The victim is likely to avoid thoughts or cues that activate memories of the event and may become withdrawn, detached or appear depressed.

Critical events are a significant cause of occupational stress for staff groups (including doctors) in this environment and this is important to recognise not only for personal and team well-being but also because operational fatigue and impaired performance may result. Awareness of stress reactions is the first step and the provision of appropriate support of colleagues and patients, largely through opportunities for discussion, will represent a significant advance in many settings. The initial aim is to provide a means for people to talk about a critical event, learning about some of the ways that people may respond and (usually) achieving an understanding that their own behaviour is within a normal range. Your hospital should be able to provide support for you should you feel particularly affected by adverse events.

## Common psychological disorders in surgical critical care

So far, the emphasis has been on specific reactions to adversity, but of course a wide range of problems may occur. Traumatic life events may trigger feelings of depression, anxiety or even relapse of certain psychoses. The assessment needs to cover the full range of psychological difficulties. In this section, brief reference will be made to four of these.

### Anxiety

Mild feelings of fear, apprehension, sadness and emotional turmoil are very common in anyone admitted to hospital with a serious condition. In general, the approach taken by the clinical team can often determine the amount of distress experienced. A team that works well together, communicates well with patients and offers appropriate emotional support will reduce these difficulties, while dysfunctional teams will exacerbate the problem.

Assessment is likely to centre on asking appropriate questions about current feelings and enquiring into any associated autonomic symptoms of anxiety (eg tachycardia, raised blood pressure) which may mislead in the assessment of physical health. Sometimes, visible overbreathing (excessive, often irregular breathing) may be a clue to the presence of the chronic hyperventilation syndrome. This can present with a multitude of physical symptoms and is often associated with anxiety or depression.

## Major depression

Depression is a common condition and is often unrecognised. It spans a wide range of severities and patterns of reaction. The core feature is a low mood, in which there is loss of pleasure and enjoyment, reduced interest, hopelessness and helplessness, and pessimism for the future. In addition, there are often biological features, such as loss of weight, impaired sleep with early-morning wakening and a diurnal variation of mood which is worse in the early morning. Finally, there may be evidence of a frank psychosis with mood-congruent delusions and hallucinations. These may include delusions of worthlessness or guilt, delusions of cancer, delusions of persecution (felt to be deserved) or accusatory auditory hallucination. All these are in keeping with the primary disturbance of mood. As a routine in the assessment of psychiatric disturbance, there should be an investigation of suicidal ideation. One way of asking about this is to combine a permissions statement with a question. For example, if someone has talked about feeling very unhappy, they may be unable to see much point in life. Then continue with something like 'I wonder if you have ever felt it would be better just to go to sleep and never wake up?' This can be followed by further questions about any suicidal thoughts, any suicidal plans (going into detail if needed) and any suicidal behaviour. In this way, the whole subject can be covered easily without causing excessive concern. There is no excuse for failing to ask about suicidal thinking in the presence of significant psychiatric disturbance.

## Alcohol dependence

This is included as a reminder that alcohol problems are common (in general, about one in five people in hospital have significant alcohol-related problems) and can cause complications for the critically ill surgical patient. The characteristic problem arises from withdrawal symptoms, which follow hospitalisation and enforced abstinence. These can include typical tremor, nausea, mood disturbances and confusion but may extend to delirium tremens and even convulsions.

## Acute organic reactions

Variously styled as confusional states, toxic confusional states, delirium, etc, these are short-lived organic disturbances characterised by confusion, clouding of consciousness (sometimes quite subtle), disorientation and often marked fearfulness. There may be delusions which are often persecutory. Common causes include alcohol withdrawal and prescribed medication (eg analgesia) but they may also occur in the context of a wide range of medical conditions. Following assessment using an ABCDE approach, further evaluation is centred on the cognitive state (ability to attend and retrieve information, awareness of environment, etc), and on the possible organic causes, and requires completion of a full assessment and review. This is an organic disorder in the psychiatric classification because it is always secondary to some physical dysfunction. It is likely to be made worse in elderly patients or those with impaired hearing and/or sight by a disorientating environment and by a failure to offer frequent and repeated explanations.

## When to refer to a psychiatrist?

This may depend on the capacity and engagement of the local psychiatric liaison service. However, there are clear indicators for referral, which are important to outline. First, there is the situation in which the diagnosis is uncertain and especially where there may be a psychiatric component. Somatisation disorder and Munchausen's syndrome are extreme examples occasionally seen in the surgical population, but there are often complex interactions between physical and psychological processes which may require assessment. It is important in these situations to make positive psychiatric assessments rather than assumptions based on the absence of signs of physical disorder.

There are situations where either the severity of the psychiatric condition or level of danger associated with the condition make referral both appropriate and often urgent. This might be following, for example, deliberate self-harm or the development of persecutory beliefs in an acute organic reaction leading to thoughts of murder.

One situation in which referral is often considered is in relation to consent for surgery. Psychiatrists have special knowledge of the legislation to do with consent to treatment for psychiatric illness. The relevant legislation has much less to say about consent to treatment for physical illness and common law principles usually apply. Nonetheless, as long as a referral is not made with overoptimistic expectations, it may still be useful to discuss difficult cases where patient consent is withheld as this is an issue which is more common in psychiatric practice.

## Transition to specialty training

Change is unsettling and it is natural for promotion within surgical training to provoke feelings of apprehension and anxiety. In 2012, Critchley introduced the concept of 'zones of change' and described how, when faced with change, people station themselves in one of three zones depending upon how confident they feel with the situation. At one extreme is the comfort zone, in which individuals are secure and competent, whilst at the other is the high-risk zone, in which huge challenges exist. Bridging the gap between these is a zone in which learning can occur. By attending the CCrISP course you have positioned yourself in this zone of development. The fundamental aim of the course is to provide you with the confidence to safely and effectively care for critically ill surgical patients, but it is also an opportunity to learn to take more responsibility for patient care, a hallmark of the step up to specialty training.

Social psychology distinguishes between a 'change', which is rapid and happens to people irrespective of their level of readiness, and a 'transition', which is a slower, developmental process occurring in people's minds when experiencing change. It is preferable to view the move to specialty training as a transition because this allows you to prepare as fully as possible by building on skills which you have already acquired during core training.

A specialist registrar will often be responsible for the daily business ward rounds, reporting as necessary to the consultant. It is unlikely that the consultant will conduct a formal ward round every day, so it is essential that the trainee actively manages the patients, looks for and identifies problems, makes decisions about management and contacts the consultant when appropriate. Initially, as a new specialty trainee you will be communicating very frequently with the consultant but, with experience, your scope for safe practice can and should expand. It is important to understand when decisions need to be made and who needs to make them at all times in your training.

Decision-making is impossible without clinical information and business ward rounds should be timetabled so that key information is most likely to be readily available from nurses and junior colleagues. As the senior trainee you need to become aware of what information you need and what is largely superfluous to any critical decision. There is a balance to be struck between hasty and unfounded decision-making and unnecessary delay waiting for tests that will add little or nothing. Getting information takes you or others time and you need to delegate and organise appropriately. The CCrISP three-stage assessment process and adherence to ward round standards will help this process.

To get the best out of a team, leadership is essential. This encompasses a range of skills including knowledge, affability, decision-making, appropriate humour, humility, acceptance of other views and firmness. All must be deployed at the right time and few, if any of us, possess all or even a majority of these attributes. You will need to work hard, praise and support your colleagues, admit when you are wrong or do not know and get timely help. Consultants will wish to be informed promptly about unwell patients (even in the middle of the night) and will expect you to have carried out an assessment, instituted immediate treatment and devised a provisional plan of action. The exception to this is the patient who clearly needs an immediate operation beyond your ability such as a collapsed patient with penetrating trauma. In this situation the consultant will want a brief, clear message and probably give you a brief and clear reply.

Role-modelling is very important and clinically you must lead by example: if you are not thorough, why will anyone else be? Reassessing patients after making decisions or instigating interventions is vitally important but is perhaps the single most neglected skill in medicine. With current working practices this is becoming more difficult, and greater organisation is required for achievement. At the end of your shift you must hand over to the duty team. A surgical handover can be a challenging task, particularly when a large number of patients need to be passed on to the duty team. A written handover list with a concise summary of each patient can be invaluable in this situation. Some hospitals may have electronic systems to support handover, and these can facilitate communication between different professional groups and enhance sharing of knowledge about patients as well as providing a permanent record of the process. This should be supplemented by a verbal reinforcement of which patients are giving cause for concern and some acknowledgement from the doctor receiving the handover that these patients have been identified and the responsibility accepted.

As the senior trainee you must be prepared to circumvent blocks to your patients' progress. At times this may require a degree of assertiveness, but caution must be exercised so that you do not appear aggressive as this may lead to alienation. Building up good working relationships between other key members of the multidisciplinary team will often help in ensuring your patients receive the treatment they need. Senior nurses, advanced nurse practitioners, outreach nurses, emergency theatre nurses and radiologists are some examples of people who can make things happen for your patient and for you.

The promotion to specialty training is associated with an increased responsibility for patient care on the wards and in the operating theatre. However, in the current climate of surgical training it is recognised that operative exposure during core training is significantly less than it has been previously. Working within your limitations is one of the key skills of being a doctor at any level of training and any feelings of dismay at perceived surgical inadequacy must be banished. You will very quickly develop new operative skills and begin to feel that you really are a surgeon.

## Summary

This chapter does not provide a comprehensive account of the field of professional behaviour but highlights those areas where further learning may be required. This learning is not readily available in text books but can be gained with experience. It does require insight and reflection on the part of the individual, the latter skill being easily neglected in a busy surgical environment. Communication skills are especially important as they help to make practice more effective and efficient. More can be achieved in less time. It is important to look at patients, relatives and staff groups and understand the ways in which we cope with the everyday workload, with adversity and how these mechanisms can be overwhelmed at times of crisis.

## Glossary

Most clinicians could improve their communication skills and surgeons are certainly no exception. The glossary outlines some principles about which you may wish to read further. The specific skills cannot be summarised in a short glossary but are included in most books on communication.

### Basic communication skills

In this section, some of the terminology will be explained. It is useful in data gathering to use an appropriate range of open, focused and closed questions. In taking a history, the open question 'Is there anything else?' is useful as a final question.

Open questions can take a wide range of responses, eg 'What is the main problem?'. Focused questions can take a limited range of responses, eg 'Which is the worst pain today?'. Closed questions must be answered 'yes' or 'no', eg 'Is the pain in the knee the worst pain that you have?'.

Some questions are likely to produce misleading answers. A leading question expects a particular response, and this may be given even if it is wrong. Multiple questions are common in checklist approaches to the history but the answer given may only relate to the final item in the list – again misleading.

A leading question expects a particular answer, eg 'The pain is worst at night, is it not?'. Multiple questions include a list, eg 'Do you have problems with chest pain, shortness of breath or ankle swelling?'. This might attract the answer 'no', which to the patient might be 'no' to ankle swelling and to the doctor might be 'no' to the three items together.

There is a skill to checking back – being prepared to check that you have the right understanding – or using a summary of the main features as a way of confirming the history with your patient.

There is also a skill to sharing a problem. If you do not know how to handle something in an interview, sometimes the best thing is to own up. For example:

'I have a feeling that you are upset but I am not sure what has caused it. Is it OK to ask you about it?'

'My problem is that I only have 5 minutes before I have to go to theatre. I really need to ask you about something. Is that alright?'

Finally, perhaps the most useful of the active steps in understanding emotional reactions is the empathic comment. This is a statement identifying an emotional reaction, eg 'That must have made you feel very frightened'. In making this statement, a great deal of care must be exercised to listen to what is being said and not simply to assume that everyone will experience fear, anger, sadness, etc, in specific situations. It is useful as a way of checking back on emotions but, more importantly, it communicates that you can appreciate at least some of what your patient is feeling. This can be a very powerful intervention and should be a skill available to all doctors.

### Blocking

This means not facing up to an issue. This occurs, or example, when a patient asks 'Are there any complications with this operation?' and the surgeon replies, 'Don't you worry, it'll all be fine'. Another example is a doctor telling a patient they have cancer and the patient says 'It can't be cancer, I feel too well'.

### Mirroring

This is reflecting what the patient is saying in terms of tone of voice and body language. For example, if a patient is talking softly and timidly, reply in similar tones. If a patient is sitting leaning forward, do the same. Doing the opposite (anti-mirroring) can adversely affect interactions.

### *Assertiveness, passivity and aggression*

In being assertive, communication allows each person to express their honest opinions without needlessly hurting the other person. In being passive, honest opinions are suppressed.

Aggression involves the use of excessive force or power, causing needless suffering. This can be active aggression (eg violent, insulting speech) or passive aggression (eg emotional manipulation).

Assertiveness is, therefore, usually the preferred option. In general, assertive statements contain the pronoun 'I' whereas aggressive statements more often include the pronoun 'you', for example, 'I feel that the patient would be better helped by this approach' versus 'You are incompetent and have got this all wrong'.

## Further reading

Beauchamp TL and Childress JF. *Principles of Biomedical Ethics*. 7th edn. Oxford University Press, Oxford; 2017. ISBN: 9780199924585.

Critchley K. Managing change. *BJMP* 2012: **5** (3): a531. Available at http://www.bjmp. org/files/2012-5-3/bjmp-2012-5-3-a531.pdf.

Royal College of Surgeons of England. 'Consent: Supported Decision-Making – a good practice guide'. Available at: https://www.rcseng.ac.uk/library-and-publications/college-publications/docs/consent-good-practice-guide/

# 16

# Assessment of surgical risk and perioperative care

## Learning outcomes

This chapter should enable you to:

- appreciate the importance of assessing perioperative risk;

- recognise the factors that contribute to increased surgical risk;

- identify patients at increased risk of a perioperative cardiac event.

## Introduction

Approximately 250,000 patients (15% of total hospital inpatients having surgery) can be considered to be at high risk of adverse outcomes during their procedure.

The presence of any comorbidity increases the risk associated with surgical procedures, and minimising that risk is vitally important to improve outcomes, as high-risk patients account for 80% of deaths after surgery. Risk assessment is also important in terms of outcome measures for comparative audit, eg the National Emergency Laparotomy Audit (NELA) and NCEPOD (National Confidential Enquiry into Patient Outcome and Death) studies. Simple scales, such as the American Society of Anaestheologists (ASA) grading system, are open to varied interpretation among experienced medical assessors, while more complex systems, such as the physiological and operative severity score for enumeration of mortality and morbidity, or POSSUM, are too complex for most daily clinical applications or have a retrospective element that makes their reliability in preoperative risk assessment limited.

Coexisting diseases can complicate even a simple operation and increase morbidity and mortality, as in the case of a patient with a heart transplant who needs to undergo surgery for a cholecystectomy. The level of care required for a particular patient needs to be anticipated and consideration given to transfer to units with appropriate facilities, and to gaining the expertise needed to advise on preoperative optimisation and perioperative management of individual comorbidities.

The concept of a 'high-risk' patient is generally understood, but the key is to recognise the factors contributing to that perceived risk and repeatedly (re)assess these patients throughout their stay in hospital to minimise the risk of developing complications.

Many of the factors that increase surgical risk are covered elsewhere in this book. This chapter will discuss risk assessment in more detail and outline the specific effects of older age and obesity. There is also a specific chapter on diabetes (Chapter 17).

## The metabolic response to injury

An understanding of the metabolic response to injury is helpful in understanding how comorbidity affects perioperative management and risk (see also Chapter 13).

Metabolic responses to major injury, surgery and severe infection have similar mechanisms. The response occurs in two phases, referred to as 'ebb and flow'. The mediators and their effects for these responses are outlined in Box 16.1. The 'ebb phase' lasts 24–48 hours and is a neuroendocrine response to tissue injury and hypovolaemia. Cardiovascular reflex activity and inhibition of central thermoregulation are reminders of the 'fight or flight' response. Energy stores are mobilised to fuel the increased metabolic demand: plasma glucose concentration increases in proportion to the severity of the injury as a result of mobilisation of liver and skeletal muscle glycogen stores and the suppression of insulin release that inhibits the uptake of glucose into cells. Lipolysis is increased but fatty acid re-esterification within adipose tissue may be stimulated by the raised plasma lactate of severe injury or impaired perfusion of fat deposits. An early rise in hepatic protein synthesis and an increase in microvascular permeability are responsible for the characteristic changes in plasma protein concentrations observed within 6 hours.

Survival beyond the first 1- to 2-day initial phase gives rise to the 'flow phase' of increased metabolic rate, principally due to muscle catabolism and resistance to the anabolic effects of insulin.

The triggers for this are similar to the first phase but with increased energy consumption. The high-energy source ATP is produced principally by glycolysis (an inefficient mechanism) and the lactate produced is reconverted into glucose in the liver in an energy-consuming process, thereby increasing hepatic oxygen consumption and blood flow. Protein catabolism predominates, principally affecting skeletal muscle, but respiratory, gut and (possibly) cardiac muscle are also affected, giving rise to problems with mobility, ventilation and enteral nutrition. There are concomitant increases in urinary excretion of nitrogen and creatinine. The increase in proteolysis provides amino acids as precursors for hepatic gluconeogenesis.

Intramuscular glutamine concentration is decreased because of increased efflux and possibly decreased de novo synthesis.

Glutamine is an important fuel for cells of the immune system and it is a precursor for glutathione (a free radical scavenger); it has a role in nitric oxide metabolism and has also been implicated in the maintenance of the gut mucosal barrier, which may be compromised after injury.

Insulin resistance after injury refers to its anabolic effects; for example, hepatic glucose production, lipolysis and the net efflux of amino acids from skeletal muscle. These effects persist as plasma glucose and insulin concentrations that are inhibitory in uninjured subjects. Uptake of glucose into skeletal muscle is also reduced, an impairment that involves glucose storage rather than oxidation. The cause may result partly from the counter-regulatory hormones cortisol, adrenaline and glucagon, although infusion in healthy individuals requires much higher plasma concentrations to cause insulin resistance than those found in injured or septic patient. The effect of these hormones can be augmented by modulation of insulin sensitivity by pro-inflammatory cytokines: IL-6 in cancer patients, IL-1 in endotoxaemia and TNF in diabetes and obesity are all correlated with the degree of insulin resistance.

## Box 16.1 Mediators of injury response and their effects

### Counter-regulatory hormones

(eg catecholamines [adrenaline], cortisol, glucagon, antidiuretic hormone)

- Breakdown of glycogen stores in liver and skeletal muscle
- Suppression of insulin release resulting in reduced uptake and oxidation of glucose

### Increased sympathetic nervous system activity

- Lipolysis

### Protein metabolism

- Increased hepatic synthesis (IL-6 induced)

- Increased microvascular permeability
- Raised plasma concentration of fibrinogen and C-reactive protein
- Fall in plasma albumin concentration

### Proinflammatory cytokines (eg TNF-α, IL-1β, -2, -6 and -8)

- Mimic some responses, but plasma levels not universally linked to injury indicating autocrine/paracrine (cf endocrine) function

### IL-6 induction of prostanoids at the blood–brain barrier

- Activation of the hypothalamus–pituitary–adrenal axis

## Perioperative medicine

There is considerable interest in the development of multidisciplinary care pathways that manage patients before, during and after their operation. Specialties such as cardiac surgery have shown that by adopting such an approach, the overall mortality of surgery can be reduced.

### Comorbidities and perioperative care

Good surgical results reflect patient selection and the quality of perioperative care. This depends on:

- surgical factors, relating to pre-, intra- and postoperative care;

- patient factors, regarding disease presentation and pre-existing comorbidities, age, gender, biomarkers and socioeconomic factors;

- systemic factors that relate to the resources available for the treatment of surgical patients and treatment of complications.

Pre-existing comorbidity increases the risk of surgery. Anticipation of risk and risk-factor modification are vital in attempting to reduce surgical morbidity and mortality. Comorbidities most commonly associated with increased surgical morbidity and mortality are:

- cardiovascular (hypertension, myocardial ischaemia, cardiac failure and cardiac arrhythmias;)

- chronic respiratory disorders;

- anaemia;

- diabetes mellitus;

- chronic renal impairment;

- obesity;

- immunocompromised states such as poor nutrition, infectious diseases, connective tissue disorders, etc;

- chronic liver disease.

Elderly patients are more likely to have coexisting medical illness and a reduced physiological reserve and much of the focus of assessment in the elderly patient should be directed towards assessing their degree of physiological reserve and any frailty. Many hospitals now have specialist geriatricians who plan the care of very elderly patients undergoing both elective and emergency orthopaedic surgery. As surgeons you will not be expected to have detailed knowledge of the long-term care of patients with chronic diseases but you are expected to understand your role within the team and act accordingly.

*Obesity*

Excessive body weight is a growing epidemic among people of all ages in the UK. The reference scale for obesity is the BMI, which is given by weight (in kg) divided by height (in m$^2$). The normal range for BMI is 20–25 kg/m$^2$. Obesity is defined as a greater than 20% increase over the ideal body weight, which equates to a BMI over 30 kg/m$^2$. A patient with a BMI over 35 kg/m$^2$ can be considered morbidly obese.

Obesity increases the likelihood of associated medical disorders including ischaemic heart disease (especially central obesity), hypertension, oesophageal reflux, diabetes, obstructive sleep apnoea (OSA), osteoarthrosis, gallstones, varicose veins and haemorrhoids. It can also result in a chronic inflammatory response driven by the excess adipose tissue.

Increased insulin resistance is strongly associated with increasing BMI. Some obese patients will develop a metabolic syndrome, which significantly increases perioperative cardiac risk: this is defined by a collection of symptoms of central obesity, insulin resistance, dyslipidaemia and hypertension. The presence of a metabolic syndrome and obesity increases complications and mortality in those with a BMI $> 50\,kg/m^2$.

OSA is frequently undiagnosed but present in 10–20% of morbidly obese patients. If untreated, heart failure and pulmonary hypertension can occur. Strong predictors of OSA include male gender, older age, diabetes, hypertension, snoring (usually reported by the partner) and large collar size.

The STOP-BANG questionnaire is a screening tool designed to pick up these predictive factors (Figure 16.1). A STOP-BANG value of 5 or more indicates the likely presence of OSA and, if OSA is identified, perioperative patient management may include admission to critical care postoperatively if general anaesthesia is required.

| | |
|---|---|
| **Do you snore loudly?** | **Yes/No** |
| **Do you often feel tired, fatigued, or sleepy during the daytime?** | **Yes/No** |
| **Has anyone observed you stop breathing during your sleep?** | **Yes/No** |
| **Do you have or are you being treated for high blood pressure?** | **Yes/No** |
| **Are you obese/very overweight – BMI more than 35 kg/m2?** | **Yes/No** |
| **Age over 50 years old?** | **Yes/No** |
| **Neck Circumference >16 inches?** | **Yes/No** |
| **Are you male?** | **Yes/No** |

Figure 16.1 STOP-BANG questionnaire.

Reaching a diagnosis of an acute problem can often be rendered more difficult in obese patients. General anaesthesia and surgical procedures are more hazardous and postoperative complications, especially those relating to cardiopulmonary events, venous thromboembolism and the wound, are more frequent.

In patients with non-life threatening conditions requiring elective surgery, preoperative weight loss should be recommended. Before all operations, at least blood glucose and ECG should be checked preoperatively, even in younger patients. Further investigations and preoperative optimisation will depend on other patient and surgical factors. The risk of an adverse perioperative cardiac event is related to the nature and severity of the underlying heart disease, associated comorbidities and the type of surgery undertaken. The need for additional cardiac-based investigations should be made on the basis of patient comorbidities, function and the planned surgery. In the immobile, morbidly obese population, many of the functional assessments, eg shuttle walk test, are not always possible. Proceeding to elective surgery requires a balance of risk versus benefit and may warrant careful discussion with the patient.

### The elderly

A social definition of elderly is all those over 65 years of age, and this group accounts about one in four patients admitted to surgical wards. Increasingly, patients over 80 years of age are being considered for major surgery, and these patients provide a special challenge.

Two main reasons for increased risk with ageing are the frequent association of age and concurrent medical problems and decreasing functional reserve in many organ systems, making the elderly less able to respond to the physiological consequences of an operation. This is especially true for the respiratory system, cardiovascular system, kidneys, nervous system and drug handling. Again, careful patient assessment, optimisation and perioperative care should reduce the surgical risk. Polypharmacy (defined as use of five of more medications regularly) is common in this patient population.

Calculated risk for elderly patients after surgery is not clearly defined. The US National Surgical Quality Improvement Programme identified events in the postoperative period as more important than preoperative patient risk factors in determining survival, but very little research has examined functional and social outcomes after major surgery. The American College of Surgeons and the American Geriatric Society have produced an evidence-based best practice guideline which provides useful guidance (see Further reading).

## Risk assessment

Defining levels of risk to patients is important, both for enhancing the outcome of surgical intervention and for managing the expectations of patients, their relatives and our colleagues. Assessment of risk is also part of the process in achieving informed consent from patients for surgery.

Assessment of clinical risk is a complex higher function that forms an integral part of training. Apart from direct clinical experience, how can we improve our risk assessment?

Evidence-based medicine provides different levels of confidence about the outcome of an intervention when examining published results. The most robust evidence comes from randomised controlled trials (RCTs) and meta-analyses of several RCTs on the same topic, while case–control series provide lower levels of evidence and case reports provide the lowest (but not always insignificant) form of evidence. These data often suffer from the constraints of carefully conducted trials but can be used in your own practice to establish criteria for audit and quality improvement. Audit aims to improve the care of patients by establishing a standard, identification of areas for improvement and implementing that improvement, then evaluating the effects of implementation. Audit can also be national with contribution of data to national databases that are being established by the surgical specialty associations, eg the National Emergency Laparotomy Audit.

In the workplace, mortality and morbidity conferences provide a forum in which factors that have contributed to adverse outcomes can be debated and strategies may be developed to improve unit outcomes. National surveys such as NCEPOD (National Confidential Enquiry into Patient Outcome and Death) allow panels of experts to analyse surgical deaths and make conclusions about their causes and recommendations for prevention. This can be around preoperative preparation, the grade and seniority of staff involved and the resources available for treatment (eg provision of emergency theatres, ICU and HDU care). NCEPOD reviewers are selected by open application and you may wish to become involved as a reviewer in an NCEPOD audit when you progress to higher training.

Measurement of risk aims to provide some objective evaluation of individual patient risk and can allow comparison of individual clinicians or units. This is a growth area for research. Scoring systems have been developed in most subspecialties and for many individual conditions or procedures to try and produce a scale that will allow an accurate prediction of outcomes for each patient. Highly complex scoring systems may be unwieldy in the clinical situation and, when found to be valid in one unit or specialty, may require modification for successful adaptation to other specialties eg POSSUM. Simple and more widely applicable scoring systems such as the ASA grading system are in wide clinical use and ASA data are frequently a feature of anaesthetic and surgical outcomes databases (Table 16.1).

Most patients will be assigned an ASA grade (I–V) by the anaesthetist assessing the patient preoperatively. Although the scale is widely used, it is recognised to be open to individual variation, and even experienced anaesthetists may vary in their assessment of the same patient. This blunts its sensitivity and ability to discern actual risk for an individual patient.

Risk management is developing in healthcare and is borrowing ideas and techniques from the aviation industry, which has practised risk avoidance with great success over many years. In addition to anticipating risk and the management of appropriate preventative strategies, a cultural change around the use of the information is developing. Using adverse incident monitoring as an education tool, rather than as a tool for apportioning blame, allows for learning appropriate lessons and putting strategies in place that minimise the likelihood of repeated failure. In addition, aviation simulators that reproduce critical incidents allow important skills to be developed that can then be put into practice at appropriate moments when real lives are at stake. In surgery, this translates to the use of courses like CCrISP, skills laboratories and simulation centres in which clinical skills and techniques can be practised in

Table 16.1  The ASA system for grading surgical risk

| Grade | Definition | Mortality (%) |
|---|---|---|
| I | Normal healthy individual | 0.05 |
| II | Mild systemic disease, does not limit activity | 0.4 |
| III | Severe systemic disease, limits activity but is not incapacitating | 4.5 |
| IV | Incapacitating systemic disease, constantly life-threatening | 25 |
| V | Moribund, not expected to survive 24 h with or without surgery | 50 |

the context of simulated patients and procedures in order that best practice can be learned and honed, for use in the clinical arena.

An international campaign to reduce harm in perioperative care has led to initiatives such as 'Patient Safety First' within the NHS. This is based on an acknowledgement by healthcare workers that events that produce harm in patients are potentially avoidable. An example of one such initiative is that of reducing surgical site infections by establishing a target reduction and examining compliance with appropriate interventions to achieve it, including appropriate use of prophylactic antibiotics, maintaining normothermia, maintaining glycaemic control in diabetic patients and using recommended hair removal methods. In addition, to increase safety in the operating theatre, the use of the World Health Organization Surgical Safety Checklist is being implemented in hospitals. This contains the team brief, sign-in, a time-out before surgery (degree of urgency permitting), sign-out at the end of the procedure prior to transfer to the recovery area and debrief after patient has gone to the recovery. The anaesthetist, surgeon, scrub nurse and other theatre staff discuss the patient preparation, any anticipated critical moments, potential complications and how these will be managed during the checklist. As champions for risk management, surgeons can demonstrate leadership in the care of patients that will improve the outcome of our treatment and operations.

## Preoperative assessment clinics

In many hospitals there are now dedicated clinics where the focus is on assessing and preparing patients for surgery, particularly assessing the cardiorespiratory system. Tests can be divided into those which are relatively static, such as resting ECG or resting echocardiography, and dynamic (stressed) tests such as exercise ECG or stress echocardiography.

Cardiopulmonary exercise testing (CPET) looks at the cardiorespiratory system in its entirety, and is dynamic, robust and replicable by progressively stressing the patient using a standardised test. CPET quantifies a patient's ability to respond to the metabolic demands of major surgery. There are considerable data to suggest that cardiorespiratory reserve absolutely correlates with probability of death and complications perioperatively. An anaerobic threshold is measured for each patient, and this is then used to triage patients into a perioperative care package that is appropriate for their degree of risk. Anaerobic threshold is the point at which inadequate oxygen delivery results in a shift to anaerobic metabolism and is not altered by patient effort. An anaerobic threshold of at least 11 ml/kg/min is considered necessary for major elective surgery, and values less than this almost certainly mark the patient out as requiring postoperative care on an ICU or HDU.

However, aside from cardiorespiratory reserve, age, nature of surgery and other physiological systems and coexisting disease are also important in terms of perioperative risk. So, for instance, concomitant renal disease or neurological disease may also impact upon perioperative risk, and there may be immunological, haematological, endocrinological, hepatic function or malnutritional considerations.

The important issue with preassessment clinics is to assess physiological reserve and consider whether any of the systems can be improved prior to surgery. There is also now growing interest in preconditioning, whereby patients are given a graded exercise programme prior to planned surgery, as this is also thought to improve outcomes.

## The role of enhanced recovery

Enhanced recovery after surgery (ERAS) programmes, initially developed in colorectal patients by Henrik Kehlet, are being increasingly used across the surgical spectrum. Evidence shows that patient outcomes, length of stay and patient satisfaction are improved by these programmes.

ERAS programmes are essentially packages of care that describe the patient journey from time of decision to operate to discharge from hospital after surgery. The basic principles are described below and all aspects of the package need to be adhered to for success. The relative effectiveness of each individual component is difficult to demonstrate but there is evidence that the catabolic phase of the surgical response earlier in this chapter can be reversed by the use of oral preoperative carbohydrate loading.

## Outline of enhanced recovery programmes

### Preoperative phase

The goal in the preoperative phase is to ensure that patients are as fit as possible so that they have the best chance of making an uncomplicated and quick recovery from their forthcoming surgery. This involves an accurate and detailed preassessment process which identifies and modifies, where possible, the patient's comorbidities. Good control over comorbidities such as diabetes, cardiovascular and pulmonary disease, as well as treating anaemia and encouraging patients to stop smoking (stopping smoking for 1 month prior to surgery can reduce the incidence of wound infection and respiratory complications) are all important considerations. Ideally, this process should start in general practice once the patient is referred. CPET is used to quantify the risk around the surgery, and may be useful in informing the discussion with the patient, and in planning postoperative requirements.

The patient needs to be actively engaged in discussing what happens around the time of surgery and goals set for them to achieve in terms of mobility and estimated length of hospital stay. Daily targets are also identified, supported by a written pathway that is actively monitored by the ward nursing staff, who, together with the physiotherapy team and any specialist nurses, play a vital role in supporting and encouraging the patient postoperatively. These expectations need to be actively reinforced by the whole of the team during the patient's journey. Having named individuals to lead and champion ERAS programmes can lead to greater compliance with the pathway.

A risk assessment for venous thromboembolic disease should be carried out and thromboembolic deterrent stockings used when not contraindicated and the appropriate dose of prophylactic subcutaneous fractioned heparin prescribed. Single-dose antibiotics are given as prophylaxis against wound or prosthesis infection in accordance with local hospital policy. The aim is to continue cardiac, pulmonary and antacid medications on the day of surgery, but a decision regarding the risks and benefits of stopping anticoagulant medication such as warfarin or dabigatran and antiplatelet medication such as clopdiogrel and dipyridamole needs to be made and may require discussion with other specialties.

## Operative phase

Medication to control postoperative nausea and vomiting is given at the time of induction. Intraoperative care includes prevention of hypothermia, goal-directed intraoperative fluid therapy using fluid boluses and stroke volume optimisation supplemented by judicious use of vasopressors. Minimally invasive techniques are preferred such as short and transverse incisions for open surgery, avoidance of postoperative drains and naso-gastric tubes, and avoidance of or short-duration use of epidural analgesia, with local blocks being preferred as appropriate.

## Postoperative phase

The postoperative phase aims to restore the patient's normal function as soon as possible. Daily goals for mobilisation and tube removal should be set and met. Good pain relief aimed at restoration of function such as deep breathing, coughing and moving rather than the elimination of all pain is important. The use of opiate medication should be minimised and other analgesics and/or local anaesthetic techniques should be used. Allowing oral intake of fluids and diet immediately after surgery, combined with the measures described above to prevent postoperative nausea and vomiting, leads to early return of gut function, another important goal in the postoperative phase. Early cessation of IV fluids contributes to this. Early removal of other tubes reduces pain and aids mobilisation. Giving patients a sense of having control over their own recovery facilitates the process.

When managing patients on ERAS programmes it is important to realise when complications may be developing. The use of a track and trigger system and the CCrISP three-stage assessment process should facilitate this. Once it is recognised that a patient has 'fallen off' the enhanced recovery pathway they need to be managed differently, especially with regard to fluid therapy which should be used in a resuscitative manner rather than in a restrictive manner.

## Summary

- It is essential to recognise the factors that contribute to surgical risk.

- All members of the surgical team have a responsibility to ensure that patients are as fit as possible prior to surgery.

- Be aware of comorbidities to predict and prevent perioperative problems and manage any that do occur in the perioperative period in a timely manner.

## Further reading

Agnew N. Preoperative cardiopulmonary exercise testing. *Contin Educ Anaesth Crit Care Pain* 2010; **10** (2): 33–37.

Khuri SF Henderson WG, DePalma RG et al. Determinants of long-term survival after major surgery and the adverse effect of postoperative complications. *Ann Surg* 2005; **242**: 326–343.

Mohanty S, Rosenthal RA, Russell MM et al. Optimal perioperative management of the geriatric patient: A best practices guideline from ACS NSQIP®/American Geriatrics Society. Available at https://www.facs.org/quality-programs/acs-nsqip

Royal College of Anaesthetists. Perioperative Medicine: the pathway to better surgical care. Available at https://www.rcoa.ac.uk/periopmed/vision-document

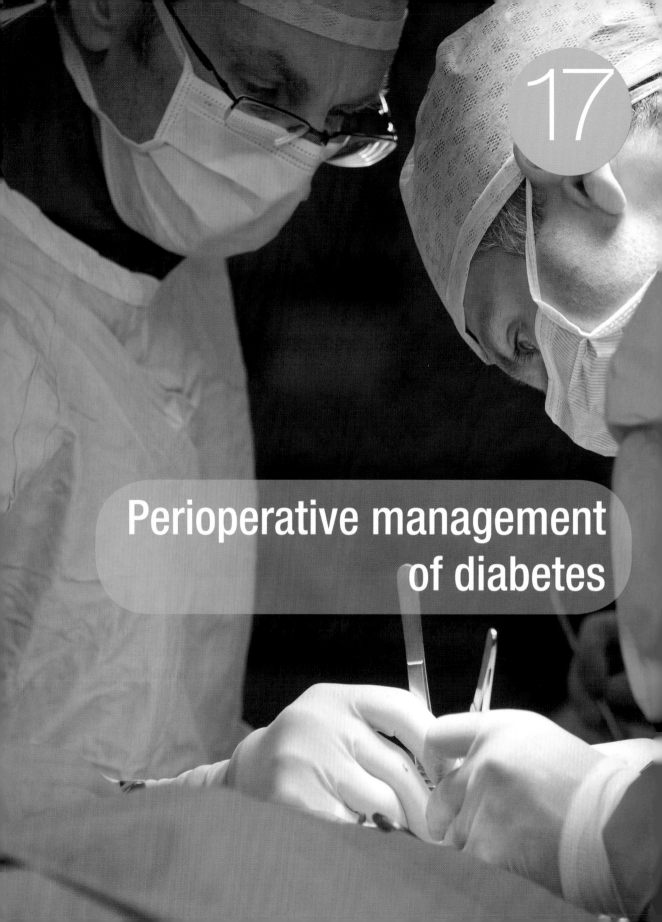

# Perioperative management
# of diabetes

17

## Learning outcomes

This chapter should enable you to:

- appreciate the importance of recognising and treating diabetes in the surgical patient;

- work through examples of management plans for surgical patients with diabetes;

- identify other clinical and metabolic states associated with poor glucose control.


## Introduction

The prevalence of diabetes mellitus is rapidly increasing and diabetes now affects 4–5% of the UK population. Diabetes is a state of impaired glucose tolerance caused by either absolute lack of insulin (type 1) or relative lack of insulin (type 2). In addition to the metabolic disturbance, micro- and macrovascular abnormalities cause retinopathy, nephropathy, neuropathy, coronary heart disease, stroke and peripheral vascular disease. Diabetic patients also develop cataracts and specific soft tissue disorders such as diabetic cheiroarthropathy as a result of exposure of the tissues to hyperglycaemia, causing accelerated irreversible biochemical and structural changes normally found in ageing. Improved glycaemic control in diabetes protects against these secondary effects.

Even the simplest surgery can be hazardous to diabetic patients. The metabolic response to surgical trauma can rapidly lead to hyperglycaemia and ketoacidosis, especially in insulin-deficient patients. Poorly controlled diabetes accelerates catabolism and delays healing. Insulin and the sulphonylureas can cause severe hypoglycaemia in fasted and anorexic patients, which can be particularly dangerous during general anaesthesia. Assessment of fitness for surgery, preoperative optimisation, an agreed management policy between specialists and ward staff and meticulous glycaemic control will greatly reduce the risks of operating on diabetic patients.

## Utility of preoperative glycated haemoglobin values

Good preoperative glycaemic control as directed by the HbA1c concentrations is associated with decreased morbidity and mortality and also shorter hospital stay (Box 17.1).

### Box 17.1  HbA1c values

Non-diabetic reference range: 4.0–6.0% or 20–42 mmol/mol

Diagnostic of diabetes mellitus: >6.5% or 48 mmol/mol on repeated testing

High risk of diabetes: 6.0–6.4% or 42–47 mmol/mol

Target HbA1c concentration for diabetic patients: 6.5–7.5% or 48–58 mmol/mol

HbA1c values of >8.6% or 70 mmol/mol are associated with four-fold mortality in cardiac surgery

Some case examples will serve to illustrate the key management issues in patients with diabetes undergoing surgical treatment. You are advised to read and review the Joint British Diabetes Societies inpatient guidelines at this point (see Further reading).

### Case scenario 17.1

A 33-year-old civil servant, admitted to the surgical unit for an open elective inguinal herniorrhaphy, is stabilised on three times daily subcutaneous soluble insulin injection and is otherwise fit and well.

#### How would his diabetes be managed perioperatively?

Such patients have absolute deficiency of insulin and require variable-rate intravenous insulin (VRIII) infusions to be instituted on the morning of surgery after an overnight fast and omission of the morning insulin dose. A protocol for infusion is given in Box 17.2, but note that most hospitals will have their own local protocols and you should make sure you are familiar with the one where you work.

The patient had an uneventful procedure under general anaesthesia on the morning list with hourly blood glucose recordings showing good control with plasma levels of glucose between 5 and 10 mmol/L. Owing to postoperative nausea and vomiting, the VRIII regimen was continued overnight. By the next morning, he was able to eat and drink normally; the VRIII infusion was discontinued and he had his normal morning insulin dose with his breakfast and was discharged home later that morning.

## Case scenario 17.2

A 67-year-old retired coach driver was seen in the preadmission clinic for workup for an elective transurethral prostatectomy for symptomatic benign prostatomegaly. He has been diabetic for 5 years and his disease is currently controlled with diet and oral glibenclamide.

### How would you manage his diabetes?

Generally, patients with type 2 diabetes that is well controlled by diet or oral agents may simply omit their oral agents and breakfast on the morning of surgery. However, long-acting sulphonylurea drugs (eg glibenclamide) should be replaced by short-acting ones (eg glicazide) some days before surgery to reduce the risk of hypoglycaemia. Blood glucose should be monitored closely in the perioperative period and persistent hyperglycaemia should be treated with a VRIII infusion. If the patient is in a steady state, the VRIII infusion will maintain satisfactory glycaemic control and prevent hypokalaemia. If glucose levels are not within the range then, as an alternative, insulin may be given as a variable-rate intravenous infusion (Box 17.2), which provides greater flexibility.

Always consider the clinical haemodynamic state and review U&Es before deciding on the type and rate at which IV fluids are prescribed and administered (Table 17.1).

Table 17.1 Fluid regime whilst on VRIII

| Patient group | Blood glucose and serum K⁺ level | Fluid recommendation |
|---|---|---|
| No concern of fluid overload | Blood glucose >14 mmol/L Serum K⁺ 3.5–5.5 mmol/L | 0.9% NaCl with 20 or 40 mmol/L KCl at 125 ml/h |
| | Blood glucose <14 mmol/L Serum K⁺ 3.5–5.5 mmol/L | 5% dextrose with 40 mmol KCl at 125 ml/h |
| | Serum K⁺ >5.5 mmol/L | No additional KCl, reassess serum K⁺ and aim to keep serum K⁺ between 3.5 and 5.5 mmol/L |
| Risk of fluid overload | | Consider whether VRIII is needed or use subcutaneous insulin regimen; consider 10% dextrose rather than 5% dextrose |
| Hyopnatraemia or serum Na⁺ falls greater than 3 mmol/L in 24 hours | | Consider whether VRIII is needed or use subcutaneous insulin regimen; high concentration NaCl can be used after discussion |

Diabetic ketoacidosis (DKA) is uncontrolled hyperglycaemia with hyperketonaemia severe enough to cause metabolic acidosis. It is caused by severe insulin deficiency that stimulates lipolysis and a massive increase in ketogenesis. It is the hallmark of poorly treated type 1 diabetes but can occur in type 2 diabetes when patients are relatively insulin deficient and there is intercurrent illness, stimulating counter-regulatory hormone secretion (especially glucagon). It carries a mortality of 5–10% (50% in elderly patients with DKA precipitated by MI or infection). Prompt diagnosis and management is essential to prevent death.

As well as hyperglycaemia, hyperketonaemia occurs due to oxidation of free fatty acids in hepatocyte mitochondria (a process stimulated by glucagon and inhibited powerfully by insulin), yielding ATP and acetyl-CoA. The latter is converted to acetoacetate, which may be oxidised to 3-hydroxybutyrate or undergo condensation to produce acetone. Ketones are transported out of the liver and used as metabolic fuels by various tissues including the brain; they provide a few per cent of the total energy needs after an overnight fast, but this rises to one-third in prolonged fasting. When produced in excess, they accumulate rapidly as uptake mechanisms become saturated. The main consequences of raised circulating ketones are:

- acidosis, both extracellular and intracellular;

▨ diuresis, as osmotically active ketones are filtered in the urine, exacerbating the osmotic diuresis caused by glycosuria, and resulting in polyuria, electrolyte losses, dehydration and hypovolaemia;

▨ nausea – by direct stimulation of the chemoreceptor trigger zone in the medulla.

Simultaneous resuscitation and investigation includes a 12-lead ECG, bacteriological cultures of all appropriate fluids including blood and urine, cardiac enzyme determination and ABG analysis. Intravenous saline and insulin should begin immediately (Box 17.2). Urgent treatment with scrupulous clinical and biochemical monitoring is essential. Correction of hypovolaemia will often improve acidosis and hyperglycaemia. However, overenergetic fluid and insulin replacement can predispose to cerebral oedema and increase mortality. CVP monitoring for the elderly and those at risk of heart failure may be required. Monitoring for response is essential and 0.9% saline (containing potassium when appropriate; see Box 17.3) is the fluid of choice. Dextrose 5% is substituted when plasma glucose has fallen to 10–14 mmol/L to prevent hypoglycaemia (insulin is still required to prevent ketogenesis and promote glucose utilisation in the tissues).

## Box 17.2  Variable-rate intravenous insulin infusion: guidance

- Start VRIII at the standard rate

- Measure blood glucose every hour and adjust VRIII to keep the glucose level between 6 and 10 mmol/L

- If blood glucose is > 14 mmol/L and not under control move to increased insulin rate scale

- If blood glucose is < 4.0 mmol/L, **stop** VRIII and treat hypoglycaemia

- If blood glucose control is too tight, ie blood glucose persistently 4 mmol/L, consider using reduced insulin infusion rate

- Monitor urea and electrolytes (U&Es) daily and adjust potassium chloride dose accordingly

- Usual diabetic medications should be omitted during VRIII

## Case scenario 17.3

A 66-year-old woman was admitted from A&E with a 6-day history of feeling unwell, with immobility and discharge from the right foot. She has had diabetes for 7 years treated with diet, glicazide and metformin. Examination revealed discharge from the instep, a necrotic heel and cellulitis extending across the ankle into the lower leg. Her pulses were all palpable, but there was diminished pedal sensation. Her Hb was 111 g/L, WCC 18.6 × 10⁹/L, blood glucose 24 mmol/L, potassium 5.8 mmol/L, urea 9.0 mmol/L and creatinine normal.

### How would you manage this patient?

She should be managed as per the CCrISP protocol, with immediate attention to ABCDE assessment and resuscitation. Her diabetes is out of control. A variable-rate intravenous insulin infusion (Table 17.2), with hourly monitoring of the blood glucose and 3- to 4-hourly potassium estimation (Box 17.3) is appropriate. She requires resuscitation with IV 0.9% saline until she has been stabilised, and her glycaemic and potassium control optimised. Administration of broad-spectrum or 'best-guess' intravenous antibiotics aids stabilisation of sepsis and the metabolic state prior to definitive treatment of foot sepsis: debridement or amputation will give the best result. Rarely, gas-forming organisms may be present; if gas gangrene is suspected, urgent surgery will be required after initial resuscitation, so urgent senior surgical review is needed.

### Box 17.3  A potassium replacement regimen

In an unstable patient with varying insulin requirements, serum potassium levels should be monitored every 3–4 hours.

Replacement should be guided by the latest serum K⁺ concentration

- if K⁺ >5.0 mmol/L, omit KCl due to the risk of cardiac arrhythmias
- if K⁺ 3.5–5.0 mmol/L, add 20 mmol KCl to each litre of IV fluid
- if K⁺ <3.5 mmol/L, add 40 mmol KCl to each litre of IV fluid.

Table 17.2 Variable rate intravenous insulin infusion

| Glucose (mmol/L) | Insulin rate (ml/h) | | |
| --- | --- | --- | --- |
| | Reduced rate | Standard rate (first choice) | Increased rate |
| <4 | 0 | 0 | 0 |
| 4.1–8.0 | 0.5 | 1 | 2 |
| 8.1–12.0 | 1 | 2 | 4 |
| 12.1–16 | 2 | 4 | 6 |
| 16.1–20.0 | 3 | 5 | 7 |
| 20.1–24.0 | 4 | 6 | 8 |
| >24.1 | 6 | 8 | 10 |

## Case scenario 17.4

A 68-year-old, overweight woman was admitted in a coma. Her family provided a history of abdominal pain, anorexia and vomiting for 1 week against a background of 15 years of diabetes mellitus. In the early years, her diabetes was controlled by diet and oral hypoglycaemic agents; however, for the past 8 years, she has required subcutaneous insulin supplementation. On admission, she appeared to be dehydrated and had a temperature of 38.3°C, a pulse of 130/min and systolic blood pressure of 80 mmHg. There was epigastric fullness and guarding and she had sighing respiration with a smell of acetone on her breath. A chest X-ray showed basal atalectasis. Blood results showed Hb 101 g/L, WCC 19.5 × $10^9$/L, $Na^+$ 152 mmol/L, $K^+$ 6.7 mmol/L, $HCO_3^-$ 15 mmol/L, $Cl^-$ 100 mmol/L, urea 22.5 mmol/L, creatinine 85 μmol/L, glucose 36 mmol/L. Her urine was strongly positive for ketones.

### What is the management of this patient?

This is a complex clinical problem that cannot be managed in a general surgical ward. The patient should be managed according to the CCrISP protocol with simultaneous immediate assessment and resuscitation. Although she probably has a surgical problem, she also has DKA and this needs to be managed jointly with critical care and endocrinology input in an HDU facility with continuous ECG monitoring and close biochemical monitoring of glucose (hourly) and potassium (3- to 4-hourly) levels (Boxes 17.2 and 17.3).

Use of bicarbonate and hypotonic solutions is contentious. Hypotonic solutions may exacerbate intracellular movement of water and could lead to cerebral oedema, while bicarbonate may improve extracellular acidosis. However, as membranes are not permeable to bicarbonate ions, intracellular acidosis may not be improved. Carbon dioxide can enter the cells to combine with water to produce $H_2CO_3$, which can worsen intracellular acidosis with an adverse impact on outcome.

A hyperosmolar hyperglycaemic state is distinguished from DKA by the absence of high ketones levels and metabolic acidosis. Hyperglycaemia may rise to higher levels but insulin levels are high enough to suppress ketogenesis. It is found in previously undiagnosed type 2 diabetes and may be precipitated by intercurrent illness, diabetogenic drugs (corticosteroids and thiazide diuretics) or fizzy glucose-containing drinks. Complications include thrombotic events such as CVA, peripheral arterial occlusion, DVT and PE, due to increased blood viscosity. Mortality exceeds 30% because these patients are often older and often have a serious precipitating illness.

Lactic acidosis is generated rapidly during tissue anoxia (eg shock, cardiac failure or pneumonia) or when liver gluconeogenesis is impaired. In diabetes mellitus, it is a rare, but fatal, complication of biguanides (phenformin, metformin), which act by inhibiting gluconeogenesis. It presents as coma with metabolic acidosis and a wide amino gap due to hyperlactataemia. Blood glucose levels are usually raised. Treatment is difficult: intravenous bicarbonate may aggravate intracellular acidosis; forced ventilation to reduce carbon dioxide levels may help; dialysis clears lactate and $H^+$ and will correct any sodium overload from bicarbonate infusion. Mortality is high (>30%) because of coexisting organ failures.

## Hypoglycaemia

This is infrequently seen as a presenting condition but still occurs as a form of iatrogenic injury on surgical wards.

Common factors that predispose to hypoglycaemia are outlined in Box 17.4.

The events as blood glucose falls are listed in Box 17.5 but without early recognition can precipitate a coma. Hypoglycaemia should be recognised and treated immediately.

# Box 17.4  Common factors contributing to hypoglycaemia

## Accelerated insulin absorption

- Exercise
- Hot environmental conditions

## Unfavourable factors relating to insulin administration

- Too early
- Too much
- Inadequate food intake

## Alcohol consumption

- Inhibits hepatic gluconeogenesis

## Weight loss

## Loss of counter-regulatory hormones

- Addison's disease
- Hypothyroidism
- Hypopituitarism
- Blunted glucagon secretion (as in long-standing type 1 diabetes)
- Intestinal malabsorption
- Renal failure (impaired insulin clearance)

## Box 17.5  Clinical events as blood glucose falls

~3.8 mmol/L: adrenaline and glucagon secretion increases

~3.0 mmol/L: onset of hypoglycaemic symptoms (note, hypoglycaemic unawareness in some patients)

~2.8 mmol/L: neuroglycopenia and cognitive impairment

<1.0 mmol/L: coma

### Practice point

Check the blood glucose with a capillary blood glucose (CBG) stick in any patient with a reduced level of consciousness as part of the initial ABCDE assessment.

## Summary

Diabetes is common, and poor management has a significant impact on outcome from surgery as well as patient quality of life and mortality. As a surgeon you should be able to identify diabetes as well as other clinical and metabolic states associated with poor glucose control.

## Further reading

Joint British Diabetes Societies for Inpatient Care. *Management of Adults with Diabetes Undergoing Surgery and Elective Procedures: Improving Standards.* Revised September 2015. Available at http://www.diabetologists-abcd.org.uk/JBDS/JBDS_IP_Surgical_Guideline_2015_Full.pdf